THI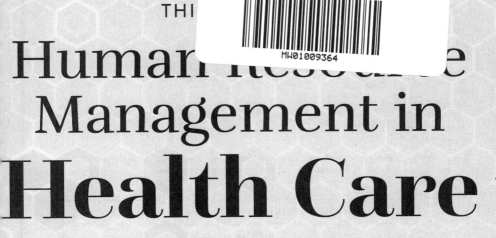

Human Resource Management in Health Care

Principles and Practice

Charles R. McConnell, MBA, CM
Human Resource and Editorial Consultant
Ontario, New York

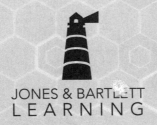

JONES & BARTLETT
LEARNING

World Headquarters
Jones & Bartlett Learning
5 Wall Street
Burlington, MA 01803
978-443-5000
info@jblearning.com
www.jblearning.com

Jones & Bartlett Learning books and products are available through most bookstores and online booksellers. To contact Jones & Bartlett Learning directly, call 800-832-0034, fax 978-443-8000, or visit our website, www. jblearning.com.

Production Credits

VP, Product Management: Amanda Martin
Director of Product Management: Cathy Esperti
Product Manager: Danielle Bessette
Product Assistant: Tess Sackmann
Product Assistant: Melina Leon
Project Specialist: Kristine Janssens
Digital Project Specialist: Angela Dooley
Senior Marketing Manager: Susanne Walker
Manufacturing and Inventory Control
    Supervisor: Amy Bacus
Composition: codeMantra U.S. LLC
Project Management: codeMantra U.S. LLC
Cover Design: Kristin E. Parker
Senior Media Development Editor:
    Shannon Sheehan
Rights & Media Specialist: Rebecca Damon
Cover and Chapter Opener Image:
    © Matejmo/iStock/Getty Images Plus/Getty Images
Printing and Binding: McNaughton & Gunn
Cover Printing: McNaughton & Gunn

Library of Congress Cataloging-in-Publication Data
Library of Congress Cataloging-in-Publication Data unavailable at time of printing
LCCN: 2019910562

6048

Printed in the United States of America
23 22 21 20 19   10 9 8 7 6 5 4 3 2 1

Contents

Chapter 13

Conducting a Successful and Legal Selection Interview 209

SECTION IV Problems, Correction, and Discipline   233

Chapter 14

Managers and Employee Problems 235

Chapter 15

Addressing Problems Before Taking Critical Action 257

Chapter 16

Terminating Employees 273

Preface

Since the initial edition of this text was published in 2007, health care has continued to change in numerous and sometimes surprising ways. The rate of change continues to accelerate with the proliferation of new technologies, social media, and changing models and contexts for providing care.

Some historical context may be useful. Human resources, known earlier as "personnel," emerged as a separate entity in business organizations in the 1930s and 1940s. The importance of human resources has steadily increased over the intervening decades. As many providers of healthcare services resist the present-day pressures calling for increased efficiency, the public continues to demand more services.

It seems clear to us that the demand for healthcare services will continue to increase as the population expands and new technologies arise. Using past behavior as a basis for predicting future actions, it is clear that the means of paying for the desired additional services will continue to lag the demand for those services. Although we do not know precisely what the future may bring, we can say with confidence that human resources will be affected.

Nonhealth businesses, manufacturing companies foremost among them, were the first to recognize the utility of human resources. Out of necessity, healthcare provider organizations began to rely increasingly on human resources professionals as legal protections for workers proliferated. Owing to characteristics of size and structure, however, some elements of health-related activity have not received the full benefit of modern human resources capabilities. For example, public health as a discipline has been slow to embrace human resources, and many smaller health-related organizations, such as independent laboratories and free-standing clinics and group practices, have too few employees to justify a full-time human resources presence.

This book introduces human resources to those who are preparing for employment in any area of health care or health services. It is written for practitioners and students in all disciplines related to health, from individual providers to major medical centers and administrators in a broad range of healthcare settings.

To accommodate a large and diverse audience, we have endeavored to provide a comprehensive yet balanced approach to the subject. Each chapter is intended to stand alone; chapters are not sequential and can be addressed in any order. Each chapter opens with a case study introducing the reader to key topics and provides questions to ponder while reading the material that follows. Each case study is resolved with commentary and suggestions that can be utilized should the reader someday become interested or involved in a similar situation. Finally, each chapter concludes with an application of customer service in the context of the chapter's subject. All chapters include learning objectives, discussion points, and listings of resources that provide supplementary materials.

The goal of this book has been first and foremost to be practical. Discussions of theory are included when needed to aid understanding of application guidelines, but pure theory runs a distant second to practicality in the pages that follow. Examples and sample forms and documents are included, drawn from our professional experiences and supplemented with input from others.

Thank you for sharing some of your time to read this book. I freely share credit with others from whom we have learned much of what is presented here and encourage your feedback.

Charles R. McConnell
Ontario, New York

Acknowledgments

First, generous thanks are owed to L. Fleming Fallon, the main author and visionary for the first two editions of this book. Without him, this book would not exist, and his contributions should not go unnoted. Additional thanks go to Mike Brown who signed the first edition of this book over a decade ago, and whose support helped me get to where I am today. I express sincere thanks and wish Mike the best in his retirement.

While spouses infrequently appear on the covers of books, they maintain a constant presence. Their contributions start with time and range to items on a list that is too long to reasonably contemplate, always accompanied by love. With humility, I thank my wife Kate, knowing that she made this project possible.

Charles R. McConnell

About the Author

Charles R. McConnell, MBA, CM

Charles McConnell is an independent healthcare management and human resources consultant. For 11 years, he was active as a management engineering consultant with the Management and Planning Services (MAPS) division of the Hospital Association of New York State (HANYS) and later spent 18 years as a hospital human resources manager. Mr. McConnell is also a freelance writer specializing in business, management, and human resource topics. As an author, a coauthor, and an anthology editor, he has published a multitude of books. He has also contributed chapters to several additional books and has contributed numerous articles to a wide range of publications. He is in his 32nd year as editor of the quarterly professional journal, *The Health Care Manager*.

Mr. McConnell received a BS in engineering and an MBA from the State University of New York at Buffalo, Buffalo, New York.

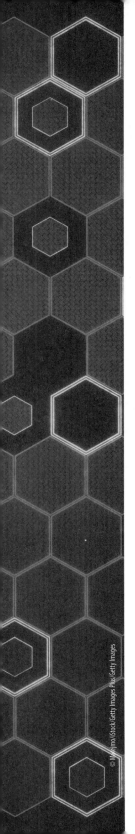

SECTION I
Fundamentals

A human resources (HR) department provides services essential to both the legal and the practical survival of an organization. This section addresses the core activities of an HR department. Chapter 1 (An Overview of Human Resources) provides a macro view of human resources, looking at the history of the function and how it evolved into what we know it to be today. Chapter 2 (How Human Resources Fits into an Organization) describes the basic services provided by the human resources department of an organization. Chapter 3 (The Legal Framework of Contemporary Human Resources) reviews the relevant laws that shape and define many of the services that a contemporary HR department is expected to provide. Chapter 4 (Human Resource Activities and Managers) discusses the interactions between HR staff and all elements of the organization's management structure. Chapter 5 (The Manager–Employee Relationship) addresses the interactions between managers and the employees they supervise, suggesting that HR sets and monitors the guidelines for effective manager–employee relationships. Chapter 6 (Position Descriptions) explains the importance of job descriptions and describes how they are written and how they are best used to serve certain purposes. Chapter 7 (Directions in Employee Relations) examines how the management of people has evolved from a largely authoritarian posture to the growing humanistic people-management outlook of today.

CHAPTER 1

An Overview of Human Resources

CHAPTER OBJECTIVES

After studying this chapter, readers will be able to:

- Understand the history of human resources in healthcare organizations and its growth from a few scattered tasks to today's all-encompassing centralized activity.
- Fully supportive of the rationale for the existence of a human resources department.
- Prepared to describe or formulate the mission of a human resources function in a healthcare organization.

▶ Chapter Summary

The human resources department provides vital services to any organization. There is no less a need for HR services in a healthcare provider organization than there is in any other business undertaking of any appreciable size.

Many contemporary human resources departments began with an overworked administrator who struggled to hire a sufficient number of employees to maintain normal operations. Organizational growth and expansion of the services that were being provided eventually far exceeded the original administrator's ability to secure employees. Delegating this task created a "personnel office," often referred to in its earliest form as "the employment office." Compensation issues were soon delegated to this newly created department, and as legal requirements were imposed, the size and complexity of the personnel office increased. The name of the department eventually became *human resources*, although the title "personnel" continues to exist in places along with other descriptive labels for the same activity (People Systems, Employee Services, Employee Affairs, etc.). Formal college-level training programs for people wishing to spend careers working in human resources have been developed in recent decades. In some quarters, contemporary human resource professionals continue to struggle for equal status within the ranks of their organizations.

🔍 CASE STUDY: Mrs. Jackson's Dilemma

In 1930, a hospital located in a prosperous town was growing along with its community. Mrs. Clara Jackson was effectively the administrator of the hospital, although it is doubtful that the title *administrator* was applied. Hospital administration had yet to emerge as a specialized field of study and a profession in its own right. This hospital had started, as many others had begun, as a private clinic owned by physicians who eventually turned their operation over to a community board that would incorporate it as a not-for-profit institution.

In 1930, few professions were represented in a typical hospital. There were physicians, most of whom were in private practice and admitted some of their patients to the hospital. A pharmacist might have been in attendance at least part of the time, as well as a few others working in occupations that later developed into the health professions known today. The dominant occupation in a hospital of that time was by far nursing. Nurses originally provided nearly all of the services required by patients. Because nurses composed the majority of the staff and the persons who were in the hospital all the time, it was natural for a senior nurse, in this case, Mrs. Clara Jackson, to oversee the operation of the facility.

Growth was accompanied by the emergence of people assigned to perform specialized tasks and activities such as housekeeping and food service. Despite their presence, Mrs. Jackson remained the principal manager in the hospital. Her administrative responsibilities, however, cut into the time she could spend where she felt she belonged, which was involved in the nursing issues of patient care. The task that especially consumed much of her time was hiring employees. Even though she was able to delegate the hiring of non-nursing personnel to other group supervisors, Mrs. Jackson was often swamped with activities related to hiring nurses. She felt trapped. If she concentrated on nursing, where she believed she belonged, jobs went unfilled and conditions worsened. If she gave her full attention to hiring nurses, however, she had inadequate time available for her professional nursing responsibilities. Her dilemma intensified when the hospital's sole bookkeeper and paymaster began to complain of having too much work to perform for a single person in keeping up with staff additions and departures. What options were open to Mrs. Jackson in 1930? What options would be available to her today? What other issues or requirements did Mrs. Jackson have to think about in 1930? With what other issues, requirements, or regulations would a contemporary hospital have to cope?

As previously mentioned, a human resources (HR) department provides essential services for any contemporary organization. Detractors claim that an HR department does not generate revenue and is thus of less value than certain other activities. While it is true that it does not produce revenue for the organization, HR does make significant indirect contributions by ensuring that the organization does not violate regulations and other requirements imposed by federal and state governments.

Beginning consideration of human resources and its operation, consider the following example.

▶ An Evolving Department

Common Origins

Many people refer to various activities when discussing the duties and responsibilities of a human resources department within a larger organization. Persons with specialized training in human resources often refer to the same activities but use the term *function* when referring to the duties and responsibilities. The word *function* is sometimes applied to an entire human resources group or organization. Using that nomenclature, a human resources department becomes synonymous with a human resources function. In this text, an effort has been made to avoid overusing the term *function*. This issue is raised at this early stage, so readers will not be surprised when encountering a reference to a human resource function. Throughout this volume, the terms *human resources* and *HR* will be used interchangeably.

The human resources department of today originated and developed in the same manner as most other areas of many healthcare organizations or any other kind of organization. That is, beginning from what now are considered to be a few fairly narrowly defined responsibilities, human resources originated and grew in the same manner as finance, purchasing, and other organizational areas. Bits and pieces of necessary work that have some characteristics in common tend to be bundled or gathered together. This occurs partly because they are related to each other and partly because their common tasks suggest the need for specialized skills and expertise. For example, the finance department evolved as activities that involve money, such as paying salaries, paying bills, receiving payments, maintaining bank accounts, and handling investments, became collected and centralized. Activities that might once have been known as accounting, keeping track of money and reporting on its movements, and payroll, dispensing compensation to workers, were bundled under this broader heading of finance, the name ultimately given to the overall managing of money.

Before the term *human resources* emerged, the bundled organizational activities related to people were called *personnel*. In what is likely a minority of organizations, these bundled activities remain known as *personnel* today. In some organizations, as the activities related to people have evolved and expanded, the change in nomenclature from personnel to human resources has indicated real changes in overall scope and direction. However, in many organizations, the change from personnel to human resources has occurred in name only, with the activities continuing unchanged in depth or breadth; in such instances, the more preferred title is being used, but the scope of activities has not changed.

Development of the Employment Office

Before personnel offices existed, there was an employment office. Before the emergence of a formal employment office, managers like Mrs. Jackson of the opening case study did their own hiring. In many instances, organizations were extremely small by contemporary standards, and the proprietor or the most senior worker was often the sole manager. As businesses grew and the manager or managers became busier, however, they acquired help. The first assistance was clerical in nature: a person to assist with hiring.

The employment office came into being in such organizations because of the growth and accumulation of tasks related to hiring. When a sufficient number of these tasks emerged, it made sense to concentrate them into a single department. One of the reasons for bringing these tasks together in one place was to relieve proprietors and managers of the growing burden of work that did not generate revenue or did not materially advance the completion of the organization's work. The two primary benefits of establishing an employment office included freeing managers from the necessity of personally having to find workers and being able to establish consistency in hiring practices.

Initially, two significant activities pertained to employees and their needs. Workers had to be hired, and they had to be paid. Before these employee-related activities became centralized, they were ordinarily accomplished by proprietors or their designees. In some instances, the task of compensating employees became centralized before hiring itself became centralized. Many proprietors established the position of *paymaster*. In many organizations, the activities of the paymaster were merged into the newly established employment office. In this way, the new area became known as the employment office. The two primary activities became known generally as "employment" and "payroll."

The responsibilities of employment and payroll grew in scope and complexity as organizations were affected by legislation at all levels of their operations. With the introduction of wage-and-hour laws by state and federal governments and the advent of income tax and Social Security with their requirements for employers to withhold monies from employees, those who hired and paid employees acquired more and more tasks to perform within a business. These new tasks were in addition to complying with the requirements of other government agencies.

In a very few organizations, payroll remains part of human resources to this day. In most organizations of any appreciable size, however, payroll has long been a subfunction of finance. The qualification "of appreciable size" acknowledges the practice by many smaller organizations of having the payroll activities provided by an outside vendor; this is an example of outsourcing. In such cases, the human resources office often retains responsibility for transmitting necessary information to the payroll service.

Tasks were added to the employment office as needs arose. These additions had one significant dimension in common: all were related to workers and the process of finding qualified people, hiring them, and maintaining them as employees. The employment office finally reached a point at which it encompassed much more than simply employment (and often payroll). Its name became less and less of an accurate descriptor of the department's activities and responsibilities.

Over time, the employment office began to be known as the personnel department; the title "personnel department" was considered to be a far more accurate description of the department's activities. All in all, the word *personnel* essentially referred to people. All of the responsibilities of a personnel department revolved around an organization's people.

The Expanding Personnel Department

Other forces emerged, and new external requirements were imposed. Employers began to offer forms of compensation in addition to wages. Some began to offer these on their own, while others were spurred by unions. However, most instituted them as a result of competitive forces. These added forms of compensation came to be called *fringe benefits*. These imposed additional responsibilities on an organization. People to support the new tasks had to be placed somewhere in the organization. Because they related to employees and their family members—that is, to people—the personnel department was a natural location for them.

In the economic boom that followed World War II, health insurance programs became part of many organizations' benefit packages or benefits offerings.

Government mandates, such as Workmen's Compensation (later changed to Workers' Compensation in the 1960s), entered the picture as statutory benefits. Statutory benefits are those that an employer is required by law to provide. These include the employer's share of Social Security taxes per the Social Security Act of 1935, participation in Workers' Compensation, and often state-mandated, short-term disability insurance programs. During this time, retirement programs also proliferated, providing more work for personnel.

A major piece of government legislation that caused a great deal of work for some organizations was the National Labor Relations Act of 1935, also known as the Wagner Act. This act provided legal protection to labor unions and made the task of organizing workers considerably easier for unions than it had been. It created a great deal of people-related work for organizations that became subject to union organizing efforts. Once one or more unions were established, their interactions with the employer had to be organized so that business could continue. Some union-related activities, such as running an anti-organizing campaign, conducting negotiations, or administering a contract, were occasionally taken on by line managers. In many organizations, these new activities fell to those who were already in the people business. In contemporary organizations that have unionized employees, an organizational entity known as *labor relations* may exist on its own or as a subsidiary operation within human resources.

Prior to the early 1960s, a typical personnel department was responsible for most activities related to employment, record keeping related to employees, some degree of compensation and benefits administration, and possibly labor relations. Over the years leading up to the early 1960s, personnel departments developed an image of a staff or service group that ran an employment office, kept records, and generally pushed paper. In the early 1960s, however, the importance of the personnel department began to expand. In 1964, personnel departments were required to adopt significantly expanded and increasingly more important roles. The pivotal event in dramatically changing the activities of the personnel department was passage of the Civil Rights Act of 1964.

Beginning in 1964, the work of the personnel department became increasingly more complex, and the level of responsibility involved significantly increased. Practitioners working in the personnel office required more significant knowledge. Specialized education began to develop, and personnel began to grow as a specific professional field. The title *human resources* came into being but did not immediately gain widespread usage.

Even as personnel work grew more complex, more requirements were imposed on the operation. More and different kinds of problems emerged, and additional but different varieties of work had to be performed. The former image of the personnel department as a group of people who recruited employees, kept files, and pushed paper continued to prevail. In many instances, this older image was reinforced by personnel practitioners who, after two or more decades in the field, were overwhelmed by the tide of change; their knowledge fell well behind the times and quickly became obsolete.

In academia, personnel administration became a specialized educational field, joining labor relations as a formal field of study. Several new subdisciplines, such as compensation analysis, benefits administration, employee testing, and selection, began to emerge. In the mid-1970s, the personnel department became responsible for interacting with a variety of external agencies and special-interest groups involved in issues such as Affirmative Action, Equal Employment Opportunity, worker safety, and social responsibility. Many new professionals came from the field of industrial psychology. Others came from programs in management or administration.

Problems with the Term *Personnel*: Real and Perceived

Most of the personnel practitioners of the mid-1900s, from approximately 1945 to 1965, lacked education that specifically prepared them to enter the field of personnel in general or for their specific jobs in particular. When the great majority of these practitioners received their education, most formal training in personnel administration consisted of one or two courses included in other programs of study.

Healthcare organizations, especially hospitals, were once seen as fundamentally low-pressure environments that offered an escape for individuals who had at times been described as industry dropouts. Many administrators, directors of finance, personnel managers, and others came to work in hospitals from businesses and industries in mid-career. Some personnel managers, for example, left manufacturing and industrial positions for hospital jobs as an escape from union involvement. Their previous experiences in healthcare working environments were extremely limited. A strong attraction for making such a career change was to escape from unions, which, at the time, were not especially common in healthcare organizations.

Many of the problems associated with the image of personnel departments and encountered by individual workers were surely due to the performance and behavior of senior personnel practitioners of the time. The lack of educational training contributed to the antipersonnel bias occasionally encountered. As the field became more complex and the pressures of the 1960s and 1970s from increasing union presence, mounting financial pressure, and the government's entry into health care via Medicare, Medicaid, and state regulations continued to mount, many of these persons found themselves in situations that far exceeded their training or experience.

Many people who spend their entire working lives in one particular job or working environment do not readily adapt to change. Some of the practitioners who entered healthcare personnel work between 1945 and 1965 fell by the wayside as the field became more complex, tougher, and considerably more demanding. Some were unable to cope with unions and the demands of labor relations. Others became frustrated by the demands imposed by Affirmative Action and other newly introduced civil rights concerns and legislation. In the 1980s, some gave up when they perceived increasing government regulation of benefits as creating a technical and legal nightmare.

Some undeniable image problems related to the personnel department still exist. A minority of senior managers continue to view personnel as a relatively unimportant staff activity that does little more than hire people and file papers. A considerable number of employees view the operations of personnel as a necessary bureaucratic activity that exists primarily for the benefit of a corporation and not for them.

What's in a (New) Name?

Today, although human resources, or HR, is the prevailing name for the department that handles personnel matters, the HR label is far from universally used. Many departments fulfilling the same overall responsibilities are still called *personnel departments.* Other names are occasionally encountered, among them, *employee affairs, employee services, personnel informatics, benefits processing,* and others. Most of the uncommon titles reflect a limited portion of the activities that are performed by a contemporary, full-spectrum human resources department.

Is the term *human resources* more descriptive than *personnel*? Some experts contend that an organization's ultimate resource is financial, and an organization uses financial resources to acquire both things (*material* resources) and people (*human* resources). Therefore, in an organizational context, *human resources* means people, as does the older, alternate title *personnel.*

Why the Change?

Most scholars of the field agree that *personnel* became *human resources* in many organizations for one or more of the following reasons: the new name more appropriately reflected the workload of the department, the change in name improved the image and elevated the status of the work being performed, and the new name enhanced the professionalism of those who were accomplishing the work.

Did the personnel department become human resources to escape the existing and often negative image of *personnel*? For some practitioners and organizations, the change was made to overcome the outmoded and limited view of personnel and to gain both professional acknowledgment and a measure of respectability.

A parallel transformation of organizational image occurred in finance. Once there was only bookkeeping, which eventually became accounting, as reporting and analytical tasks were added to the simple business of keeping track of money in and money out. As organizations grew, there developed the necessity to raise money, invest money, and generally manage money well beyond the needs of day-to-day operations, so the finance function developed. In most instances, those narrower money-related activities, such as payroll and accounting, were brought under the umbrella of finance. This particular transformation is incomplete and far from being universally accepted; many contemporary accounting and finance practitioners are dismissed as number-crunchers or bean-counters. Marketing professionals incur a similar lack of professional respect or identity. Despite extensive efforts to modify their image, many marketing departments are stereotypically referred to simply as *sales,* a term that has existed for decades and frequently carries derogatory connotations.

Practitioners in every field are required to learn and grow. The alternative is to fall behind and eventually fail. Change occurs at various rates in different occupational fields. In the field of personnel or human resources, several bursts of change occurred within a sufficiently brief period to impact the career spans of many practitioners.

Bias, whether real or perceived, cannot be overcome by a simple change of name. Neither can respectability be acquired by a change of name. Respect, however, can be earned over time as a new image emerges, one that has nothing to do with the department's title other than shedding the negativity that some associate with the name *personnel.* Human resources is taking its place among those activities now viewed as being essential to the success and survival of a modern organization. It required decades to form and solidify the image of personnel as being neither especially difficult nor demanding. The transformation of that image has been under way for years, yet it is far from complete.

Not everyone associated with the field has been enthusiastic about the name change to human resources. One personnel director described the trend to change the name of the company personnel office to the department of human resources as "an excellent example of corporate pomposity" (Hoey, 1987). The article argued that employees are human and special, not just another resource similar to real estate or spare parts. As an interesting side note, not long after the article appeared in the professional journal *Personnel*, the publication changed its name to *HR Magazine*. Regardless of whether or not one approves of the name change, no title alone will confer respect. That is a commodity that must be earned through performance. When performance is forthcoming, respect will follow.

Here to Stay

For a number of years, *human resources* has been the growing name of choice for this service activity of an organization. The *HR* name has been adopted by professional organizations, academic programs, and publications formerly designated as serving personnel. This is a fairly good sign that the title *human resources* will probably dominate for the next few decades.

The changeover of name was most evident during the 1980s. Surveys indicated that in 1986, some 40% of such departments used the HR designation. Just 42 months later, the proportion using the HR designation was at 60% and still climbing. Also, the HR title was more prevalent in larger organizations, in use in 80% or more of organizations having 2500 or more employees (Stier, 1989).

The title *human resources* is more prevalent in larger organizations. Professional organizations have also changed their names. The American Society for Personnel Administration has become the Society for Human Resource Management.

A number of additional surveys conducted by professional HR organizations during the 1980s and 1990s seemed to focus primarily on the degree to which the name change from *personnel* to *human resources* had affected the status of the department within its organization. Historically, the position of the head of HR has carried the title *director* or *manager* among supposed peers who enjoy the title *vice president*. The head of HR frequently reports to a vice president rather than directly to the president or executive vice president.

The component duties and responsibilities of HR are not uniform across organizations. Changes are being made, but the relative status of HR within most organizations is improving only slowly. Many HR departments remain in stages of transition, and some have made little progress. However, they are changing and continuing to evolve to be better able to address new and more complex responsibilities.

Experts disagree as to the present status of an HR department within the healthcare industry. Most do agree on several broad points, however. First and foremost, HR must continue to evolve so that it can remain current with the changing needs of healthcare organizations. Next, HR must strive to transcend its traditional reactionary role and adopt a more proactive outlook and approach. Human resources should be available to minimize undesirable occurrences to an organization through the systematic identification of potential problems. The next step is working to avoid them or similar ones in the future.

In addition to performing all of the expected duties in support of an organization's employees, an effective contemporary HR department serves as a full-fledged partner on an administrative team, participates in organizational strategic planning as a full-fledged member, guides succession planning for an organization, and works as an agent for necessary and healthy change.

Throughout the remainder of this text, the term *human resources* (or simply HR) will be used as the prevailing name for the department or functional area. This use is not to be construed as claiming that any group that is called *personnel* or another name is any less legitimate than a human resources department. True differences do not reside in labels.

▶ The Focus Broadens

For all practical purposes, during the 1900s, human resources in the healthcare industry essentially meant human resources in hospitals. Until the 1960s, acute-care hospitals were perceived as being the center of the American healthcare system. Virtually, all healthcare services provided to people were delivered in a hospital. Those that were not provided in hospitals were rendered in physicians' personal offices. One has only to look briefly at the different healthcare provider organizations in existence today to appreciate that human resources in health care is now practiced in a variety of settings and organizations that are both large and small.

Identifying only a small sample of organizations that deliver healthcare services will help to make an important point. Contemporary components of the healthcare system include free-standing surgical centers; urgent care providers; community health centers; public health agencies; long-term care providers; groups specializing in imaging, physical therapy, laboratory testing, and other activities; and several forms of medical and surgical group practices of varying sizes. All of these organizations, from the smallest partnership or group practice to the largest acute-care hospital, require the presence of human resources knowledge and expertise. In larger organizations, this expertise is provided by a human resources department. In a small organization, HR expertise may be provided by an in-house individual whose time and duties wholly or partly focus on personnel-related activities. Human resources needs may be outsourced or met by an external consultant who provides them on an hourly basis or whose services are shared among several small health provider offices. Regardless of size, however, human resources needs are essential to the operation of organizations in today's healthcare environment.

▶ Conclusion

The typical human resources department has grown from a single-person operation into a multifaceted, complex organization. In some organizations, a single person continues to perform all of the needed tasks, although this has become an exception rather than the rule. The volume of government regulations has greatly increased in recent decades. The scope of duties performed has also increased. Changing the departmental name from *personnel* to *human resources* reflects these developments. People are now receiving specialized training in colleges and universities for subsegments of human resource activities. However, they continue to struggle for professional recognition and equal status with their organizational counterparts.

🔍 *CASE STUDY: Resolution*

Returning to the dilemma posed in the initial case study, the first step that Mrs. Jackson took in lightening her load of non-nursing responsibilities was to hire a helper. The selected person was a combination secretary and general assistant who coordinated most of the hiring activities for the hospital. In effect, this helper was the hospital's first personnel worker. It is likely that the first personnel records section was a drawer in this individual's desk or file cabinet. At the time, employee hiring was the only element of a personnel worker's position description or list of job duties. No government regulations had yet been introduced in 1930; the Social Security Act, with its automatic withholding of employees' contributions, was not created until 1935. Affirmative Action and Equal Opportunity legislation was not enacted until the mid-1960s. The Americans with Disabilities Act added additional duties in 1990.

Mrs. Jackson's helper was a staff of one that became the hospital's employment office. Within a few years, this office evolved into a personnel department. Mrs. Jackson was extremely relieved to be able to delegate the growing burdens of securing employees and looking after many of their needs. She continued to be involved in employee acquisition to the extent of interviewing potential employees for her own area, but she no longer assumed the responsibility to find and screen all job applicants. Furthermore, she did not have to process them into and out of the organization.

SPOTLIGHT ON CUSTOMER SERVICE

Customer Service: An Introduction

Customer service has become a buzzword in contemporary organizations. The good news is that organizations are waking up and beginning to recognize the importance of customer service. The bad news is that many of the same organizations treat customer service as little more than a passing fad.

Customer service is important. Critics may be correct when they say that customer service is only a single factor among many that contribute to an organization's success. However, poor customer service alone has the potential to cause organizational failure. Consider a restaurant that employs servers with poor attitudes. Conventional wisdom asserts that all dissatisfied customers tell as many as 20 additional actual or potential customers about their unsatisfactory experience. Satisfied customers typically share their experiences with only one or two other persons.

Quickly, the reputation for poor customer service spreads through a population and buries perceptions of good service. The main cost associated with customer service is remembering to provide it.

Modified from Hoey, J. T. (1987). Human resources versus personnel. *Personnel, 64*(5), 72–75; Stier, D. (1989). More use of the human resource title. *Resource, Society for Human Resource Management (SHRM), 10*, 2–4. (SHRM was formerly ASPA, the American Society for Personnel Administration.) Townsend, R. (1970). *Up the organization*. New York, NY: Alfred A. Knopf.

Questions for Review and Discussion

1. Describe how you believe the business of locating, hiring, and maintaining employees was accomplished before the establishment of an employment office. List the activities that were probably performed, and who was most likely to have performed them.

2.   With specific reference to activities found within healthcare organizations, describe how three departments or functional areas *other than human resources* might have evolved in a manner similar to the evolution of HR. In each instance, describe the activities that might have initially existed and then accrued to form the basis of each activity as it is known today.

3.   In your opinion, what did senior managers in the past believe were the primary benefits of gathering a variety of employee-related tasks together to form an employment office?

4.   In your opinion, what were the two or three earliest changes that influenced the development of a centralized operation to address matters related to employees? Why?

5.   Why might some people consider the term *fringe benefits* to be misleading at best or completely erroneous at worst? Why is the value of these benefits most appropriately included as part of total compensation?

6.   Comment concerning the industry dropout phenomenon as it concerned earlier full-time human resources managers in health care. Is the somewhat derogatory label of "industry dropout" reasonably or unreasonably applied? Why?

7.   Do you personally agree with changing the name from *personnel* to *human resources*? Why or why not?

8.   Do you support or oppose the abolition of a central personnel department in favor of having individual managers assume the responsibility for all such activities for their own departments? Why?

9.   Do you believe that changing the name of *personnel* to *human resources* substantially improved the image of the department or service area? Why?

10.   Comment on the following quotation from *Up the Organization* (Townsend, 1970): "Fire the whole personnel department. Unless your company is too large (in which case break it up into autonomous parts), have a one-girl people department (not personnel department)." Keep in mind that this passage was written in the late 1960s.

References

Hoey, J. T. (1987). Human resources versus personnel. *Personnel, 64*(5), 72–75.

Stier, D. (1989). More use of the human resource title. *Resource, Society for Human Resource Management (SHRM), 10,* 2–4. (SHRM was formerly ASPA, the American Society for Personnel Administration.)

Townsend, R. (1970). *Up the organization.* New York, NY: Alfred A. Knopf.

Resources

Books

Bashford, A. (2004). *Imperial hygiene: A critical history of colonialism, nationalism, and public health.* New York, NY: Palgrave Macmillan.

Flynn, W. J., Langan, P. J., Jackson, J. H., & Mathis, R. L. (2003). *Healthcare human resources and management.* Mason, OH: South-Western Publishing Company.

Ljungberg, J., & Smits, J. P. (2005). *Technology and human capital in historical perspective.* New York, NY: Palgrave Macmillan.

Martocchio, J. J. (2005). *Research in personnel and human resources management.* Burlington, MA: Elsevier.

Mathis, R. L., & Jackson, J. H. (2005). *Human resource management* (11th ed.). Mason, OH: South-Western Publishing Company.

McConnell, C. R. (2019). *The effective health care supervisor* (9th ed.). Burlington, MA: Jones & Bartlett Learning.

Niles, N. J. (2012). *Basic concepts of health care human resource management.* Burlington, MA: Jones & Bartlett Learning.

Phillips, J. J., & Phillips, P. P. (2012). *Proving the value of HR: How and why to measure ROI* (2nd ed.). Alexandria, VA: Society for Human Resource Management.

Renckly, R. B. (2004). *Human resources.* Hauppauge, NY: Barrons.

Stredwick, J. (2005). *Introduction to human resource management* (2nd ed.). Burlington, MA: Butterworth-Heinemann.

Periodicals

Anand, S., & Barnighausen, T. (2004). Human resources and health outcomes: Cross-country econometric study. *Lancet, 364*(9445), 1603–1609.

Armstrong, G. (2005). Differentiation through people: How can HR move beyond business partner? *Human Resources Management, 44*(2), 195–199.

Bowen, D. E., & Ostroff, C. (2004). Understanding HRM-firm performance linkages: The role of the "strength" of the HRM system. *Academy of Management Review, 29,* 203–221.

Boxall, P. (2003). HR strategy and competitive advantage in the service sector. *Human Resource Management Journal, 13*(3), 5–20.

Butler, T., & Waldroop, J. (2004). Understanding "people" people. *Harvard Business Review, 82*(6), 78–86, 136.

Clark, I., & Colling, T. (2005). The management of human resources in project management–led organizations. *Personnel Review, 34*(2), 178–191.

Ellem, B. (2005). Putting work in its place: The making of ideal workers and social contracts. *Asia Pacific Journal of Human Resources, 43*(2), 238–251.

Knouse, S. B. (2005). The future of human resource management: 64 thought leaders explore the critical HR issues of today and tomorrow. *Personnel Pathology, 58*(4), 1089–1092.

Marchal, B., & De Brouwere, V. (2004). Global human resources crisis. *Lancet, 363*(9427), 2191–2192.

Meisinger, S. R. (2005). The four Cs of the HR profession: Being competent, curious, courageous, and caring about people. *Human Resources Management, 44*(2), 189–194.

Mendenhall, M., Jensen, R., Black, J. S., & Gregersen, H. (2003). Seeing the elephant: HR challenges in the age of globalization. *Organizational Dynamics, 3*(4), 261–274.

Phillips, P. P., & Phillips, J. J. (2004). ROI in the public sector: Myths and realities. *Public Personnel Management, 33*(2), 139–149.

Roehling, M. V., Boswell, W. R., Feldman, D., Graham, M. E., Guthrie, J. P., & Morishima, M. (2005). The future of HR management: Research needs and directions. *Human Resources Management, 44*(2), 207–216.

Ryan-Nicholls, K. D. (2004). Preceptor recruitment and retention. *Canadian Nurse, 100*(6), 18–22.

Zapf, D. (2002). Emotion, work and psychological well-being: A review of the literature and some conceptual considerations. *Human Resource Management Review, 12,* 237–268.

CHAPTER 2

How Human Resources Fits into an Organization

CHAPTER OBJECTIVES

After studying this chapter, readers will be able to:

- Understand the placement of human resources within an organizational hierarchy.
- Distinguish between line and staff activities and classify human resources as an essential staff operation.
- Describe several models for organizing a human resources department.
- Describe how the human resources operation is commonly organized to best serve an organization.
- Appreciate the relationship between human resources and executive management and other organizational departments.
- Understand the role of human resources when implementing changes within an organization.
- Understand the effects of reengineering on services provided by human resources.
- Appreciate contemporary trends regarding outsourcing human resource services.

▶ Chapter Summary

Ideally, the person heading a human resources (HR) department should report to an organization's chief executive officer (CEO). A variety of organizational structures are used in HR departments. These include models based on clerical tasks, counseling, industrial relations, control, and consulting. Some HR professionals have proposed using similar approaches when establishing an HR organization.

Line and staff employees perform different tasks for an organization. Line operations advance the work of an organization. Staff operations support and enhance the work of an organization by making it possible to continue producing products or delivering services as intended.

The degree of effectiveness of HR depends on a chief executive officer's attitude toward that activity. As a staff operation, HR does not issue commands and is

🔍 CASE STUDY: What Shall It Be and Where Do We Put It?

"Things were much simpler when we were just a small-town hospital with a four-person personnel department," said personnel director Sharon Kelly to her immediate superior, chief operating officer Don Thomas. "But now that we're a so-called health system, it's almost impossible to tell who is supposed to be doing what for whom on any given day."

Sharon's allusion to a system was in reference to the recent merger of their facility, Community Hospital, with a somewhat smaller rural facility located 15 miles away. At the time of the merger, Community Hospital, newly renamed the Affiliated Community Health and Education System (ACHES), acquired an organization consisting of three primary care centers that became satellite facilities for the system and became affiliated with an additional two sizable group practices, one medical and one surgical.

Sharon continued, "And now, as I understand it, we're going to be called human resources, not personnel. Is that right?"

Don nodded. "Yep, it'll be Human Resources from now on." He grinned and added, "We might as well call it HR. That's what every other place is doing."

"Don't get me wrong," Sharon said. "I'm not complaining. I'm really pleased with being named personnel—that is, HR—director for the system. But look at what we've got to work with. There are four of us here at Community. Two people are in the department at the other hospital and one personnel person at the biggest of the satellites, with just a secretary taking care of personnel stuff at the other two satellites. Office managers at the group practices are overloaded trying to take care of personnel matters along with a dozen other concerns. And now we've got such a far-flung setup that if I were to get in my car and make a circuit of all of our facilities, I'd travel more than 60 miles. What can we do with all of this?"

Still smiling, Don said, "That's what we want to know. We want to know how to organize the new HR department to best serve the Affiliated Community Health and Education System. Every essential base has to be covered, but keep in mind that nothing is forever, given that we'll probably continue to grow and change."

"But what does the CEO want from Pers . . . ah, Human Resources?"

Don shrugged. "In some respects your guess is as good as mine. You know how she's been about your area since she's been here. She expects us to recruit good employees for the hospital system and keep good records. Keep the system out of legal trouble, but don't make waves."

At that moment, Sharon had very little idea of the direction she should recommend.

How would you respond to Don's request? How should the new HR department be organized? What issues should the HR department focus on first? What aspects may change over time? Why?

vulnerable to changes that result from reengineering. Outsourcing human resource services is relatively common.

▶ Human Resources in the Organization: The Macro View

In healthcare facilities, the individual in charge of HR usually reports to one of the organization's two top executives, generally the president or chief executive officer, referred to in some healthcare organizations as administrator or director. Alternatively, the head of the HR department may report to the number two executive in the organization, the executive vice president or chief operating officer (COO), who may hold the title of associate administrator or assistant administrator. In many large, contemporary healthcare organizations, people heading HR departments report to the top executive. In a small facility, there may be no second level of executive management, so the head of human resources will likely report directly to the CEO.

Having HR report to a level other than executive management is inappropriate; reporting at a lower level has the potential to weaken HR's effectiveness. Even reporting to the second executive level, COO, or associate administrator can result in conflict with other organizational departments that report to the CEO. The COO has responsibility for all of the operating departments, which includes the majority of employees. Other staff operations (for example, finance) typically report directly to the president or CEO. Instances can arise in which finance and HR are in disagreement. It can seem like HR "belongs to" operations alone when HR reports to the COO. In such an arrangement, HR might be incapable of fair and equitable dealings with others in the larger organization or at least be perceived as such. If HR reports at any level lower than CEO, in instances of conflict there is always the possibility that this function will be seen as favoring the division that "owns" it.

▶ Line and Staff

Two important distinctions must be made when using the terms *line* and *staff*. How do people in these different positions operate within an organization, and how do they differ? Although the actual relationships may be different, how does organizational authority—that is, the chain of command—apply to both?

Doing Versus Supporting

Simply stated, the difference between line and staff in an organization is as elementary as the difference between doing and supporting. Line departments actually perform an organization's work, while staff departments facilitate the work, striving to enable overall efficiency and effectiveness.

Another way to describe a line operation is to say that it advances the work of the organization. In the manufacture of a physical product, each line activity that is performed changes the physical shape or state of a product and brings it closer to completion. When a service is being provided, each activity advances the state of completion of the service. If a line operation is ignored or omitted, the final physical product remains incomplete or unfinished; if a service is not delivered in a satisfactory manner or if an activity that should have been performed along the way is omitted, then the service is incomplete. In the food service area of a hospital, for example, if one station on a tray assembly line is missing, then the meals that are assembled on that line will be incomplete. In another example, if a nurse neglects to administer a particular medication when scheduled, then the services delivered to the affected patient will be incomplete.

A staff operation does not advance the work of an organization or hasten its completion. Rather, it supports and enhances the work of an organization by making it possible to continue producing products or delivering services as intended.

Staff positions may be removed and the productive work of an organization will usually continue, at least for a time. However, the organization is likely to become inefficient and will eventually cease working without the necessary staff support. Staff areas within a healthcare organization include HR, finance, housekeeping (or environmental services), and maintenance (or plant engineering). While none of these activities directly advance the provision of services, if they are not performed, then patient care will eventually experience both inefficiencies and deteriorating quality. The primary role of staff or supporting areas is to maintain an organization's service environment and capability, making it possible for line operations to continue in an optimal manner.

In most instances, it is possible to determine whether an activity is line or staff by imagining what would happen to the workflow if the activity were to cease. If an activity or position is abandoned and the workflow is immediately disrupted, then it is a line operation. If there is no apparent short-term effect on workflow, then it is a staff operation.

What happens when individuals engaged in line activities disagree about how services should be provided or supported with those who perform staff operations? If a conflict between line and staff cannot be resolved by the managers of the respective departments, then it is ordinarily referred to higher management.

The Chain of Command

The concept of line and staff can become somewhat confusing when considered in conjunction with the chain of command. In every department, whether line or staff, there is a line of authority that runs downward from the department manager. This line includes all subordinate supervisors and eventually all rank-and-file employees. The line of authority is known as the chain of command. A manager of a staff activity is also a line manager, but only within that particular area. For example, the director of finance has line authority over the employees in finance, but that authority does not extend beyond the boundaries of the department. The director of finance can exercise line authority within but not outside of finance. Every staff activity has a limited chain of command embedded within it, but this line of authority does not extend outside of the department. In line operations, the chain of command can extend through several organizational levels and include more than one department. For example, the CEO has authority over the COO, who, in turn, has authority over the director of materials management, who has authority over others, and so on, to the final link in the chain of command. The line of authority extends through all levels.

As described earlier, the HR department is a staff organization. The line and staff distinction is extremely important when considering where HR is located in the organizational structure and how it operates. The person in charge of HR has line authority only within HR. As a staff operation that provides services, HR has no authority over any employees outside of its departmental boundaries. The HR department may be an organization's expert and official voice regarding personnel policies, compensation, benefits, and many of the legalities of employment, but HR has no power of enforcement. However, a limited minority of HR professionals object to this contention; they operate within a control model under which HR assumes some enforcement authority.

Occasionally, an operational area straddles the boundary between line and staff. An obvious example is dietary services, which has the responsibility to feed patients, administer therapeutic dietetics (both line activities), and prepare cafeteria and snack shop meals (both staff activities).

Managers working in a healthcare organization must understand that although HR may ultimately report at or near the top of an organizational structure, it is a staff operation. Its role is largely providing service and rendering advice. As such, HR has no authority over any other operational areas or departments in an organization. The HR department exists to provide advice, guidance, assistance, and whatever other services may be deemed appropriate according to the mission of the organization and the needs of other departments.

▶ The Appearance of Human Resources

Perceived Human Resources Models

Human resources may be viewed in a variety of ways depending on the department's position in an organization's hierarchy. Relevant aspects include how it is perceived by other employees, the behavior of HR management and staff, and the expectations of senior HR managers. Other influences include the traditional role of HR within an organization, the demands placed on HR by the larger organization, and the education, training, and experience of the HR staff and personnel. Previous perceptions of an HR department are often viewed as models for HR service delivery. One author discussed five recognizable models of HR organization: clerical, counseling, industrial relations, control, and consulting (Andrews, 1986).

The Clerical Model

The clerical model represents the long-held and unflattering stereotypical view of personnel. Under this model, an HR department exists to process and file paper, maintain records, track statistics and key dates, and administer employee benefits plans. Under the clerical model, the top manager of HR is likely to be experienced as a benefits administrator or have a similar practitioner orientation. In organizations where this model still exists, HR is rarely called upon to go beyond these expectations.

The Counseling Model

This model is relatively common in hospitals and other service organizations where the total cost of employees represents a relatively large proportion of the budget, and where an organization places an emphasis on maintaining employees as effective producers. Under this model, HR is likely to act as an advocate for employees, provide a resource to managers for addressing people problems, resolve disputes and disciplinary issues, place a high priority on preserving privacy and confidentiality, stress training and development throughout the year at all levels of an organization, lag behind the state of the art in effective compensation and benefits administration, and maintain a posture that is primarily reactive.

The Industrial Relations Model

The industrial relations model typically develops in organizations in which the workforce is unionized and there are periodic contract negotiations. Another aspect of this model is considerable activity having to do with grievances, arbitrations, and similar confrontations. Under this model, an HR group is likely to have its activities and procedures specified by contract and performed automatically with little innovation. Because employees are directed by a contract, they have few opportunities to display flexibility or judgment as they perform their job duties. HR employees are viewed as powerless within an organization's structure. Such a view is usually limited and not especially positive.

The Control Model

Infrequently encountered in American organizations, under the control model, HR has substantial power. This usually stems from the charisma, personality, or individual strength of its top manager and key staff. A control-model HR department usually exerts dominance over any aspect of operations having HR implications. Consistent with this model, many managerial decisions are made only following clearance by HR personnel. HR staff members must be current and knowledgeable concerning applicable legal requirements and must understand policies and procedures. Other work rules must be consistently applied. Under the control model, an HR departmental executive is a key member of an organization's administrative team. With this model in place, managers of other departments may feel stifled and see the larger organization as being inflexible, bureaucratic, and rule-bound. Under the control model, employee involvement activities receive minimal if any support.

The Consulting Model

This model is ordinarily found in larger organizations. Here, HR practitioners are usually expert resources. Employees, department managers, and executive management rely upon them. The services provided by HR personnel are determined by demand. However, this is primarily a reactive model that provides effective service wherever an apparent need is identified but leaves some organizational needs either unmet or unidentified.

The models previously discussed describe some dominant perceptions of HR. These models are unlikely to exist in their pure forms. Rather, most organizations feature a mix of the characteristics of two or three models. This commonly prevails because of differing philosophies introduced by a succession of HR department heads. However, one particular model will usually prevail in the perceptions of employees and their department managers. Most HR professionals agree that an effective HR department is best utilized as a consultant or advisor. Ineffective HR departments are relegated to providing clerical services.

The greatest single problem with all of the foregoing models is that they are primarily reactive. All of the HR services provided by the models are needed. These services should be delivered without any single model dominating or overwhelming an organization. However, managers at all organizational levels must constantly work to make HR a true strategic partner in the achievement of an organization's mission.

Alternative Human Resources Models

In the late 1980s, another approach to providing human relations services emerged. Driver, Coffey, and Bowen (1988) created alternate models based on the operational areas of an organization. Organizations would, in theory, adopt the model that best reflected the most dominant aspect of their mission or core business. The next models to be described are similar to those already discussed. However, they reflect different points of view. The HR activities and services of an organization can be accurately described by using a combination of the foregoing classic models and the next revised models. The next models include approaches based on alternative clerical approaches, the law, finance, management, humanism, and behavioral science.

The Alternative Clerical Model

This is similar to the clerical model described earlier. According to this model, the primary role of HR is to acquire data, maintain records, and file required reports. Human resources personnel perform routine tasks, process paperwork, comply with regulations, provide a steady pool of prospective employees, and meet the needs of existing and retired workers. This model presents HR as passive and relatively weak.

The Legal Model

Under the legal model, an HR department derives its primary strength and reputation from its knowledge and expertise concerning legislation that affects various aspects of employment. Compliance with all applicable laws is the overriding concern of all who work in such a department. Others in an organization may view HR as a bureaucracy. Occasionally, others may judge it to be intrusive, obstructive, or both. The legal model is frequently present when part of a workforce is unionized. An advantage of the legal model is its expertise and ability to negotiate contracts, monitor contract compliance, and address grievances.

The Financial Model

An HR department operating under the financial model displays maximum attention to human resource costs. Particular attention is paid to indirect compensation costs such as health and dental insurance, life insurance, retirement plans, paid time off, and other benefits offered to employees. Successful human resource practitioners working under this model are frequently well versed in matters of finance. A potential hazard of this model is placing financial matters above all other employee relations issues.

The Managerial Model

Under a managerial model, HR personnel often work within the same bottom-line productivity-oriented framework as do most line managers. They share the same goals and values as line managers and make decisions in accordance with organizational managerial objectives. This model lends itself to decentralization of HR activities and services, under which line managers perform many of the tasks typically reserved for HR personnel. This model sometimes results in inconsistency in the application of HR practices because of having organizational guidelines interpreted by so many different persons. A potential drawback of the managerial model is that an organization may end up having no particular strategic outlook or involvement in long-range planning.

The Humanistic Model

The central tenet of the humanistic model of HR is that it exists primarily to foster human values and potential within an organization. Individual employees are the primary focus of HR practitioners. Individual development and career planning are emphasized. The model assumes that enhancing the working life of each individual enhances the overall effectiveness of an organization. Experts claim that the rising level of education and the general sophistication of employees and their expectations of a high-quality work experience provide support for this model.

The Behavioral Science Model

The behavioral science model assumes that disciplines such as psychology, social psychology, sociology, and organizational behavior provide the foundation for most HR activities. This model is frequently used when designing performance appraisal systems, job evaluation classifications, reward and incentive programs, employee development plans, and employee interest and attitude surveys. Increasing sophistication of both managers and employees provides some support for this approach.

As with the first set of models introduced, the alternative HR models are unlikely to be found as pure types. For example, many managers continue to assume that HR provides clerical services. Despite how modern and sophisticated HR becomes, organizations will continue to maintain a significant number of records. In the highly unlikely event of a marked change or reversal in the amount of legislation impacting employment, the legal model will appear to prevail. Nevertheless, for many HR departments, one or two particular models will predominate, or at least seem to according to the perceptions of line managers and rank-and-file employees.

Internal Organization of Human Resources

An HR department will customarily be organized according to an organization's expectations, reflecting the prevailing goals and structure of the organization that it serves. Smaller organizations typically employ HR generalists. The usual reason for such a decision is staffing limitations. The requirements of a small organization can usually be satisfied by a single person, sometimes working less than full time. Larger organizations employ a mix of specialists and generalists. Their requirements cannot be met by a single person, and they have the resources to employ several individuals. In larger healthcare organizations, specialists are most often used. These specialists are listed in descending order of the frequency with which they are most likely to be encountered.

1. Employment
2. Compensation and benefits
3. Employee relations
4. Training and development

5. Labor relations
6. Equal Employment Opportunity (EEO)
7. Security
8. Safety

The individuals or customers served by an HR department vary. Internal customers include all existing or former employees at all organizational levels. External customers include potential employees or applicants for employment.

Human Resources and Senior Management

The attitude of an organization's CEO toward HR usually sets the tone for the rest of the employees. Tone includes attributes such as the relative standing of an HR department within the larger organization and the respect that is accorded to HR by others throughout the organization. Translated tone determines how much power or influence an HR department will be able to exercise. Human resources departments that have power or influence are respected; the reverse is also true. Respect leads to involvement and interdependence throughout an organization. The respect is fundamentally based on the expectations of the CEO.

What CEOs Expect from Human Resources

Chief executive officers have some common expectations of HR departments. Most want their HR department to supervise recruitment, administer compensation and benefits programs, and maintain personnel records. These are the activities that HR experts include as the minimum or basics of the profession. While many other activities can be assumed or provided by an HR department, some senior managers demand only the basics.

A considerable number of CEOs expect their HR departments to provide advice and counsel on employee matters. Many expect the head of HR to serve as a personal adviser for personnel issues. In unionized working environments, CEOs may expect someone in HR to monitor activities related to labor relations.

Occasionally, a CEO wants to have an HR department that provides the basic services but does so in an unobtrusive manner. In other words, such an HR department should not make waves. It should be seen but not heard. In reality, this is a difficult assignment. Human resources is expected to meet basic personnel expectations in a competent and professional manner but must not advocate for innovation or positive changes. The CEOs making such demands on an HR department often have large or oversized egos.

Many CEOs say that they want a professional and innovative HR department. However, those that mouth the words are more numerous than individuals who truly desire, appreciate, and utilize competent and professional HR services and advice.

The personal and organizational priorities of CEOs influence their expectations of an HR department. If senior managers are content with simply maintaining the status quo, then few changes are likely to emerge from HR. Such executives are not oriented to the future or instituting changes. They usually overlook HR's potential value in business and strategic planning, personnel and career path preparation, and development of different or innovative HR strategies.

Human resource-related tasks have dramatically expanded over the past several decades. Most of these additional requirements have been mandated by legislation that began with the Civil Rights Act of 1964 and received added impetus from the Equal Employment Opportunity Act of 1972. Human resources departments have become much larger as they attempt to keep pace with legal demands, to create and update necessary systems, and to add and expand services. Because of this reactive posture, the discipline of HR has missed an opportunity to become more of a full partner in organizational management. Many critical observers have wondered whether HR is a full planner and decision maker or simply a firefighter.

This distinction is related to the attitudes of senior management. Human resources becomes a more integral and important member of a management team to the extent that senior managers regard HR as a professional specialty. Furthermore, they ensure that the HR department is staffed and led by competent people who have been appropriately educated and trained. They provide support for an HR department in an open and continuous manner.

How does a department whose responsibilities are continually changing and evolving remain current? Further complicating this question is the widely held perception that HR is an entity to be tolerated rather than embraced because it does not generate revenue. Expressed differently, how does an HR department become a strategic organizational partner with its leader a full-fledged member of senior management? The field of HR has been wrestling with this question for decades without reaching any satisfactory conclusions. It has gained status in some healthcare organizations, but in many this has yet to become a reality.

▶ Human Resources in Relation to Other Departments

From the perspective of departmental personnel, HR has traditionally been viewed as more administrative than advisory, more as an enforcer of policies than a policy maker. Many individuals throughout almost every organization regard HR as a group of paper pushers. It acquired this sobriquet by virtue of its employment-related activities. Increasing governmental reporting requirements have reinforced this perception. In short, in the minds of many people, HR merely hires people and files papers.

The proliferation of laws and regulations governing almost all aspects of employment relationships has been a major factor in the changing role and relative organizational position of an HR department. However, organizational managers outside of the HR department often cannot see or appreciate the legal and regulatory obstacles that must be avoided. Rather, they see only the portion of HR that applies to their own departments. Furthermore, they often lack the perspective to appreciate why HR makes the demands that it imposes on other organizational units. For many, HR appears to be a rule-bound, bureaucratic group that, in their opinions, is trying to prevent them from accomplishing tasks they feel are necessary. Even persons who have a partial appreciation of the regulatory environment in which HR must operate often come to view HR as little more than a necessary evil.

Many of the prevailing views or, more accurately, stereotypes of an HR department prevent managers from seeking appropriate counsel or assistance until their needs or problems have become critical. The time to call upon experts from HR for assistance is when the earliest signs of a problem appear. When personnel-related issues involve discipline or legal action, many opportunities for intervention have already been lost. Full-blown problems can be resolved, but the cost is usually far greater than it could have been if advice had been sought at an earlier juncture.

If an HR department exists to serve an organization, then why is it still often viewed as an obstacle? Resistance sometimes emerges as a result of a particular department's approach or the attitude of its practitioners. When individuals in an organization perceive a group as a miniature bureaucracy, the reasons for the perception can usually be found in the behavior of the group's staff. In addition, the reasons why persons in an HR department may offer recommendations that are contrary to the expectations of department managers are not clearly communicated. Consider the following example.

A department manager has had a key position open for several weeks, and the lack of a person to fill the position is impacting the department's output. It is affecting other staff members who have been obliged to cover the vacancy through mandatory overtime. An ideal candidate appears, is referred to the manager by HR, is interviewed, and is immediately offered the position. This ideal candidate accepts and indicates an ability to begin work at any time. The manager responds to HR by saying, "I want this person to start work tomorrow."

However, protocols used by HR call for a delay. The recruiter in HR responds to the departmental manager by saying, "We must have time to check references and properly clear this candidate. Even on a fast track, the earliest starting date we can give you is in a week." Although the manager understands that proper clearance means conducting reference checks and completing a pre-employment physical examination, the manager insists on a next-day start and says, "The reference checks and the physical can be concluded next week. In the meantime, we can get a start on attacking the backlog of work that has accumulated."

Because HR refuses to authorize the immediate start, the department manager proceeds to complain to other peer and senior-level managers about HR's inflexibility and unwillingness to cooperate. The involved HR representative stands firm, without appreciating the fact that the complaining department manager may not be aware that regulations (at least in some states) legally prohibit a new employee from starting work in a healthcare position before being medically cleared, or that the organization, reinforced by personnel policy, has an obligation to make a good-faith effort to check references before accepting an individual as an employee.

In this example, the HR representative is bound by state regulations and corporate personnel policy. If this is not fully understood by the other department manager, then HR's opposition will appear as arbitrary resistance. It does little good for staff from the HR department simply to cite organizational policies and regulations to a manager. Such an approach, coming from HR, usually sounds like more HR rules and generates division. Education of line managers concerning existing legal and regulatory restrictions that affect aspects of an employment relationship and have an impact on their activities is required.

It is helpful to remember that the HR department does not issue orders, commands, or directives. Rather, it merely advises or makes recommendations. As in the previous example, however, HR has the responsibility not only to make a recommendation in favor or against a specific action but also to advise others of the possible consequences of the proposed action. An HR department manager should never expect to issue mandates and should avoid allowing HR to command by default.

"This was really personnel's decision," or "HR made me do it," are two laments commonly heard by executives or senior-level managers when lower-level supervisors are unhappy with a recommendation made by HR. These defensive reactions can transform an HR recommendation into an HR command. Human resources managers must explain the reasons for their recommendations and be sure that they are clearly understood. Human resources is purely a staff activity that operates by advising, counseling, suggesting, recommending, and occasionally by negotiating, persuading, or convincing—not by issuing commands.

▶ Healthcare Human Resources and the Changing Scene

As with any other organizational activity, HR must adapt to a frequently changing environment. Changes external to the healthcare industry and changes within the industry itself affect the ways that health care is being delivered. In turn, these changes affect how the services of HR are provided. Three kinds of changes are faced by a modern healthcare organization: technological, financial, and social. Not only are the three interrelated, but these major areas of change have also resulted in many specific modifications of the ways in which health care is organized and delivered.

Technological change encompasses advances being made in methods of diagnosis and treatment, including all new or improved equipment, new procedures, and new or improved drugs. In short, this encompasses most advances made in any dimension of restoring health and preserving life. But technological changes collide with considerations of finance because the cost of having the benefits of the latest and best equipment and the information that such resources generate can produce conflict with the pressures experienced to stem the rapid increase of healthcare costs. Social change becomes a strong influence as the population ages and society experiences the changing attitudes of contemporary generations.

The three major categories of change mutually affect each other. The results of this interplay can be seen in a number of changing forces within the healthcare industry. Financial pressure increases as revenues are constrained from growing in a manner consistent with actual cost increases. In some instances, available funding is being reduced. Competition is increasing as elements of a rapidly changing hospital system struggle to acquire or retain a share of the available business in a particular area.

There is a growing emphasis on outpatient care. Technological advances and financial pressures are continually conspiring to transfer more modes of treatment to outpatient settings. Free-standing specialty centers that perform some of the same services provided by hospital departments are proliferating. Corporate restructuring is occurring as provider organizations consummate mergers or other affiliations and form ever-larger health systems.

Turnover rates among healthcare executives are increasing. Some organizations are folding under mounting pressures, while others are discovering that mergers result in fewer executive positions. Medical entrepreneurship is increasing as individual providers establish specialty practices or attempt to tap into specific market segments.

Emphasis on productivity is growing, and getting more output from the same or less input becomes necessary as financial constraints and other shortages occur.

Chronic shortages of critical caregiving staff are occurring as occupational and professional groups react to the combination of financial pressures that restrict earning potential and the stresses associated with working under increasing demands while short of critical staff. An increasingly better educated and more sophisticated workforce of employees is finding that they are less likely than members of earlier generations to accept what they are offered without expressing what they want.

Change within a healthcare organization or in any enterprise occurs in one of two ways. Change is either intentional, being planned and executed for some specific purpose, or forced, coming about in response to circumstances beyond the control of an organization. Healthcare organizations, especially hospitals, experience far more reactionary changes than planned changes.

Several reasons contribute to these developments. Change is often difficult to promote unless it is driven by a crisis. Few organizations engage in planning that creates significant change. Because of workload and other continuing problems, top managers have little time to focus on change. Resistance to change is often prevalent throughout many organizations. Middle managers and department managers do not view themselves as agents of change. Finally, few managers are skilled or effective at creating and managing change.

Experts often suggest that managers at all levels should be agents of change. In HR departments, fostering a climate that is conducive to constructive change is especially important. This belief should be communicated in all of HR's interactions with organizational managers and employees. Contemporary healthcare organizations benefit from a culture of change that encourages innovation, rewards risk-taking, and values employee participation and input. Human resources can best communicate its belief in a change process by implementing up-to-date policies and procedures that convey respect for the capabilities of every employee.

Job descriptions should be flexible and should allow room for innovation and employee participation and input. A modern performance appraisal process that permits employees to set objectives for themselves and participate in their own growth and development fosters change. Opportunities for promotion and transfer from within reinforce employees' personal growth and development. A compensation structure that includes the opportunity to influence earnings through performance and a flexible benefits structure that recognizes the divergence of individual needs also support change.

Given its unique relationship with all line and staff operations and its mission to provide service for all employees, an HR department is ideally positioned to be a healthcare organization's primary driver of internal change. Whether it is used as such is up to executive management and HR's leadership.

▶ Human Resources Reengineered

A Process by Any Other Name

Reengineering is intended to make work processes easier and more productive. *Reengineering,* a term used to describe many improvement-oriented activities, is far more complex than many people realize. The term literally means engineered again. It involves addressing something that is currently being done and redesigning a process so that a different objective related to the same result is achieved—for example, savings in time or labor or direct savings in money. Practically, this may be a reduction in materials or supplies consumed or an improvement in quality without an increase in cost. As applied to an entire organization or significant sub-unit, reengineering is the systematic redesign of a business's core processes, starting with desired outcomes and then establishing the most efficient possible processes to achieve those outcomes.

At the heart of traditional methods-improvement or problem-solving processes is the way that something is currently being done. These processes begin with the present method and look for ways to eliminate steps or make improvements. By contrast, reengineering ignores how something is currently done and focuses only on desired outcomes. Abandoning a familiar routine is difficult; overcoming the comfort of familiarity is the challenge of reengineering.

Reengineering is a business term that has replaced a number of other buzzwords, such as reorganizing, downsizing, repositioning, rightsizing, revitalizing, and modernizing. The term *reengineering* has evolved as the intent has gradually clarified. It is now the preferred term because it connotes more of a focus on process and thus less of a focus on people. Despite this meaning, an announcement of impending reengineering has come to be synonymous with the likely loss of jobs.

Human Resources Meets Reengineering

As organizations change, the need to improve services and reduce costs is the driving force behind most reengineering efforts. Reengineering consistently results in reductions of staff. Many instances of reengineering have been undertaken specifically to reduce the cost of services by reducing staff. Human resources is so labor intensive that, with the exception of reducing employee benefits, there is no way to achieve significant cost savings other than reducing staff. As a consequence, HR is often unaffected by staff reductions driven by reengineering programs.

Effects on Human Resources Staffing

Human resources staffing ratios in different areas of organizational activity vary. Healthcare organizations have approximately half of the number of staff persons per 1000 employees compared with HR departments in industries such as manufacturing or finance. Human resources departments in contemporary healthcare organizations have approximately one staff member for every 100–150 total employees.

The Flatter Organization

Organizational flattening, the elimination of layers of management such that the institution's organization chart becomes flatter, often accompanies reengineering. As many managers have discovered, when an organization is flattened, middle managers are often eliminated. The responsibilities of remaining managers, usually first-line supervisors, are increased.

A typical HR department, even in a mid- to large-size healthcare organization, has only three layers. The middle layer, usually composed of specialist-managers for activities such as employment or compensation and benefits, may vanish, leaving only HR staff and a departmental supervisor. When this occurs, an organization's department managers must then relate directly with several staff-level individuals rather than with two or three specialist-managers.

Centralization Versus Decentralization

Reengineering can lead to changes in an organization's degree of centralization as it seeks more cost-effective ways of getting its work done. Decentralization is a more common outcome of reengineering than is centralization. Whichever outcome occurs affects not only HR personnel and how they do their jobs, but also department managers.

When HR's activities are decentralized, individual managers must be more aware of HR concerns because decisions must be made closer to an organization's lowest levels. For example, if some aspects of employment are decentralized, then a department manager may have to screen incoming applications and decide which applicants have the qualifications for a particular open position. Such tasks were handled by HR before decentralization.

Some forms of technology—for example, computerized communication systems—have led to the centralization of question-and-answer protocols and other systems for geographically scattered organizations. When using newer communication systems, employees at multiple locations have been able to transact business about their benefits without having to travel to an HR office. In turn, this can enable an organization to maintain a smaller HR presence at satellite locations while handling all business centrally. For widely dispersed organizations, toll-free numbers for employees who have benefits questions provide an effective and financially viable partial replacement of HR staff with technology.

Outsourcing

Outsourcing is defined as having an external vendor provide, on a continuing basis, a service that would normally be provided within an organization (Harkins, Brown, & Sullivan, 1995). Although outsourcing is frequently linked to staff reduction in HR departments, budget cuts and staff reductions are not always the leading reasons for outsourcing. **EXHIBIT 2-1** lists common reasons for outsourcing in approximate descending order of their frequency of occurrence.

EXHIBIT 2-1 Common Reasons for Outsourcing Selected Human Resource Services

- Use the expertise of specialists (for example, payroll, pension plan administration, and Workers' Compensation administration)
- Conserve staff time when addressing required tasks
- Reduce administrative costs
- Allow staff to focus on needs more relevant to an organization's purposes
- Compensate for overload caused by increasing responsibilities
- Reduce human resources staff
- Make organizational and departmental budget cuts

EXHIBIT 2-2 Human Resources Activities Frequently Subject to Outsourcing

- *Payroll.* Payroll is often a responsibility of the finance department. Payroll input often flows through HR. Where payroll is processed has an effect on HR staff.
- *Outplacement services.* These services are outsourced because they are needed intermittently or infrequently.
- *Employee assistance program administration.* This is outsourced to maintain confidentiality for employees.
- *Employee training and development.* Many organizations contract with training specialists or consultants for services because they are needed intermittently.
- *Relocation services.* These are outsourced because the need for them is intermittent or infrequent.
- *Benefits administration.* Many benefit programs are internally administered. Pension plans and self-funded insurance programs, such as dental and short-term disability, are often administered by external trustees.
- *Compensation planning and administration.* This is occasionally outsourced, especially when executive incentive compensation plans are involved.
- *Recruitment and staffing.* Some elements are outsourced. Organizations experiencing rapid expansion or adding a significant service may outsource application and résumé screening and initial interviews.
- *Candidate background checks and credential verification.* Very few healthcare organizations attempt to perform their own background checks or verify credentials. These activities are frequently outsourced.
- *Safety and security.* Few organizations entirely outsource these activities. Many organizations contract with specialists to supply such services.

Cutbacks related to economic pressures and reengineering have created opportunities for companies that specialize in HR services. **EXHIBIT 2-2** lists a number of activities that are commonly outsourced and the reasons for so doing.

Payroll is the most commonly outsourced activity, although it is now normally based in the finance department. Payroll processing requires considerable detailed knowledge of the Fair Labor Standards Act and related regulations that affect payroll deductions and other aspects of payment. Firms that specialize in payroll have created automated systems that fully account for all of the detailed requirements of wage payment. Users submit input information. The payroll service creates paychecks or direct deposits and generates all necessary records. This particular form of outsourcing has eliminated a great deal of frustration for businesses. It is usually less expensive than an internal payroll operation. Because many smaller healthcare organizations have small payrolls, purchasing an automated payroll system is cost efficient.

Some of the downsizing of HR operations has resulted in outsourcing to save money. At the end of the 20th century, 58% of all companies were outsourcing at least one HR activity. In 2002, this number had increased to 74% (Knight Ridder News Service, 2002).

Many small facilities lacking the resources to employ adequate full-time HR staff rely heavily on outsourcing, particularly on firms known as professional employer organizations (PEOs). A PEO takes over and provides all HR services. When an organization or business contracts with a PEO, its employees become co-employees of the PEO. A PEO charges a percentage of payroll, typically 2%–4%, for its services. These ordinarily include benefits administration as well as payroll. In one instance, for example, by contracting with a PEO, a small healthcare provider organization reduced its costs of personnel administration from 9% of payroll to 3% of payroll.

Reengineering aside, HR departments have outsourced activities because doing so often makes economic sense. Activities such as administering a self-funded health insurance or disability program or coordinating an employee assistance program are frequently provided by nonorganizational employees for reasons of confidentiality. This prevents the company from having to reveal employees' personal and medical information to the persons administering the programs.

Additional outsourcing of HR activities is often one of the results of reengineering. As HR staff members are eliminated, adjustments are made in the HR workload. However, essential tasks that remain may occur so infrequently that it is inefficient to retain and pay staff to perform them. Almost any HR operation can be a candidate for outsourcing. Commonly outsourced HR activities include payroll, insurance claim processing, employee assistance program (EAP) administration, retirement and savings plan administration, employee education, and employment candidate background checks.

Effects on Corporate Culture

Corporate culture is made up of the shared basic assumptions and beliefs developed by an organization over time. It requires time for an organization's culture to develop to the extent that those entering can tell the kind of organization they have entered in a relatively short time.

It also takes time for an organization's culture to mature. Time is also required for an organization's culture to adapt to change. Reengineering is inevitably accompanied by change. For an organization's culture to successfully absorb and accommodate, change should occur in increments that can be absorbed without trauma. The pace of change should allow full assimilation of one significant modification before another is introduced. In many healthcare organizations, the pace of change has been so rapid that the corporate culture has had no opportunity to reach a new equilibrium before once again being thrown off balance.

Reengineering inevitably introduces turmoil into an organization's culture. Mergers; acquisitions and other forms of affiliation; downsizing, rightsizing, and other forms of reorganization; increasing external regulation; and all forms of cost cutting involve organizational turmoil.

▶ Conclusion

To ensure maximum effectiveness in all organizational relationships, the individual in charge of HR should report to the CEO. Line and staff tasks are different. Line and staff employees perform different tasks for an organization. Line operations advance the work of an organization. Staff operations support and enhance the work of an organization by making it possible to continue producing products or delivering services as intended.

A variety of organizational paradigms are used in HR departments. These include organizational models based on clerical tasks, counseling, industrial relations, control, and consulting. Alternative models are recognized by some HR professionals.

The degree of effectiveness for HR depends on the attitude of a CEO toward HR. For the most part, however, human resources is no longer a "second-class citizen" in contemporary organizations. Human resources does not issue commands. It is vulnerable to changes because of reengineering. Outsourcing HR services is relatively common.

🔎 CASE STUDY: Resolution

Returning to the opening case study, Sharon, the HR director for the newly designated health system, reports to the COO. This is but the second best of the two acceptable reporting relationships for HR. Her organizational standing is compromised from the outset.

Sharon was wise enough to realize that she could not immediately establish the kind of HR department that she would like to have. Despite a change in name, the CEO still thinks of HR as personnel. Uniting all of the scattered elements of personnel into an HR department to serve the new health system's needs was a significant challenge. Her present HR structure, a combination of the clerical and counseling models, would have to prevail until she could get HR properly organized and transform it into a full-fledged business partner. She realized that this might not occur until the current CEO left.

Sharon's initial recommendations included opting for partial decentralization of some HR activities, with the senior person at the smaller hospital, a single HR person at the largest satellite, and the office managers at the other satellites and the group practices handling local matters. These included making changes to the employee information and benefits databases and addressing employee matters as they arose. In addition, they would serve as channels for policy interpretation.

Sharon decided to keep recruiting centralized, primarily to maintain consistency in such matters as formulating salary offers, explaining benefits, checking references, and initiating background checks. She was concerned about organizational consistency in pre-employment activities. She opted to maintain all personnel files centrally, but created a procedure to ensure quick access by managers at any location when necessary. Finally, she established a helpline for employees to call at any time. Through this service, employees could learn where and how they might access HR or benefit information or secure assistance in addressing problems related to benefits.

Sharon realized that she would have to provide direct support to her HR staff by visiting the satellite facilities in person. She planned to ensure that all of her HR managers were trained. She would send them to local colleges or universities for instruction by HR experts. Supervisors having the least HR experience would be the first to receive training. Sharon established a personal goal to make HR activities as easy as she could for the managers who had only part-time involvement in HR matters.

SPOTLIGHT ON CUSTOMER SERVICE

Integrating Customer Service into an Organization

This chapter has focused on integrating human resources into an organization. Contemporary human resources departments are very complex, with a myriad of responsibilities. While customer service is similar, its functions are spread across an organization more than the functions of human resources are. Every employee should contribute to the customer service effort in an organization. Three important concepts relate to customer service:

1. The single goal of addressing customer needs is clearly expressed in the program's name: customer service.
2. An organization requires only one formal customer service program.
3. Customer service is a priority activity that should be shared by all employees.

Modified from Andrews, J. R. (1986). Is there a crisis in the personnel department's identity? *Personnel Journal, 65*(6), 86–93; Driver, M. J., Coffey, R. E., & Bowen, D. E. (1988). Where is HR management going? *Personnel, 33*(1), 28–31; Harkins, P. J., Brown, S. M., & Sullivan, R. (1995). Shining new light on a growing trend. *HR Magazine, 40*(12), 75–81; Knight Ridder News Service. (2002, February 17). Outsourcing human-resource tasks. *Democrat & Chronicle*, Rochester, NY.

Questions for Review and Discussion

1. Describe a specific outsourcing practice about which you are knowledgeable, and explain what you believe are the primary benefits achieved by having the services provided by outside persons rather than keeping them within an organization.
2. Why do experts contend that a primary characteristic of line personnel is present within a clearly defined staff activity such as HR or finance?
3. What is the fundamental difference between a line activity and a staff activity? Provide two examples of each in a healthcare setting.
4. What problems develop when the head of HR reports to any executive other than the chief executive officer?
5. Describe under what organizational circumstances the following models of HR could be successful in a healthcare organization: Clerical Model, Control Model, Industrial Relations Model, Legal Model, Consulting Model, and Financial Model.
6. Which of the HR models appears most appropriate for managing personnel in a healthcare organization? Why?
7. Describe how an HR department in a healthcare organization might evolve through different organizational models as the department grows and matures.
8. How do the expectations of an organization's CEO shape the model or manner in which HR services are delivered?
9. What are the primary areas of conflict between HR and department managers? How might these conflicts be reconciled?
10. What are the advantages of a decentralized organization for delivering HR services? What are the risks?
11. What is organizational flattening? Why is it practiced?
12. What are the primary shortcomings of reengineering as it is practiced in contemporary healthcare organizations? How does reengineering differ from minor modifications of existing practices?

References

Andrews, J. R. (1986). Is there a crisis in the personnel department's identity? *Personnel Journal, 65*(6), 86–93.

Driver, M. J., Coffey, R. E., & Bowen, D. E. (1988). Where is HR management going? *Personnel, 33*(1), 28–31.

Harkins, P. J., Brown, S. M., & Sullivan, R. (1995). Shining new light on a growing trend. *HR Magazine, 40*(12), 75–81.

Knight Ridder News Service. (2002, February 17). Outsourcing human-resource tasks. *Democrat & Chronicle,* Rochester, NY.

Resources

Books

Barbeito, C. L. (2004). *Human resource policies and procedures: For nonprofit organizations.* New York, NY: John Wiley.

Learning Initiative. (2005). *Human resources for health: Overcoming the crisis.* Cambridge, MA: Harvard University Press.

Manion, J. (2005). *Create a positive health care work place: Practical strategies to retain today's workforce and find tomorrow's.* Chicago, IL: Health Forum Publishing.

Niles, N. J. (2012). *Basic concepts of health care human resource management.* Burlington, MA: Jones & Bartlett Learning.

Shiver, J., & Cantiello, J. (2016). *Managing integrated health systems.* Burlington, MA: Jones & Bartlett Learning.

Society for Human Resource Management. (2005). *SHRM Health care survey report: A study by the Society for Human Resource Management.* Alexandria, VA: Society for Human Resource Management.

Thomas, M., & Keagy, B. (2004). *Essentials of physician practice management.* New York, NY: John Wiley.

Walburg, J., & Bevan, H. (2005). *Performance management in healthcare.* London: Taylor & Francis.

Periodicals

Anonymous. (2005). Excess, shortage, or sufficient physician workforce: How could we know? *American Family Physician, 72*(9), 1670–1675.

Burritt, J. E. (2005). Organizational turnaround: The role of the nurse executive. *Journal of Nursing Administration, 35*(11), 482–489.

Chen, L. C., & Bouford, J. I. (2005). Fatal flows—Doctors on the move. *New England Journal of Medicine, 353*(17), 1850–1852.

Desselle, S. P. (2005). Job turnover intentions among Certified Pharmacy Technicians. *Journal of the American Pharmacy Association, 45*(6), 676–683.

Greene, J. (2005). Should ASCs hire RNs from the hospital? *OR Manager, 21*(11), 25–26.

Higginson, L. A. (2005). Profile of the cardiovascular specialist physician workforce in Canada, 2004. *Canadian Journal of Cardiology, 21*(13), 1157–1162.

Lucas, A. O. (2005). Human resources for health in Africa. *British Medical Journal, 331*(7524), 1037–1038.

Mannion, R., Davies, H. T., & Marshall, M. N. (2005). Cultural characteristics of "high" and "low" performing hospitals. *Journal of Health Organization Management, 19*(6), 431–439.

Northam, S. (2005). Views on the nursing faculty shortage. *Journal of Nursing Education, 44*(10), 440–442.

Sox, H. C. (2006). Leaving (internal) medicine. *Annals of Internal Medicine, 144*(1), 57–58.

Thorgrimson, D. H., & Robinson, D. H. (2005). Building and sustaining an adequate RN workforce. *Journal of Nursing Administration, 35*(11), 474–477.

Yamamoto, L. G. (2005). We have a shortage of specialists. *American Journal of Emergency Medicine, 23*(7), 895–896.

CHAPTER 3

The Legal Framework of Contemporary Human Resources

CHAPTER OBJECTIVES

After studying this chapter, readers will be able to:

- Understand the evolution of the regulated environment in which human resources must work in serving a healthcare organization.
- Trace the chronology of legislation affecting employment with a brief explanation of each pertinent law.
- Agree that 1964 was a pivotal year in legislation affecting human resources.
- Understand the highlights of legislation enacted in 1964 and beyond.
- Acknowledge the 1964 as the beginning of an effort by the federal government to shift considerable social responsibility to employers.
- Describe the cumulative effects of employment legislation to date.

▶ Chapter Summary

This chapter is intended to provide readers with sufficient background and knowledge of employment legislation to enable them to develop an understanding of the effects of employment law on the activities of a department manager. It provides a review of the laws affecting aspects of the employment relationship. To the maximum extent possible, these laws are described using nonlegal terminology. In each instance, how the pertinent piece of legislation approaches its subject is reviewed. The importance of each law is reviewed, along with the extent to which each has addressed a societal need through the legislation's stated intent. Effects of the more significant laws are reviewed, along with descriptions of some apparently unintended outcomes.

🔍 CASE STUDY: Does Weight Constitute a Disability?

Susan J. applied for a position as a licensed practical nurse at County Memorial Hospital. She had generated an impressive record during her training, possessed good references from prior employment in two different private duty situations, and interviewed well. After the interview, Helen Harding, director of nursing at County Memorial, extended a tentative offer of employment to Susan. The offer was contingent on passing the hospital's pre-employment physical examination. Susan was clearly very heavy. Helen estimated her weight to exceed 300 pounds. An average weight for her 5-foot, 5-inch body was 120–140 pounds.

The County Memorial employee health physician examined Susan but declined to approve her for employment unless she could first achieve a safer weight, in her case less than 275 pounds. Susan failed to get the job because of her overweight condition. She then filed a complaint with the State Division of Human Rights charging discrimination based on disability, citing Title VII of the Civil Rights Act of 1964 and the Americans with Disabilities Act of 1990. She claimed that her only responsibility was to demonstrate that she was capable of doing the job, and that in spite of her physical handicap she could still adequately perform all required duties of the job. Her obesity, she claimed, was due to a medical condition over which she had no control.

County Memorial moved for dismissal of the complaint on three grounds. First, it argued that obesity was not a true physical impairment under the law. Second, it claimed that Susan's condition resulted from her own voluntary actions. Finally, the hospital claimed that she could reduce and control her weight if she so chose.

How might the foregoing situation be resolved? Is obesity truly a disability, or will a different argument prevail? Do you believe that the hospital will be successful in getting the complaint dismissed, or will Susan successfully persuade the Division of Human Rights to act on her complaint? Why?

▶ A Regulated Environment

An important disclaimer is in order before proceeding further with this chapter. Nothing in this chapter constitutes legal advice, and no such advice should be inferred from its contents. Individuals with questions about the applicability of any particular point of law should take those questions to the appropriate people in their organization. These may be persons in human resources (HR), administration, risk management, or perhaps even in-house legal counsel who can provide or secure appropriate responses.

The pivotal year when HR began to change to its current incarnation was 1964. Internal operations that addressed issues related to employees were still called "personnel" in most organizations. Sweeping civil rights legislation came into being with the passage of the Civil Rights Act of 1964; the specific turning point was the appearance of Title VII. This legislation marked the beginning of significant changes in relations between government and business. It marked a change in philosophy that resulted in a completely new direction for government in its concern for the citizens of the United States.

Pre-1964: Regulation Minimal and Tolerable

Before 1964, businesses were free to treat employees essentially any way they chose to treat them, with only two exceptions: wage-and-hour laws and labor-relations laws. Prior to 1964, the only laws that had noticeable impact on the employment relationship were the Fair Labor Standards Act (FLSA) and related state laws, and the National Labor Relations Act (NLRA).

The FLSA and its numerous amendments govern the payment of wages and other related conditions of employment. This and similar laws existing in some of the states are commonly referred to as wage-and-hour laws.

The NLRA governed relationships between work organizations and labor unions. Similar laws existed in some but not all states. They were relevant only to organizations in which employees were unionized or where active union organization efforts were under way.

Prior to 1964, managers did not have to be knowledgeable of more than a scant few regulatory requirements. Few legal restrictions impinged on HR operations or on managers in general. The majority of business organizations complied with the wage-and-hour laws as a matter of operating routine. Leaders of organizations having a union presence, either being organized or already under contract, generally expected to comply with all applicable labor laws.

Other applicable legislation was in place before 1964, but the FLSA and the NLRA were the only ones having a visible influence on HR operations and department management. These two are discussed more fully in the chronology of legislation that follows.

The turning point of 1964 heralded a change in philosophy concerning government's relationship with business. For years, the governing philosophy had largely been one of hands-off to the maximum practical extent. Employers were expected to concern themselves only with wage-and-hour requirements and restrictions imposed by labor relations legislation. Since 1964, however, the government has been addressing many of the perceived needs of individuals by involving employers in meeting those requirements. President Lyndon Johnson's signature on the Civil Rights Act in 1964 initiated a significant change in the actions that government would be taking over after on behalf of its citizens. This trend continues to the present day.

The Growing Regulatory Environment: Chronology of Legislation

Some of the legislation included in the following chronology receives little more than a brief description because it is addressed more thoroughly in subsequent chapters. These laws will be so identified. For others, implications for HR and department managers are briefly reviewed.

Norris–LaGuardia Act (1932)

The first significant piece of legislation to address the growing organized labor movement in the United States was the Norris–LaGuardia Act of 1932. This law reflected an important shift in public policy concerning labor unions, from a posture of legal repression of unions and their activities to one of actual encouragement of union activity. Although the Norris–LaGuardia Act legalized union organizing activities and affirmed workers' rights to organize for collective bargaining purposes, it did little or nothing to directly restrain employers in their conduct toward labor organizations. During the first three decades of the 1900s, many workers who attempted to organize for collective bargaining lost their jobs because of their involvement with the organizing process and other union-related activities. Often, their organizational efforts were countered with violence. The impact of the Norris–LaGuardia Act is essentially long past; it is mentioned here simply because of its role as a forerunner to subsequent labor legislation.

National Labor Relations Act (1935)

Also known as the Wagner Act, the NLRA established a number of rules for the conduct of both unions and employers in labor organizing and collective bargaining situations. Although it seemed largely to favor unions and encourage their presence, the NLRA established some boundaries on what unions could do in their organizing activities. In addition to affirming the right of employees to organize, the NLRA made it illegal for an employer to refuse to negotiate with a union. This requirement assumed that the union had conducted a legal organizing campaign and had won a proper representation (certification) election.

The NLRA created the National Labor Relations Board. This body was charged with administering the Wagner Act by conducting representation elections to determine whether employees in particular groupings (called bargaining units) wished to have union representation. The NLRA specified that a union chosen by a majority of the employees in an appropriate unit would be the exclusive representative for all employees in the unit. The NLRA delineated a list of unfair labor practices that were punishable by fines. Many unfair labor practices pertain to management reactions to union organization activities. The NLRA was subsequently modified by the Taft–Hartley Act and the Landrum–Griffin Act.

Social Security Act (1935)

The Social Security Act established a basic system of contributory social insurance and a supplemental program for low-income elderly persons. In 1939, it was expanded to provide benefits to survivors of covered workers and dependents of retirees. The Social Security Act has been further expanded to cover workers who become permanently disabled. Coverage under the Social Security Act was again expanded in 1965 to provide Medicare health insurance coverage for the elderly.

Fair Labor Standards Act (1938)

In part, the FLSA was intended to reduce the high unemployment rate that typified the years of the Great Depression. Congress intended to reduce the length of a work week to a uniform standard, thus spreading available work among a greater number of workers. In addition to defining a normal work week, the FLSA set minimum pay rates, established rules and standards for the payment of overtime, and regulated the employment of minors. Over the years, FLSA has been amended many times, most recently in 2016 addressing new overtime eligibility rules, dual job codes, exempt employee compensation, employee status (exempt vs. nonexempt), the minimum wage, payment of overtime, and other emerging concerns. The FLSA remains as the country's basic wage-and-hour law and has served as the model for the wage-and-hour laws of many states.

Labor–Management Relations Act (1947)

The Labor–Management Relations Act, commonly referred to as the Taft–Hartley Act, amended the NLRA. As passed in 1935, the NLRA clearly favored unions over employers. The principal intent and subsequent effect of the Taft–Hartley Act was to level the playing field to some extent by more appropriately balancing the responsibilities and advantages of both unions and employers. Taft–Hartley listed additional unfair labor practices. Although many experts still view it as a law favoring labor unions, the Taft–Hartley Act was clearly a change in the direction of management's rights.

Two points are of immediate interest concerning the Taft–Hartley Act. Today, most mentions of the NLRA are in fact referring to the NLRA as amended by Taft–Hartley. The Taft–Hartley Act was itself amended in 1975 specifically to address not-for-profit hospitals by removing the exemption that had been in place since its original passage in 1947.

Labor–Management Reporting and Disclosure Act (1959)

The Labor–Management Reporting and Disclosure Act, more commonly known as the Landrum–Griffin Act, further amended the NLRA. Because it actually amended the NLRA as amended by Taft–Hartley, it is sometimes jokingly referred to as an amendment to an amendment. Among its numerous provisions, the Landrum–Griffin Act required employers, including not-for-profit hospitals and other nonprofit healthcare facilities, to report any financial arrangements or transactions that were intended to improve or retard the process of unionization in detail to the Secretary of Labor. Reporting and disclosure requirements were imposed on unions.

Equal Pay Act (1963)

The Equal Pay Act was an amendment to the FLSA. It prohibited the payment of unequal wages for men and women who worked for the same employer in the same establishment performing equal work on jobs requiring equal skill, effort, and responsibility, and performing under similar working conditions. Simply put, people doing the same work in the same place in the same way have to be paid equally regardless of gender. Although the Equal Pay Act came into being before 1964, it had no noticeable impact on the activities of HR and no effect on the roles of department managers. To this day, it remains evident that equality of pay rates is not universal; many men continue to earn more than women for comparable jobs.

Civil Rights Act (Title VII) (1964)

This legislation has led to greater regulation of the employer–employee relationship by the government. Title VII provided the legal basis for all people to pursue the work of their choosing and to advance in their chosen occupations subject only to the limitations imposed by their own individual qualifications, talents, and energies. This legislation defined unlawful employment discrimination as the failure or refusal to hire or to otherwise discriminate against any individual with respect to compensation or other terms, conditions, or privileges of employment because of that individual's race, color, religion, sex, or national origin. The act prohibits setting limits, segregating, or classifying employees or applicants for employment in any way that deprives them of employment opportunities or otherwise adversely affects their status as employees because of race, color, religion, sex, or national origin.

The Civil Rights Act of 1964 established the Equal Employment Opportunity Commission (EEOC) to enforce the antidiscrimination requirements of Title VII. This act was amended in later years to compensate for perceived erosion of its strength and effectiveness owing to a number of Supreme Court decisions.

Age Discrimination in Employment Act (1967)

The Age Discrimination in Employment Act (ADEA) legally established the basic right of individuals to be treated in employment situations on the basis of their ability to perform the job rather than on the basis of artificial age limitations. The ADEA prohibits discrimination in employment on the basis of age in hiring, job retention, compensation, and all other terms, conditions, and privileges of employment. Originally enforced by the Department of Labor, in 1978 enforcement of the ADEA was transferred to the EEOC. The threshold for defining age discrimination is 40 years. Therefore, workers aged 40 years and older constitute a protected class for EEOC purposes.

The ADEA has had a direct effect on retirement. Before ADEA, employers were free to mandate retirement at a specific age. The most commonly mandated age for retirement was 65 years. When passed in 1967, the ADEA raised the limit such that employers could no longer mandate retirement at any age younger than 70 years. When the ADEA was again amended in 1986, the limitation of age 70 years was removed. This means that retirement can no longer be required by any specific age. The sole legal criterion for continuing employment is an individual's ability to fulfill the requirements of the job.

Some exceptions exist under which retirement by a stated age can be mandated for a limited number of specific occupations. These include police officers, firefighters, airline pilots, surgeons, and some policy-making executives—generally all occupations for which it can be established that age is a *bona fide occupational qualification (BFOQ)*. In many instances, the ADEA has permitted people who wished to keep working to do so. This has ensured the continuing employment of some workers who might otherwise have to depend on government assistance. It must be stressed, however, that an older worker's continued employment depends on the person's ability to perform all aspects of the job in the same manner of, for example, a considerably younger employee engaged in the same work; no accommodation for the older worker's advanced age is to be expected.

Occupational Safety and Health Act (1970)

Passed in 1970 and effective in 1971, the Occupational Safety and Health Act (OSHA) is a highly influential piece of legislation concerning employee safety in the workplace. Before this law was passed, efforts to ensure health and safety in the workplace were minimal. The "A" in OSHA indicates either Act or Administration, depending on the specific situation and reference. The intent of Congress in establishing the OSHA was to provide all persons with workplaces free from recognized hazards that have the potential to cause serious physical harm or death to employees. The OSHA is authorized to promulgate legally enforceable workplace safety standards, respond to employee complaints, and, as necessary, conduct on-site inspections to follow up on employee safety complaints or on lost-workday injury rates that are considered excessive. The act also created the independent Occupational Safety and Health Review Commission to review enforcement priorities, actions, and cases and established the National Institute for Occupational Safety and Health (NIOSH).

On May 25, 1986, OSHA began enforcement of the second phase of an elaborate set of rules known formally as *Hazard Communications*. These rules provide workers with the right to know about any hazardous substances to which they are exposed or handle in the course of performing their job duties. According to OSHA's hazard communication rules, health facilities are required to create and deliver programs for informing and training employees about hazardous substances in their workplace, ensure that warning labels on all incoming containers are intact and clearly readable, and inform and train employees in the nature and appropriate handling of hazardous substances at the time of initial assignment. Suppliers are required to create and distribute a material safety data sheet (MSDS) for all products containing a hazardous substance that they produce. These must be provided to all purchasers of their product. The OSHA hazard communication rules mandate that employers maintain copies of MSDSs for all hazardous substances in the workplace, supply copies of MSDSs to employees upon request, and maintain current copies of MSDSs for all products so that they are accessible to any employee on all work shifts.

Under OSHA regulations, more than 1000 substances are considered to be hazardous. A number of the states have enacted right-to-know laws with requirements that are similar to OSHA regulations. Federal and state standards for the handling of hazardous substances require that employers distribute MSDSs, ensure that warning labels are always in evidence on workplace containers, and be able to produce a written employee orientation program at any time. Department managers are typically assigned the responsibility for ensuring that these regulations are followed and all requirements are fully satisfied within the department or areas under their direct supervision. Personnel from HR usually supply training materials and provide supportive services to department managers.

A section of the act permitted and encouraged states to adopt their own occupational safety and health regulations, providing that state standards and enforcement are at least as effective as the federal act in cultivating a safe and healthful workplace.

This particular legislation is expanded and updated almost annually. For example, update activity for the period 2016 through 2018 included the following: Final Rule to Protect Workers from Exposure to Respirable Crystalline Silica; Final Rule to Improve Tracking of Workplace Injuries and Illnesses; Final Rule to Update General Industry Walking-Working Surfaces and Fall Protection Standards; and numerous other updates, some affecting the country as a whole and some relevant to individual states.

Health Maintenance Organization Act (1973)

This legislation was passed as part of a Nixon administration cost containment initiative, preempting all state regulations that posed any barriers to health maintenance organization (HMO) formation. It set conditions for HMOs to become federally qualified and mandated that most employers offer an HMO option if a federally qualified HMO in the area requested inclusion in their benefits offerings (this condition was eliminated in 1995). In theory, the act was intended to reduce costs by eliminating regulatory barriers to HMO development and encouraging the proliferation of what was seen as a more cost-effective healthcare delivery system.

Rehabilitation Act (1973)

Although disabled persons were mentioned in the Civil Rights Act of 1964, they were addressed separately for the first time in the Rehabilitation Act of 1973. Congress recognized that the handicapped were subject to cultural myths and prejudices similar to those biases that existed against women and ethnic minorities. However, this law applied only to employees of the federal government and to employers doing a specified amount of business with the government.

One portion of the Rehabilitation Act prohibited discrimination in the hiring, promotion, and other employment of the handicapped, essentially paralleling Title VII of the Civil Rights Act of 1964. Another portion required employers doing more than $2500 in business with the federal government to apply affirmative action guidelines so as to employ and promote qualified handicapped individuals. Employers having more than 50 employees and fulfilling government contracts worth $50,000 or more were required to have written affirmative action programs as required by the Office of Federal Contract Compliance Programs. These employers were required to make reasonable accommodations for the physical or mental limitations of employees or applicants. The Rehabilitation Act is significant because it was a precursor of the Americans with Disabilities Act (1990).

Employee Retirement Income Security Act (1974)

The Employee Retirement Income Security Act (ERISA) established four basic requirements governing employee retirement plans. The ERISA mandated that employees must become eligible for retirement benefits after a reasonable length of service (also known as vesting or being vested), adequate funds must be reserved to provide the benefits promised under the plan, the persons who administer the plan and manage its funds must meet established standards of conduct, and sufficient information must be made available on a regular basis, so plan participants, auditors, or other interested parties may determine whether ERISA requirements are being met. The provisions of this act were later reinforced by legislation included in the Retirement Equity Act of 1984 that greatly increased the complexity of ERISA and added multiple layers of Internal Revenue Service regulations.

Taft–Hartley Act Amendments (1975)

The Taft–Hartley Act, as noted earlier, which was an amendment to the NLRA, was itself amended in 1975. This "amendment to an amendment" was created specifically to address not-for-profit hospitals by removing the exemption that had been in place since Taft–Hartley's original passage in 1947. Beginning in 1975, not-for-profit hospitals could no longer be considered beyond the reach of labor unions. The exemption was removed, but specific rules were created in recognition of the special circumstances of this vital service that deals in matters of human life. For example, written notice must be provided by a union to the healthcare institution and the Federal Mediation and Conciliation Service 10 days prior to engaging in any picketing, strike, or other concerted refusal to work. No such notice is required prior to similar actions in other industries.

The 1975 amendments preempt all state labor laws that previously applied to nongovernmental hospitals. Also, the 1975 amendments apply to healthcare institutions previously covered by the act, such as proprietary hospitals and nursing homes, as well as to all those institutions brought under federal law by these amendments to the act.

A significant element of Congress's intent in passing the amendments was to provide time to transfer patients from a struck or threatened institution to another facility and to obtain limited assistance from another facility without risking secondary strikes or boycotts against the assisting institution.

Pregnancy Discrimination Act (1978)

The Pregnancy Discrimination Act declared that discrimination on the basis of pregnancy, childbirth, or related medical conditions as unlawful sex discrimination under Title VII of the Civil Rights Act of 1964. From this point forward, pregnancy has been considered to be a medical disability and is treated accordingly as a disability of some 6–8 weeks' duration. The exact length varies and depends on whether federal or state guidelines are applied.

Consolidated Omnibus Budget Reconciliation Act (1986)

The Consolidated Omnibus Budget Reconciliation Act (COBRA) is a complex piece of legislation that addresses many concerns. However, most pertinent to employment is the provision that COBRA allowed for the extension of group insurance coverage to employees and their dependents on a self-pay basis for set periods of time for those who would otherwise lose group health or dental benefits due to a loss of employment, change in employment status, or other defined events. The maximum period for COBRA benefits is 36 months. The length of the period depends on the qualifying event or the reason for accessing COBRA. By making it possible for these employees and dependents to remain on the group contracts under which they had been covered, COBRA shifted to employers a portion of the cost of health coverage for many individuals who would otherwise be uninsurable except under government programs. As far as health insurance is concerned, COBRA simply provides temporary or stopgap coverage. Persons who continue coverage under COBRA must secure other insurance after the eligibility period expires. Insurance coverage can be continued up to 18 months for laid-off employees, up to 29 months for disabled individuals, and up to 36 months for dependents following separation, divorce, or the death of the previously covered employee. Should the employer go out of business or for some other reason terminate its health insurance plan, however, all rights under COBRA immediately cease.

Immigration Reform and Control Act (1986)

The Immigration Reform and Control Act (IRCA) requires employers to review and, as necessary, modify their hiring practices; they must institute procedures to verify that all job applicants are U.S. citizens or otherwise legally authorized to work in the United States. This law established civil and criminal penalties for knowingly hiring, recruiting, referring, or retaining in employment persons designated as unauthorized aliens. The act prohibits employers from discriminating against job applicants on the basis of citizenship status or national origin.

Much initial business reaction to IRCA was strong, vocal, and negative. Because IRCA forces employers to take steps to screen out illegal immigrants (the majority of whom enter this country with employment as a goal), many organizational heads have expressed the belief that businesses are being made to perform a function that more correctly belongs within the purview of the federal government. Skrentny (1987) provided the following early assessment of the act: "This onerous piece of legislation for business turns every employer in the country, whether he or she hires a lone housekeeper or 10,000 auto workers, into an arm—an agent or a cop, if you will—of the Immigration and Naturalization Service (INS)." The Homeland Security Act of 2002 required the INS in 2003 to be dismantled and separated into three components: the U.S. Citizenship and Immigration Service (USCIS), Immigration and Customs Enforcement (ICE), and Customs and Border Protection (CBP). As of this writing there is growing political pressure, largely partisan, to eliminate the ICE component established by the Homeland Security Act; however, this suggested change is far from certain.

Most employment legislation specifies the minimum-size organization to which it applies. For example, the Family and Medical Leave Act (FMLA) applies only to employers with 50 or more employees. The IRCA pointedly applies to all employers of one or more employees. The basis for this requirement is the premise that a significant number of undocumented aliens find work as household help.

This legislation has created work in the form of a document known as the Employment Eligibility Verification Form I-9, which is ordinarily completed in HR as part of the hiring process. Each new employee or employee-to-be must furnish specified proofs of identity and, in the instance of legal aliens, proof of authorization to work in the United States. After examining (and usually copying) the appropriate proofs, a representative of the employer signs the I-9 attesting to having seen the documents. An employer has 3 business days from the date of hire to complete an I-9 form. This requirement changes to the first day of employment if the term of hire is to be less than 3 days. Completed I-9 forms are retained in employees' personnel files, where they are subject to inspection and audit by ICE. Forms may also be inspected by the Department of Labor and certain immigration-related branches of the Department of Homeland Security other than ICE. Financial penalties may be imposed for missing or incomplete I-9 forms. Significant penalties can be imposed if illegal aliens are discovered in the workforce.

Some critics have claimed that the IRCA has resulted in increased employment discrimination. Employment applicants who look or sound foreign, especially Asians and Hispanics, are often faced with an increased likelihood of discrimination by employers who may shy away from hiring them because they fear inadvertently hiring illegal aliens and thus exposing themselves to action by the ICE. Laws affecting employment have proliferated to such an extent that some of them occasionally come into conflict with each other. For example, Title VII of the Civil Rights Act declares that discrimination on the basis of race or national origin is illegal, while the Immigration Reform and Control Act encourages closer scrutiny of applicants on the basis of national origin.

Pension Protection Act (1987)

This act requires organizations with underfunded pension plans to make additional payments to the Pension Benefit Guaranty Corporation (PBGC). The PBGC is a government agency established to guarantee benefit payments to participants of legally qualified defined-benefit pension plans. In addition to increasing employers' payments to the PBGC, this legislation reduces or eliminates the deduction of contributions by employers for better-funded plans.

Drug-Free Workplace Act (1988)

The Drug-Free Workplace Act requires organizations having $25,000 or more in federal contracts or grants to make good-faith efforts to maintain a drug-free workplace and to establish drug education and awareness programs for their employees. As a precondition to receiving a contract or grant, the law requires an organization to certify that it will provide and maintain a drug-free workplace. The manager of any department involved in the fulfillment of any portion of an appropriate federal contract or grant will be involved at several points in the following process. An organization must notify all employees in writing (via a published statement) that the possession, use, manufacturing, or distribution of a controlled substance in the workplace is prohibited. The statement must include the penalties that will be imposed for violations of company rules. Each organization must establish a drug-free awareness program to inform employees of the dangers of drug abuse in the workplace; comply with the external requirement of a drug-free workplace as a condition of seeking and accepting contracts and grants; note drug counseling, rehabilitation, or employee assistance programs that may be available to them; and enumerate the penalties to which the organization may be exposed for violations that occur in the workplace.

An organization must require that each individual employee who is to be involved in the fulfillment of an appropriate contract or grant possess a copy of the organization's published statement concerning controlled substances. Furthermore, the organization must notify all employees receiving the controlled substances statement that they are expected to abide by all terms of the statement and notify their employer of any criminal drug statute conviction for a violation in the workplace no later than 5 days after conviction. Within 10 days of receiving such a notice of criminal drug statute conviction, the granting or contracting agency must be notified of the conviction. Within 30 days of receiving notice of an employee's criminal drug statute conviction, an employer must take appropriate disciplinary action against the employee, or require the employee to complete an approved drug-abuse assistance or rehabilitation program in a satisfactory manner. Finally, each employer must make a good-faith effort to maintain a drug-free workplace through implementation of the foregoing procedures and requirements.

All healthcare institutions have an interest in keeping their work environments free from dangers to patients, visitors, and employees created by the use of illegal drugs or controlled substances. For a number of years, drug abuse in the workplace has made it necessary for employers to develop and implement different means of addressing this growing problem. Although the requirements of the Drug-Free Workplace Act apply only to employees receiving federal contracts and grants, conscientious management practices suggest that a comprehensive policy and drug-free awareness program be implemented for all employees. Conscientious departmental managers should have a strongly vested interest in displaying a high level of concern for maintaining a drug-free work environment whether or not there are external requirements for doing so.

Employee Polygraph Protection Act (1988)

The Employee Polygraph Protection Act (EPPA) prevents most private-sector employers from requiring job applicants or current employees to take polygraph (lie detector) tests. Under EPPA, the routine use of polygraph tests is permitted only in organizations that produce and distribute controlled substances and in those concerned with nuclear power, transportation, currency, commodities, or proprietary information.

In most organizations, an employee may be asked to submit to a polygraph when other evidence gives management reason to suspect an individual of wrongdoing. This is sometimes referred to as reasonable suspicion or, somewhat inaccurately, as reasonable cause. However, an employee may not be disciplined or discharged solely on the results of a polygraph test. Under EPPA, an employer may not ask an employee or job applicant to submit to a polygraph test other than in the situations already delineated. Furthermore, an employer may not take any adverse action against an employee or applicant for refusing to take a polygraph test. Finally, the results of a polygraph test to which a person has submitted for one specific reason cannot be used for a different purpose.

There are limited exceptions under which certain individuals may be subject to pre-employment polygraph examination. Among these are applicants for armored car and security alarm and security guard firm positions, as well as prospective employees of pharmaceutical and other firms involved in manufacturing, distributing, or dispensing controlled substances.

Worker Adjustment and Retraining Notification Act (1988)

The Worker Adjustment and Retraining Notification Act (WARN) requires employers with 100 or more employees at any individual site to provide advance notification of major reductions in force. An employer must provide 60 days' notice of an impending layoff of 50 or more employees, and must notify local government and the appropriate state agency, bureau, or unit responsible for dislocated workers that provides employment and training services.

Americans with Disabilities Act (1990)

The Americans with Disabilities Act (ADA) provides individuals with disabilities with the same protections afforded to minorities and other protected groups under the Civil Rights Act of 1964. The ADA calls for access equal to that available to others in regard to employment, transportation, and telecommunications, and ensures that all services and facilities are available to the public, whether under private or public auspices.

Disabilities are broadly defined under the ADA, including, in addition to physical limitations ordinarily thought of as disabilities, hearing and visual impairments, paraplegia and epilepsy, HIV or AIDS, and literally dozens of other conditions. The list of recognized disabilities is long, and it continues to expand as legal challenges continue over what constitutes a disability.

The ADA prohibits potential employers from asking about a job applicant's medical conditions, if any, and imposing major limitations on pre-employment physical examinations. Under the law, a physical examination cannot be conducted until after a job offer has been extended. If a physical examination reveals a medical condition that does not affect the person's ability to perform the major functions of the job being sought, an employer may be expected to make a reasonable accommodation to the needs of the applicant. The key to applicability of the ADA lies in an individual's ability to perform the major functions of a job satisfactorily. Thus, an individual cannot be denied a job because an impairment prevents performance of a minor or nonessential activity. The employer may find it necessary to make a reasonable accommodation for the condition, providing such accommodation does not cause unreasonable expense or hardship.

From time to time each department manager may have reason to be familiar with some aspects of the law concerning disabilities. Involvement surely will be required should a need arise to make a reasonable accommodation for one or more employees in the department. However, it is not always possible to identify an individual who is disabled. Unlike race or gender, some disabilities may not be visually apparent.

Managers should not be concerned unless they know factually that a disability exists. To obtain protection available under antidiscrimination laws, employees must identify themselves as being disabled. If a disability is neither apparent nor declared, then the employee in question should be treated the same as any other worker. Managers who suspect the presence of a disability that has not been declared are advised not to inquire about the situation with the employee in question. Furthermore, they should not offer unsolicited advice to an employee about a possible but undeclared problem. Such a course of action has been ruled as treating an employee in a different manner and is against the law.

The ADA has frequently been in the news. A decade after its passage, lawyers argued before the Supreme Court that the ADA went too far in allowing disabled public employees to sue state and local governments in federal court (Hearst News Service, 2000). States and localities generally have immunity against such lawsuits unless Congress has documented sufficient discrimination in the states to deny them that immunity. The federal government must invoke its power under the 14th Amendment to ensure that people have equal protection under the law. States have contended that Congress has been lax in demonstrating that individual states were not enforcing their disability laws.

In a 2002 decision, the Supreme Court unanimously narrowed the number of people covered by the ADA. The opinion held that "merely having an impairment does not make one disabled for purposes of the ADA," that a person's ailment must extend beyond the workplace and affect everyday life, and that the ability to perform tasks that are of central importance to most people's daily lives must be "substantially limited" before an individual can qualify for coverage under the original legislation that was intended to protect the disabled from discrimination because of physical impairments (Newsday, 2002). In other words, the court ruled that individuals who could function normally in daily living could not claim disability status because of physical problems that limited their ability to perform some manual tasks on the job.

In another opinion that was viewed by some as a defeat for disabled workers, the Supreme Court ruled that disabled workers are not always entitled to premium assignments intended for more senior workers (Associated Press, 2002a). The practical implication of this ruling is that, in the majority of instances, seniority can take precedence over disability. In continuing its series of clarifications and rulings limiting rights under the ADA, the court ruled that disabled workers cannot demand jobs that would threaten their lives or health (Associated Press, 2002b). This ruling arose from a case in which a worker with a particular medical condition wanted to return to his original position although it was considered medically risky for him to do so. The ADA's requirement for reasonable accommodation has always made exceptions for those who may be a threat to the health or safety of others on the job. This decision interpreted the exception as applying to workers who may present a risk only to themselves.

In September 2008, Congress passed the Americans with Disabilities Act Amendments Act (ADAAA), intended to provide broader protections for disabled workers and reverse a number of court decisions that Congress considered too restrictive. The ADAAA added to the ADA a number of examples of "major life activities" and overturned a Supreme Court case that held that an employee was not disabled if the impairments could be corrected by mitigating measures, specifically providing that an impairment must be determined without considering corrective measures. It also overturned the interpretation that an impairment that substantially limits one major life activity must also limit other activities to be considered a disability.

Case law continues to influence the ongoing implementation of the ADA. A number of cases are still pending, and it is likely that the ADA will continue to be refined through Supreme Court decisions over the next several years.

Older Workers Benefit Protection Act (1990)

The Older Workers Benefit Protection Act (OWBPA) amended the ADEA by clarifying the authority of the ADEA relative to employee benefits. Although still requiring equal benefits for all workers, as a result of several legal decisions, the ADEA allowed reductions in benefits for older workers in situations where added costs were incurred to provide the benefits. The OWBPA removed employers' option to justify lower benefits for older workers. It requires that any waivers or releases of age discrimination must be voluntary and part of an understandable, written agreement between employer and employee. In other words, this law prohibited an employer from unilaterally providing a reduced benefit to an employee on the basis of age.

Civil Rights Act Amendments (1991)

Adding to the original Civil Rights Act of 1964, the 1991 amendments allowed employees to receive compensatory and punitive damages from employers who committed violations with malice or reckless disregard for an individual's protected rights. They allowed women and disabled workers to sue for compensatory and punitive damages, a right they previously did not have. This legislation provided for jury trials in such discrimination cases. Previously, these had been handled with nonjury processes. For employers, the overall impact of these amendments was to increase the likelihood of longer and costlier legal processes and to increase potential penalties. The effect of this act was to add "teeth" to portions of the Civil Rights

Act of 1964, expand certain other parts, and generally make possible more and larger damage awards.

Family and Medical Leave Act (1993)

The FMLA applies to eligible persons in organizations having 50 or more employees. The FMLA defines eligible employees as those having been employed for at least 1 year and having worked at least 1250 hours during the previous 12 months. These persons are permitted to take up to 12 weeks of unpaid leave during any 12-month period when unable to work because of a serious health condition, or to care for a child upon birth, adoption, or foster care, or care for a spouse, parent, or child with a serious health condition. Under specified circumstances, leave may be taken intermittently or on some reduced time schedule. This has the potential to extend any given leave over a period longer than 12 calendar weeks. Employees who are entitled to a set amount of paid time off are ordinarily required to use that time as part of their 12 weeks. Most employees on leave ordinarily use up their available paid time off rather than experiencing their entire leave without pay.

The FMLA does not take precedence over any state or local laws that happen to provide greater leave rights. Some states mandate a threshold lower than 50 employees. For example, in Maine the threshold is 15 or more employees for private employers and 25 or more for public employers; in the District of Columbia the threshold is 20 or more employees. Several states have their own definitions of "family." Some, for example, include "domestic partners," and a number include grandparents and parents-in-law. With FMLA, as with all instances in which federal and state governments have passed laws addressing the same issue, it is the more stringent law—that is, the one that is more generous to employees—that applies.

While on approved leave, employees must continue to receive healthcare benefits but are not entitled to accrue vacation, sick time, or seniority. The employer must guarantee that, upon returning from leave, an employee will be reinstated to the previous position held or placed in a fully equivalent position with no loss of benefits or seniority.

In many situations, the FMLA has made life considerably more difficult for department managers. When an employee in an essential position takes leave, that position and its responsibilities must be covered. Some positions cannot be left vacant for a few days, let alone for a 12-week period. Filling the position and later returning the employee to an equivalent position is not readily accomplished. Courts and other external agencies have repeatedly interpreted equivalent as essentially the same in all aspects: pay, benefits, tasks, and responsibilities. Some courts have ruled that equivalent extends to reinstating similar hours and shifts. Because equivalent has been so strictly interpreted, the safest course of action for managers is to preserve the original position of the person on leave. Managers are often advised to juggle coverage until the employee returns from leave. This often requires the use of temporary employees, overtime, reassignments, and other means. The practical result of the FMLA is that staffing and scheduling has become more difficult, time-consuming, and expensive for some managers.

Some critics of the FMLA suggest that the law mandates various forms of leave that are used more often by female employees than by males and thus renders women more expensive to employ than men (the same criticism has been leveled at the Pregnancy Discrimination Act of 1978), arguing that this will encourage employers to engage in subtle discrimination against women in the hiring process. Supporters point out that since FMLA applies to both women and men, it encourages both men and women equally to make use of family-related leave.

Along with the ADA, the FMLA continues to be subject to frequent clarification and adjustment. In late 2009, Congress acted to provide alternate eligibility criteria for airline flight crew members with some additions specific to that employee group. Also, a section of the National Defense Authorization Act of 2010, passed in October 2009, expanded the definition of "serious injury or illness" to specifically include aggravation of existing or preexisting injuries or illnesses incurred in the line of military duty. Also in late 2009, the Department of Labor (DOL) updated its regulations to provide better understanding of workers' rights and responsibilities. The DOL expanded FMLA coverage for military family members, and revised employee notice rules to minimize workplace disruptions due to unscheduled FMLA absences.

Several states have expanded access to leave through state FMLA laws, but federal legislation has not followed the states' lead. Possibilities for amending the FMLA include expanding the number of employees covered by the FMLA; updating the definition of "family" to include more family caregiving relationships; providing FMLA protections for grieving parents, spouses, and adult children; ensuring that leave can be used to address domestic and sexual violence; and providing unpaid time off to attend school events or medical meetings. It is unclear at this time which of the foregoing possibilities will receive serious consideration.

Retirement Protection Act (1994)

The Retirement Protection Act strengthens and accelerates funding of underfunded pension plans and increases PBGC premiums for plans that pose the greatest risk. It improves the flow of pension-related information for workers and increases the PBGC's authority to enforce compliance with pension obligations.

Small Business Job Protection Act (1996)

Despite the title of this legislation, its provisions are not restricted to small businesses. This legislation included the 1996 increase in the minimum wage. It increased pension protection and makes it easier for workers to roll over (change to another fund or plan) their retirement savings upon changing employment. It simplified pension administration to an extent and reduced the vesting period for selected multiemployer plans from 10 years to 5 years. The act allows specified smaller employers to establish simplified 401(k) plans for their employees.

Health Insurance Portability and Accountability Act (1996)

When the Health Insurance Portability and Accountability Act (HIPAA) came on the scene in 1996, as far as most persons working in health care were concerned, HIPAA had little effect. At the time, the most visible portion of HIPAA addressed "portability and accountability" in reference to employee health insurance. The intent was to enable workers to change jobs without losing coverage. This let workers move from one employer's plan to another's without gaps or waiting periods and without restrictions based on preexisting conditions. A worker could move from plan to plan without interruption of coverage.

Not a great many managers in health care concerned themselves with HIPAA in 1996. Human resource managers were the ones who became most aware of this new legislation because it affected their benefit plans. However, even many HR managers had little involvement with HIPAA. In most instances, the required notifications were handled by the employers' health insurance carriers, so there was little for HR to do other than answer employee questions. At that time, nothing about HIPAA affected the role of individual non-HR managers. In the minds of many who did not look beyond the simple implications of the law's title, the organization had little more to do than to ensure the portability of health insurance. However, the real impact of HIPAA was yet to come, and its arrival was a surprise to many.

HIPAA consists of five sections or "titles," each addressing different topics and different areas of responsibility:

- Title I: Healthcare Access, Portability, and Renewability
- Title II:
  - A. Preventing Healthcare Fraud and Abuse
  - B. Medical Liability Reform
  - C. Administrative Simplification
- Title III: Tax-Related Health Provisions
- Title IV: Group Health Plan Requirements
- Title V: Revenue Offsets

The Contentious Title II

The portion of HIPAA having the most far-reaching implications for many healthcare managers in the performance of their jobs is C, Administrative Simplification (which for many has proven to be anything but "simple").

Managers within health care, some to a greater or lesser extent than others, are finding or are yet to find their jobs affected by portions of HIPAA. Eleven separate "Rules" have been designated. Not all of them have yet been released for implementation, so for healthcare managers, HIPAA implementation will be a continuing process for some time to come.

The controversy over the intent versus the reality of HIPAA primarily concerns the requirements of the Privacy Rule. The intent was to strike a balance between ensuring that personal health information be accessible only to those who truly need it and permitting the healthcare industry to pursue medical research and improve the overall quality of care. Essentially, patient privacy is at the center of most current interest in HIPAA.

HIPAA has impacted not only HR but also nearly every department and division of all healthcare organizations. Although there may be future modifications to some of its rules and mandated procedures, the heightened emphasis on personal privacy and the confidentiality of patient information is here to stay.

Patient Protection and Affordable Care Act (2010)

The Patient Protection and Affordable Care Act (PPACA) was signed into law on March 23, 2010, and was immediately amended by the Health Care and Education Act of 2010, which became law on March 30, 2010. The PPACA is, of course, the still-controversial "healthcare reform" undertaking of the Obama administration. The law included provisions intended to take effect over several years, including expanding Medicaid to cover more lower-income people, subsidizing insurance premiums for persons of a certain income level, providing incentives for businesses to provide healthcare benefits, prohibiting denial of claims or coverage because of preexisting conditions, and other fixes aimed at expanding coverage to include greater numbers of people, controlling costs, and reducing the deficit.

Passage of the PPACA did not stem the continuing controversy over how the nation should address the widespread problems of health insurance cost and availability. If anything, controversy increased as the law came under criticism from several quarters, and some in Congress and elsewhere began advocating its repeal.

Some of the changes called for during the first year of enactment (2010–11) included the following: insurance companies were barred from dropping people from coverage because of illness, young adults could remain on their parents' plans until age 26, coverage was made possible for uninsured adults with preexisting conditions, insurers were forbidden to deny coverage to children with preexisting conditions, and a number of changes were made that affected Medicare. Changes targeted for 2011 included Medicare bonus payments to primary care physicians and general surgeons, Medicare coverage of annual wellness visits, and other changes to Medicare and Medicaid.

The legislation stipulated that additional reforms would be implemented annually between 2012 and 2015. Some new requirements had been scheduled for 2018. One extremely controversial feature originally scheduled for implementation in 2014 was the requirement for most people to obtain health insurance coverage or pay a tax if they do not so.

The PPACA is likely to affect most healthcare managers in two ways. First, the manager may be affected as a participant in the employer's health insurance plan. Depending on the nature of the plan and its features, there could be changes that affect coverage for all employees, including the manager. Second, the individual manager is likely to be asked questions by employees who want to know how the plan's changes will affect them and what will happen to their present coverage. The manager will need to be knowledgeable enough to respond to general questions and to know where in human resources to go for more complete answers. For the most part, the interpretation of the features and effects of plan reform on the organization's health insurance plan will reside with the benefits-management area in the HR department.

Greater Responsibilities and Increased Costs for Organizations. In addition to the laws described in the preceding pages, there are state laws that often vary from state to state. The closing decades of the 1900s saw the federal government spreading its influence over an increasing number of aspects of the employment relationship. Fortunately, the proliferation of employment legislation has slowed since 1999. In addition to creating added work for HR personnel by designating what cannot be done or by imposing new requirements, many of the laws affecting employment have created new or tighter boundaries in which managers must operate.

Overall, the effect of employment legislation has been to compel employers to be more socially responsible for their employees. This is especially evident in significant pieces of legislation such as the ADA and the FMLA. Legislation affecting social responsibility and rules of conduct for interactions between employers and their employees imposed added work responsibilities on organizations. These requirements have increased the cost of doing business and thus increased costs are passed on to the ultimate consumers of all goods and services.

While some new laws have required only minor changes in procedures or modest alterations in recordkeeping practices, most have clearly increased the cost of doing business because provider organizations and their customers are the only entities available to pay the increased costs. Legislators know very well that costs are associated with implementing any new law. Legislators and senior managers are often far from agreement concerning the costs of implementing new legislation. When elected officials create new programs, they are undoubtedly aware that only three options exist to cover the costs associated with implementation. Legislators can discontinue an existing program to free up funds. This rarely occurs because it is politically unpopular. Legislators can raise taxes, but suggesting this is even more unpopular. Finally, legislators can find other parties or organizations (someone else) to bear the costs of new legislation. The entities that have been paying to implement most of these laws affecting the employment relationship are businesses and other commercial enterprises. Ultimately, the costs are passed along and paid by individual consumers.

A Cumulative Effect: Some Comments. EXHIBIT 3-1 presents a list of all of the laws discussed earlier by decade of passage. It is not difficult to see the shift from the pre-1964 concerns with collective bargaining and wage-and-hour issues to the growing post-1964 concerns with social responsibility.

A simple comparison of the pre-1964 years with the present day demonstrates how significantly the employment environment has changed. Although very few of the laws reviewed replaced features of earlier legislation, most of the legislation enacted since 1964 has exerted new and often different influences on how work organizations treat employees and how managers can direct their own departments. The accumulation of more than four decades of legislation affecting the employment relationship has transformed personnel from the days of an employment office to the modern HR department. A contemporary department manager must comply with countless rules for supervising and directing employees. Although the accumulation of new legislation seems to have slowed somewhat, most experts agree that the future is likely to bring more, not less, regulation.

Discrimination cannot be legislated out of existence. Discrimination is extremely personal, as it resides in individual attitudes, likes, and dislikes. It is the product of both home and culture. Therefore, no job is completely immune from the possibility of discrimination.

A new law can come into being in a relatively brief period, yet it can take a very long time for the changes in human behavior required by that law to come about. Title VII of the Civil Rights Act of 1964 provides a useful illustration. Employment discrimination has been prohibited by law for five decades, but problems of discrimination continue to exist in many organizations. However, the workforce in the United States is becoming increasingly diverse. Organizations that eliminate discrimination will be the ones best able to value and manage this diversity.

For five decades, employee rights have been an extremely active legal topic in the federal and state legislatures and thus in the courts. We can expect this interest in individual rights to continue, probably even to intensify from time to time. The employment environment has changed and will continue to change. Those who manage within this environment must either change with it or be left behind.

EXHIBIT 3-1 Employment Legislation by Decade

1930s

- Norris–LaGuardia Act (1932)
- National Labor Relations Act (1935)
- Social Security Act (1935)
- Fair Labor Standards Act (1938)

1940s

- Labor–Management Relations (Taft–Hartley) Act (1947)
- 1950s
- Labor–Management Reporting and Disclosure (Landrum–Griffin) Act (1959)
- 1960s
- Equal Pay Act (1963)
- Civil Rights Act (Title VII) (1964)
- Age Discrimination in Employment Act (1967)

1970s

- Occupational Safety and Health Act (1970)
- Health Maintenance Organization (HMO) Act (1973)
- Rehabilitation Act (1973)
- Employee Retirement Income Security Act (1974)
- Taft–Hartley Act Amendments (1975)
- Pregnancy Discrimination Act (1978)

1980s

- Consolidated Omnibus Budget Reconciliation Act (1986)
- Immigration Reform and Control Act (1986)
- Pension Protection Act (1987)
- Drug-Free Workplace Act (1988)
- Employee Polygraph Protection Act (1988)
- Worker Adjustment and Retraining Notification Act (1988)

1990s

- Americans with Disabilities Act (1990)
- Older Workers Benefit Protection Act (1990)
- Civil Rights Act Amendments (1991)
- Family and Medical Leave Act (1993)
- Retirement Protection Act (1994)
- Small Business Job Protection Act (1996)
- Health Insurance Portability and Accountability Act (1996)

2010s

- Patient Protection and Affordable Care Act (2010)
- Health Care and Education Act (2010)

▶ Conclusion

The legal aspects of HR have changed dramatically over the past 80 years. The emphasis on the right of workers to form unions and establishing basic parameters such as length of a work week and establishing a minimum wage has changed. The emphasis of most recent legislation has been grounded in social

🔍 *CASE STUDY: Resolution*

Returning to the initial case study, it is reasonably certain that County Memorial's request for dismissal of the complaint will be unsuccessful. The ADA prohibits potential employers from imposing major limitations on pre-employment physical examinations. Concerning Susan and her complaint, the potential employer should attempt to negotiate a reasonable agreement and offer her employment in some capacity, rather than allow the State Division of Human Rights to conduct a full investigation and run the risk of imposing a costly settlement. The division might consider Susan to be a handicapped person (anyone who has a physical or mental impairment that substantially limits one or more major life activities). If it so rules, the division can then sue County Memorial Hospital on Susan's behalf.

Susan's case is far from cut and dried, however. Different jurisdictions have rendered varying decisions related to any disability. For example, a New York state court ruling declared obesity to be a handicap, but a Pennsylvania decision stated that obesity can be but is not always automatically a handicap. As is often the case with disputes that arise under some aspect of employment law, clarification of the law in its application is left to the courts. Courts in different jurisdictions and locations do not always see the same situation in the same light.

SPOTLIGHT ON CUSTOMER SERVICE

Customer Service, the Law, and Creators of Laws

The legal system, through many pieces of legislation enacted over the past 80 years, makes many demands on human resources departments. Many statutory programs require HR departments to collect money or information or both. Some HR insiders joke that they have been turned into bill collectors.

Customer service has been exempted from the pieces of legislation that have affected HR. No statutes outline how customers should be treated. Statutes do not stipulate that customers should receive any particular treatment.

How customers are treated is determined locally. Often, supervisors of employees that interact with the public have the responsibility to establish norms for interaction and treatment. Many managers choose not to exercise their responsibilities.

A small number of companies have made customer service an organization-wide priority. The phrase "The customer is always right" was an early attempt (1909) to establish norms for customer service. Harry Gordon Selfridge is generally credited with originating the phrase for the London department store that bears his name. In the United States, F. W. Woolworth adopted the approach for his company. Today, the Disney Company has a reputation for training its employees to provide excellent customer service.

The bottom line for the first part of this story is that customer service cannot be legislated. It must emerge because individuals and organizations care about their customers.

What about the individuals who actually create the legislation? Many elected officials claim that they have devoted their lives to public service. An important question then becomes, "Does a relationship exist between public service and customer service?"

(continues)

Maybe.

For most lawmakers, the answer is likely to be determined using the following logic. Customer service often (usually) requires putting the welfare and satisfaction of customers first. When discussing lawmakers, constituents can be substituted for customers. Lawmakers put themselves first, ahead of constituents, because lawmakers must be reelected if they want to continue their present employment.

Programs that increase taxes or fees provide convenient examples. In order to curry favor with constituents, most lawmakers are reluctant, often to the point of refusal, to vote for legislation that openly requires constituents to spend money.

Lawmakers like to claim that they enact legislation that benefits their constituents without the constituents having to pay increased taxes or fees to the government. When affected businesses raise prices to recover additional costs required to comply with requirements of the new legislation that benefits constituents, lawmakers can claim that they are not responsible because they did not raise the prices. Whether money to cover the costs associated with a new program is paid to a governmental unit or to a company, constituents ultimately bear the costs.

Back to public service and customer service. For individuals willing to overlook payment realities that are not discussed and the fact that this allows lawmakers to put their own welfare ahead of their constituents, the answer to the question is yes, lawmakers do provide customer service. For individuals who understand the deception of the undiscussed connection, the answer to the question becomes no, lawmakers do not provide customer service.

Customer service is, or should be, synonymous with openness.

Modified from Associated Press. (2002a, April 30). Seniority outweighs disability, court says. *Democrat & Chronicle*, Rochester, NY; Associated Press. (2002b, June 11). Top court disallows dangerous jobs for disabled. *Democrat & Chronicle*, Rochester, NY; Hearst News Service. (2000, October 12). High court scrutinizes Disabilities Act. *Democrat & Chronicle*, Rochester, NY; Newsday. (2002, January 9). High court limits disability law. *Democrat & Chronicle*, Rochester, NY; Skrentny, R. (1987). Immigration reform—What cost to business? *Personnel Journal, 66*(10), 53–59.

responsibility. As government has compelled employers to become more socially responsible, the costs of those government-mandated changes have been shifted to consumers.

American workers can expect equal access to employment and to receive equal pay for similar jobs. They can expect to work in safe surroundings without being discriminated against on the basis of age, gender, race, religion, national origin, or personal preference. Persons with disabilities must be treated like any other workers. They can expect to work in an environment that is free of drugs and harassment. American workers can take time off during a pregnancy or illness. They can expect access to healthcare benefits after losing their jobs. To a degree, pension rights have been established. Information related to one's health is now protected and considered to be private.

HR personnel must be familiar with the requirements of the legislation discussed in this chapter. This task has made the jobs and activities of HR employees more complex and challenging. Compliance with the legal requirements has imposed additional costs on organizations. Most experts expect that this trend will continue, although the pace of implementing changes is likely to slow.

Questions for Review and Discussion

1. Why is 1964 and the passage of the Civil Rights Act (Title VII) a turning point in the evolution of HR? Stated differently, other than 1964 representing the beginning of a steady flow of regulations to follow, what occurred that constituted a change of direction? Why?

2. Define and describe a contemporary bargaining unit as defined by the National Labor Relations Act. How, if at all, does it differ from a bargaining unit in 1935?

3. When and how was the Equal Employment Opportunity Commission established? What is its purpose?

4. What is a bona fide occupational qualification? Provide at least two specific examples.

5. What is the intended goal of the right-to-know laws? In your opinion, have they been successful? Why or why not?

6. Well before the passage of the Americans with Disabilities Act, in some instances employers were required to provide reasonable accommodation of the limitations of an employee or applicant. When did this occur, and what were the conditions under which this requirement applied?

7. What appears to have been the primary intended purpose of the Employee Retirement Income Security Act? Why was this legislation deemed to be necessary?

8. What have been the primary effects of the Immigration Reform and Control Act on businesses?

9. Pose two hypothetical examples of situations in which a healthcare employer might legally require a polygraph (lie detector) test as a condition of either initial or continued employment.

10. Viewing the Family and Medical Leave Act from the perspective of a working department manager, describe the ways in which this legislation has affected a supervisor's ability to manage.

References

Associated Press. (2002a, April 30). Seniority outweighs disability, court says. *Democrat & Chronicle*, Rochester, New York, NY.

Associated Press. (2002b, June 11). Top court disallows dangerous jobs for disabled. *Democrat & Chronicle*, Rochester, New York, NY.

Hearst News Service. (2000, October 12). High court scrutinizes Disabilities Act. *Democrat & Chronicle*, Rochester, New York, NY.

Newsday. (2002, January 9). High court limits disability law. *Democrat & Chronicle*, Rochester, New York, NY.

Skrentny, R. (1987). Immigration reform—What cost to business? *Personnel Journal, 66*(10), 53–59.

Resources

Books

Buckley, J. F., & Green, R. M. (2004). *State by state guide to human resources law, 2005*. Frederick, MD: Aspen.

Guerin, L. (2005). *Create your own employee handbook: A legal and practical guide with CD* (2nd ed.). Berkeley, CA: NOLO.

McConnell, C. R. (2011). *The health care manager's legal guide.* Burlington, MA: Jones & Bartlett Learning.

McConnell, C. R. (2019). *The effective health care supervisor* (9th ed.). Burlington, MA: Jones & Bartlett Learning.

Shilling, D. (2004). *The complete guide to human resources and the law.* Amsterdam: Wolters Kluwer.

Periodicals

Koen, C. M., Jr., Carmichael, A. J., & Koen, K. E. (2017). Attention deficit disorder and the Americans with Disabilities Act: Is anyone paying attention? *The Health Care Manager, 36*(2), 116–122.

O'Brien, G. V., & Ellengood, C. (2005). The Americans with Disabilities Act: A decision tree for social services administrators. *Social Work, 50*(3), 271–279.

Popovich, P. M., Scherbaum, C. A., Scherbaum, K. L., & Polinko, N. (2003). The assessment of attitudes toward individuals with disabilities in the workplace. *Journal of Psychology, 137*(2), 163–177.

Ritchie, A. J. (2002). Commentary: Implementation of the Americans with Disabilities Act in the workplace. *Journal of the American Academy of Psychiatry and Law, 30*(3), 364–370.

Schiff, M. B. (2004). A primer on case law under the Americans with Disabilities Act. *Tort Trial and Insurance Practice Law Journal, 39*(4), 1141–1196.

Takakuwa, K. M., Ernst, A. A., & Weiss, S. J. (2002). Residents with disabilities: A national survey of directors of emergency medicine residency programs. *Southern Medical Journal, 95*(4), 436–440.

Weill, P. A., & Mattis, M. C. (2003). To shatter the glass ceiling in healthcare management: Who supports affirmative action and why? *Health Services Management Research, 16*(4), 224–233.

Westreich, L. M. (2002). Addiction and the Americans with Disabilities Act. *Journal of the American Academy of Psychiatry and Law, 30*(3), 355–363.

CHAPTER 4

Human Resource Activities and Managers

CHAPTER OBJECTIVES

After studying this chapter, readers will be able to:

- Identify the services that are almost always, often, and occasionally provided by a human resources department.
- Subdivide human resource services according to the major tasks of acquiring, maintaining, retaining, and discharging or separating employees.
- Identify the activities for which a department manager can expect contact and involvement with human resources, and the likely extent of that contact and involvement.
- Compare and contrast line management and human resource management as to background.
- Interpret perspective and other characteristics for the purpose of explaining some of the tensions that develop between the two groups.
- Understand and eventually overcome the apparent differences between human resources personnel and line managers.

▶ Chapter Summary

A human resources (HR) department is involved in a number of activities that together compose four major groupings: acquiring employees, maintaining employees, retaining employees, and separating employees. Within these groupings, the specific activities of employment and recruitment, compensation and benefits administration, and employee relations are undertaken. Also to be found in many HR departments are labor relations (if unions are present), training and development, employee health and safety, security, child care, and other employee services. Generally, all of the activities that may be found within a given HR department relate in some way to acquiring, maintaining, retaining, or separating employees.

🔍 CASE STUDY: Who Has a Recruiting Problem?

Jane Cassidy is director of nursing at Community General Hospital. The institution recently completed an expansion that included, among other additions, a new 36-bed medical/surgical unit. Until recently, Jane had worked in conjunction with HR employment manager Carrie Smith and had fared reasonably well in keeping her nursing staff up to required levels in spite of a general shortage of nurses in the local area. The opening of the new unit, however, has strained the nursing department's resources to the extent of leaving the department short several registered nurses.

Community General's nursing shortage is particularly evident on the evening shift (3:00 P.M. to 11:30 P.M.). There are more than enough people willing to work days, and Jane has been fortunate in having a thoroughly stable crew of nurses who prefer to work nights.

Employment recruiter Carrie has regularly gone out of her way to do everything possible to locate candidates for nursing positions. Being extra cautious about the possibility of scaring good candidates off before they can be interviewed, Carrie has been deliberately vague with candidates concerning available shifts and hours. Unless specifically asked, she has not mentioned to anyone that new graduates being hired are expected to work day–evening or day–night rotations.

In response to the long-running recruiting efforts of Jane and Carrie, a well-qualified registered nurse applies for employment. Both are impressed with this nurse. She seems energetic and personable and is immediately available. She is quite willing to take a position on the evening shift.

Unfortunately, although this candidate is willing to work 3:00 P.M. to 11:30 P.M., she stated during her initial screening interview with Carrie that she cannot work weekends. She will say only that weekend work causes severe inconvenience in her family life, and she repeats her willingness to work evenings, straight evenings, but only Monday through Friday. Nevertheless, Carrie refers this candidate to Jane, quietly suggesting that Jane see if she can talk her into rotating weekends. The applicant has yet to learn that scheduling practices in Community General's nursing department require everyone below the level of day, evening, or night supervisor to work every other weekend, although Carrie has become aware of a few situations that might constitute quiet exceptions to the scheduling policy.

Considering the critical need for nursing help on evenings as well as weekends, what can Carrie and Jane tell this applicant? If Jane has to adhere rigidly to her scheduling policy and the candidate refuses to accept the job, what problems might Jane face? If Jane alters the scheduling policy and offers the applicant a Monday through Friday position without requiring weekends, a position that she accepts, what problems might Jane then face?

How can Carrie, as an HR professional, provide further help to Jane, a supervisor in nursing services, as she attempts to recruit sufficient staff for the nursing department?

Human resources services are provided by a staff (as opposed to line) activity. This means that no individual in HR has direct authority over employees in any of the other departments of a healthcare organization. As such, HR is oriented toward service. It exists to provide services to employees at all levels of an organization.

▶ The Activities of Human Resources

Finance, operations, and sales and marketing are examples of organizational subdivisions that are encountered in companies or businesses of any appreciable size. The tasks performed within these functional areas are similar in most organizations, as are the tasks performed within each functional area of a healthcare organization. Human resources, however, differs in that the tasks performed by HR personnel may be quite varied. Only within the past 2–3 decades have educational programs been created to prepare people for careers in the field of human resources.

Regardless of the form or operational purview of a particular healthcare organization, whether hospital, long-term care facility, free-standing clinic, urgent care center, physician group practice, or other entity, all HR departments have similar goals and pursue similar overall missions. These working groups exist to provide service to an organization and its employees. Not all HR departments are organized in the same fashion, however, and not all provide the same services or perform exactly the same tasks or activities. Under some organizational structures, activities that are often associated with HR may be performed by other departments or may even be separate departments in their own right.

In the sections that follow, the activities of HR are subdivided into three categories or levels. The first encompasses activities that are commonly associated with HR and usually part of the HR department. The second includes tasks that are often but not always performed by people from an HR department. The third discusses activities that are occasionally associated with HR or sometimes found outside of an HR department structure.

Category I: Typical HR Activities

Of the four groups of activities that follow, the first three are invariably components of HR. The fourth is usually part of HR if a union is present in an organization.

Employment or Recruitment

This activity addresses the original function of what was previously described as the employment office. Different names may survive from the past, but employment or recruitment or some variant of either word is usually part of the organizational designation for this activity. The heart of this activity is concerned with finding or identifying prospective employees, screening them, and arranging for them to be interviewed by supervisors and managers throughout the larger organization. The same HR employees extend official offers of employment and perform a number of other tasks that are necessary to bring new hires into an organization.

With a diminishing number of exceptions, employment for an entire healthcare organization is centralized in HR. The few exceptions that may still be encountered, especially in hospitals of medium to large size, typically involve nursing departments that continue to conduct their own recruiting. In the past, this was a much more common practice than at present, although some nursing departments maintain a designated nurse recruiter who frequently works closely with HR. Physician recruiting is often coordinated by an institution's medical director, although the paperwork is usually delegated to HR.

Compensation and Benefits Administration

Historically, administration of benefits was the second significant area of responsibility to be assigned to HR. Depending on an organization's size and mode of operation, compensation and benefits may be combined as a single activity or may be pursued separately by individuals who specialize in each. The separation of these activities is often the case in larger organizations.

The activities associated with benefits administration ordinarily include explaining benefits and related policies to employees and answering questions related to benefits. These people assist employees in accessing their benefits. They maintain relationships with benefits providers such as insurance carriers and pension overseers. These HR employees must stay current with regulations that concern benefits and must maintain employee benefits records. They participate in periodic assessments of the appropriateness of benefits. When necessary, they become involved in designing and implementing changes to benefits programs and packages.

Compensation activity is, by definition, concerned with wages and salaries. Primarily, this includes recommending starting pay for new hires consistent with their education and experience as well as taking into account the compensation of existing employees. Compensation encompasses answering questions related to wage and salary issues and recommending corrective action when necessary. Specialists in compensation monitor an organization's wage structure to ensure that pay equity exists throughout an organization. They recommend changes in the wage structure that are consistent with pay changes in the local community, industry, and individual occupations as necessary.

Employee Relations

Some may refer to an activity such as employee relations as being on the soft side of HR. This is in contrast to elements that are on the hard side, such as compensation and benefits. The distinction is based on the relative ease with which matters can be quantified. Hard issues generally refer to compensation and benefits that can be quantified using dollars and cents or other numerical measures. Soft issues encompass relations with people. An employee relations practitioner is likely to be involved, for example, in advising supervisors and managers on how to proceed in addressing selected employee problems or monitoring applications of the organizational disciplinary process. They may listen to troubled employees and refer them to sources of assistance as needed. Experts in employee relations counsel individual employees as needs arise and serve as employee advocates when necessary. They may represent the organization in relations or negotiations with external advocacy agencies such as the State Division of Human Rights. (Names of similarly charged agencies vary from state to state.)

Labor Relations

Labor relations exist as a separately identified entity in larger organizations, but only when some or all of an organization's nonmanagerial employees are unionized. The emphasis is on larger organizations because in a smaller setting, even with a union present, there may not be enough continuing activity to justify having a specialist in labor relations. When this is the case, labor relations activities become part of another HR practitioner's job. For example, an employee relations specialist or the HR director may take on labor relations activities when this becomes necessary.

The scope of labor relations includes continuing contact and ongoing relations with elected officials of one or more unions representing some or all of an organization's eligible employees. A majority of labor relations activities consist of hearing and resolving complaints. A collective bargaining agreement defines steps for processing grievances. A labor relations specialist represents the employer in related matters such as arbitration hearings and other formal processes. Many organizations have personnel who are actively involved in promoting labor relations or trying to prevent unionization when additional union organizing occurs. After a union is formed, specialists in labor relations participate in contract negotiations and other related activities when necessary.

Category II: Frequent HR Activities

Depending on the size of a particular institution, the way in which it is organized, and how its activities are distributed, some of the following may exist as separate departments. Others may be housed within HR. Some may not require a solely dedicated individual, so the few duties are incorporated into the job descriptions of other HR practitioners.

Employee Health and Safety

These may be separate activities; employee health is often located separately from safety. In small organizations, however, they are frequently combined. Either or both may be components of HR. Almost as commonly, they may be contained within other organizational units. Employee health is often found within one of the organization's medical divisions. However, such a reporting arrangement can create problems with confidentiality of records. In theory, employee health should be a subsidiary component of HR, with the director of employee health reporting directly to the chief of HR. The rationale for such an arrangement is that employee health renders service to employees by performing pre-employment physical examinations. This activity is clearly related to HR's employment section. Because physicians render the services, however, they should report to an institution's medical director or chief of medicine. This is just as clearly not a section of HR.

Training and Development

Training and development is often a subsidiary activity of HR. However, depending on organizational size, it is frequently situated as a separate, free-standing entity with a reporting relationship to another department. In healthcare settings, training and development is often a component of a nursing department or an equivalent group with a more broadly encompassing name, such as patient care services. Many nursing departments have developed and maintained educational capabilities. These evolved long before spreading to other disciplines because activities of long-standing continuing education (in-service) requirements that were developed by the nursing profession. As a result, in some quarters training and development has long been the province of nursing alone. When educational needs of other professions emerged, nursing simply attended to them. Thus, in many healthcare organizations, this remains the norm: education originates in nursing and is provided by nurses but easily crosses departmental boundaries. Sometimes training and development are split. Clinically oriented education remains in the nursing department, originating and being presented by nurses. Other training that is not clinically based often originates and is presented by personnel from HR.

Security

The security department is typically self-contained. The exception occurs in small organizations where it may have a reporting relationship to plant maintenance or building services. A distinctly separate security department with a manager of its own may report to the head of HR. Equally likely is a reporting relationship within the plant facilities chain of command or directly to the administrator who oversees general services for an entire organization.

Child Care

If a healthcare organization operates a child-care center or program, it is equally likely that the individual who manages child care will report either to the chief human resource officer or to another person such as the administrator for general services. Because a child-care center is subject to unique state licensing arrangements that govern staffing and facilities, it usually appears as a distinct and separate entity. The rationale for attaching it to HR is the service to employees' aspect of the activity. There are differences in how healthcare organizations having child-care programs define their scope of services. Some limit themselves exclusively to an employee clientele, but many are open to any member of the community. Often, child-care programs give priority to employees, but after meeting employees' needs, they fill the remaining capacity from other persons in the community.

Award and Recognition Programs

Responsibility for award and recognition programs will ordinarily be part of some department or group's assigned duties rather than being a separate entity. Exceptions occur in extremely large organizational settings. The most common exception is a large teaching institution that is an element of a university and thus served by the parent organization's award and recognition group. In smaller healthcare organizations, awards are often coordinated by a member of a public relations or community relations department or, occasionally, by an administrative assistant. For the majority of healthcare organizations, award and recognition programs are the responsibility of HR and often fall to an employee relations practitioner.

Equal Employment Opportunity/Affirmative Action

If separate offices for Equal Employment Opportunity (EEO) or Affirmative Action (AA) exist within an organization, they will usually, although not always, be found within the HR department. A person who is designated as responsible for compliance with EEO regulations is frequently an employee relations practitioner or HR executive. This person has the primary responsibility for monitoring the organization's compliance with all applicable antidiscrimination laws. The individual in this position will be charged with some of the responsibilities that were described within the realm of employee relations, particularly those that relate to external advocacy agencies such as a state Division of Human Rights and the local branch of the federal Equal Employment Opportunity Commission (EEOC).

AA programs are no longer actively mandated for the organizations to which they formerly applied. As a result, HR personnel who had responsibility for AA programs have been assigned to other duties. AA required organizations holding government contracts to demonstrate that positive efforts were being made to align the composition of an organization's workforce with the demographic characteristics of those living within the organization's labor market area. In other words, the goal of an AA program was to achieve a workforce in which the percentages of women and minorities mirrored those of women and minorities in the labor market area. Most of the compliance requirements have been reassigned and are now included in EEO mandates. EEO monitoring of workforce composition and compliance with regulations continues.

Category III: Infrequent, Occasional, or Outsourced HR Activities

The following activities are sometimes found within the structure of an HR organization.

Risk Management

Risk management is present in most healthcare organizations—indeed, in most organizations of any size or type. Interests of risk management include monitoring malpractice and liability actions brought against the organization while overseeing and constantly evaluating forms of insurance coverage. Risk managers study loss trends such as costs associated with Workers' Compensation. The goal of these activities is to manage risk in an effort to achieve an appropriate balance between costs of doing business and potential exposure to a variety of legal risks.

Although formerly a component of HR in some organizations, risk management is currently more often found elsewhere in the administrative structure. With its increasingly significant legal implications, risk management is frequently coordinated by a person who reports to the organization's legal counsel. Increasingly, if risk-management duties are assigned to more than one person, then risk management may become a separate department, and its manager often has a legal background.

Executive Compensation Administration

This activity is rarely left to persons in HR. More commonly, it is undertaken at the executive level within finance. If executive managers are not included in an organization's payroll system, then executive compensation is most likely to be accomplished through an external confidential payroll service. Such an arrangement is quite uncommon in healthcare organizations; it is far more likely to be encountered in other businesses. Executive compensation is almost certain to be externally administered if an organization's top executives are under individual contracts or their salary arrangements include incentive compensation.

Organizational Development

Organizational development encompasses a wide variety of tasks. In some organizations, it is little more than management development under a different label. True organizational development, however, goes beyond simply providing the continuing education necessary to keep managers current with developments in health care as well as to helping them cope with the changing times. Organizational development encompasses the changing requirements of an entire organization. It asks an ongoing question: How should this organization be changing its philosophy, mission, and vision, and its organizational structure, to meet the demands brought on by changing social and economic environments and the changing healthcare delivery milieu? In many organizations, organizational development is considered a luxury. It is often among the first departments to be cut when budgetary limitations arise or economic hard times occur.

A comprehensive approach to organizational development needs should include succession planning. Succession planning complements management development and expands upon it by preparing managers and other individuals at all levels not only to keep current but also potentially to advance within the organization. This facet of organizational development emphasizes the internal development of managerial talent. A comprehensive approach to organizational development usually includes some means of identifying and educating potential supervisors and managers from among nonmanagerial employees.

Organizational development exists as a separately identified activity in a minority of healthcare organizations. The work is typically coordinated by a person reporting directly to the director of HR. Organizational development activities are often conducted in parallel with employment, compensation and benefits, and other HR work. In rare situations, typically in very large healthcare provider entities, organizational development may be found as a separate office parallel to HR. In such a situation, its head reports to the same executive as the director of HR.

Employee Assistance Program

An employee assistance program (EAP) is intended to assist employees in addressing particular personal problems that can affect their work performance. It is ordinarily described as an employee benefit. An EAP is primarily a referral program that helps individuals to identify and focus on their own needs and problems. EAPs help to secure professional referrals for troubled employees. A capably functioning EAP can help control absenteeism, tardiness, and other circumstances that can affect job performance. Addressing such personal problems usually contributes to improvements in quality and productivity. EAPs commonly address alcohol and drug abuse, family and marital difficulties, legal and financial problems, compulsive gambling, and other personal problems and issues.

A majority of healthcare organizations have EAPs. The initial referral point within a healthcare organization is usually an office located in HR or in employee health. The latter may itself be a component of HR. The professionals who provide assistance to workers are often employed by an outside entity and provide their services on a contract or retainer basis. Employees may use EAP resources with the assurance that no one within their organization has to know about their personal problems. This improves confidentiality and reduces the opportunities for embarrassing situations to develop in the workplace. The HR role is limited to simply putting an employee who expresses a need in touch with the external EAP coordinator.

Outplacement Services

Outplacement involves assisting displaced employees in finding new employment. Outplacement services are offered and provided in instances of reductions in the workforce or elimination of specific management positions. Occasionally, they are offered to individuals as part of a severance or termination package. Because outplacement is costly and not needed on an ongoing basis, outplacement usually does not exist as a permanent component of HR or any other organizational element. However, something that may resemble formal outplacement occasionally occurs when someone in HR or elsewhere in an organization is able to assist a displaced employee in finding a position with another employer.

Payroll

The activities of payroll were once a common adjunct to the employment activities of early personnel departments in many organizations. Both of these basic needs impact all employees. Before benefits became common, the only activities required in support of employees were hiring them and paying them. There was a compelling logic in having these two activities located in adjoining offices and coordinating their activities. However, as time passed, payroll requirements became increasingly more complex.

Financial activities have steadily become more sophisticated. As a result, payroll has been organizationally relocated.

In some organizations, it is still possible to find payroll attached to HR. However, these instances are uncommon, and their number is steadily declining. Today, most payroll activities are performed in one of two locations. In the majority of organizations that process their own payrolls, this activity is part of the finance department. Another department, such as data processing or information systems, which may or may not be part of finance, will make electronic transfers or actually print and distribute checks and reports. A growing number of organizations, especially those of small to medium size, utilize external contractors that specialize in providing payroll services. When outside payroll services are used, the input information from which they work is usually submitted to them by the finance department. Only occasionally is such information supplied by HR.

The foregoing activities are summarized in **EXHIBIT 4-1**.

Outsourcing

Outsourcing is the business term currently used to describe the practice of having services that were once performed by the organization's employees done by outside parties or vendors. Outsourcing sometimes becomes necessary because of changes in organizational structure, reduction in number of employees, or mergers. Reengineering encompasses these circumstances. Reengineering is not the only reason that organizations seek outsiders to perform needed services. A business organization might consider outsourcing for several reasons, including the following: the services

---

EXHIBIT 4-1 Human Resource Department Organizational Areas or Activities

Category I: Typical HR Activities

- Employment or recruitment
- Compensation and benefits administration
- Employee relations
- Labor relations (if one or more unions are present)

Category II: Frequent HR Activities

- Employee health and safety
- Training and development
- Security
- Child care
- Award and recognition programs
- Equal Employment Opportunity/Affirmative Action

Category III: Infrequent, Occasional, or Outsourced Activities

- Risk management
- Executive compensation administration
- Organizational development
- Employee assistance programs
- Outplacement services
- Payroll

---

to be performed require special skills or expertise; the demand for such services may not be sufficient to justify hiring one or more skilled persons to supply them; or a particular need is expected to be temporary in nature. A convenient example is managing pension fund investments, a task that is most always placed with dedicated specialists.

An outside supplier is often able to perform a task more economically than company employees can do so. This is one reason why outplacement services for displaced executives are provided on a contract basis by an external entity. Reductions in staff sometimes create needs that must be met for which no time is available among remaining employees.

Infrequent but necessary organizational requirements are sometimes referred to as "orphans"; a particular necessary task may occur irregularly and require insufficient time to justify training and retaining someone to do it. Preparing, publishing, and printing an employee newsletter provides a relatively common example. Finally, some work is of a sufficiently sensitive nature that confidentiality is best served by having it performed by an outside vendor. EAPs and executive compensation programs are two examples of sensitive programs.

The decision to outsource any particular task will ordinarily involve considerations of cost, capability, and confidentiality. Many outplacement decisions are driven by staff reductions brought about by reengineering or organizational downsizing. Often when a decision is made to eliminate a position, many of the responsibilities associated with that job may be eliminated, modified, or transferred to other persons. Remaining essentials may have to be outsourced.

Among the HR activities described in this chapter, the most likely candidate for outsourcing is outplacement services. This is not only logical but understandable because it is a specialized activity that is only occasionally required. The next most likely activity to be outsourced is an EAP. This is done to maintain employee privacy and confidentiality. Other commonly outsourced HR services are pension plan administration and Workers' Compensation and disability programs administration.

External vendors (outsourcing) are being used for two other important services: payroll and legal services. Increases in complexity of compensation programs, changes in tax withholding requirements, concern for security, and the desire to achieve economic savings are driving the trend to use outside vendors for processing payroll. Finally, most healthcare organizations are not sufficiently large to justify employing a full-time attorney, so legal services are most commonly provided by a law firm engaged on a retainer.

▶ Human Resources from a Different Perspective

The earlier discussion of HR analyzed the services by categories. Each category included services on the basis of their likelihood of being included in a typical HR department. Alternatively, the services supplied to an organization by HR can be discussed by dividing them into groups on the basis of how they relate to an organization's employees. These generalized activities include employee acquisition, support or maintenance, retention, and separation (see **EXHIBIT 4-2**). This section reflects such organizational groupings.

Employee Acquisition

This category of activities includes every task undertaken to find employees and bring them into an organization. In most healthcare organizations, this means all employment or recruitment activities. Human resources personnel may attend job fairs at local colleges and training facilities or travel to regional or professional meetings to recruit prospective employees. Placement of advertisements for employees is coordinated by HR, although other persons in the organization may provide input on the copy or text of such ads. Pre-employment testing is usually coordinated by HR even if the actual services are provided by persons elsewhere in the organization or external to it. A critical HR activity is checking references and verifying credentials. All new employees are given the same initial organizational employee orientation by HR. In general, HR coordinates or supplies any activities that are undertaken, from locating employees to successfully situating them in their positions within the organization.

Employee Support or Maintenance

Many HR activities are intended to support or maintain employees by addressing needs relative to their employment. These activities include administering compensation and benefit programs, enforcing personnel policies and procedures for the entire organization, and coordinating disciplinary and other corrective processes as needed. In unionized environments, the latter includes formal grievance procedures as outlined in the collective bargaining agreement. Human resources maintains or

EXHIBIT 4-2   Major Activities of the HR Department

Employee Acquisition

- Employment and recruitment activities (representing the organization at job fairs and professional meetings, placing job advertisements, etc.)
- Pre-employment testing
- Checking and verifying of references
- Initial organizational orientation

Employee Support or Maintenance

- Compensation administration
- Benefits administration
- Personnel policies and procedures
- Performance appraisal programs
- Disciplinary and corrective programs
- Coordinating grievances (in unionized environments)
- Personnel record keeping
- Workers' Compensation programs
- Disability programs
- Employee assistance program
- Labor relations (in unionized environments)
- Parking
- Communication programs
- Employee health clinic
- Cafeteria
- Savings and investment programs

Employee Retention

- Retirement plans
- Performance appraisal and management programs
- Award and recognition programs
- Education, training, and development
- Tuition assistance
- Child-care assistance
- Succession planning programs
- Career development opportunities
- Career ladders and parallel path progression

Employee Separation

- Discharge and dismissal procedure documentation
- Unemployment compensation
- Outplacement services
- Retirement counseling
- Exit interviews
- Terminal benefits processing

coordinates personnel record keeping. This includes ensuring that employee records are maintained in a secure location for long periods of time. Human resources may administer Workers' Compensation and disability programs or coordinate them if the services of an external vendor are used. Other ongoing activities related to employees often provided or coordinated by HR include EAPs, labor relations activities, security and parking, communications with large groups of employees, and any other services that may be provided for the purpose of supporting or maintaining employees as effective producers. Services that are sometimes coordinated by HR include operating an employee health clinic, maintaining a cafeteria for employees and members of the general public, and coordinating savings and investment programs.

Employee Retention

Significant overlap can exist between the tasks of maintaining and retaining employees. Compensation and benefits administration provides a convenient example. If compensation for a particular position is not perceived as fair or equitable when compared with other positions or with community standards, then compensation alone will provide little incentive to retain employees in the organization. Likewise, if the contents of a benefits package are clearly less than other employers are providing, benefits will have minimal to no effect in retaining employees. The importance of compensation and benefits in retaining employees is embodied in the need to keep them competitive so that valued employees will be encouraged to remain loyal to the organization.

Immediate monetary compensation, such as pay and benefits, is not sufficient to motivate good employees. Numerous other incentives, activities, or perquisites are offered to help retain employees. The variety of such incentives is limited only by the imaginations of organizations offering them or employees requesting them. However, some are fairly common. These include retirement plans, performance appraisal and performance management programs, and award and recognition programs. Other noncash incentives that organizations may offer include opportunities for training and development, tuition assistance programs, and career development and succession planning programs. Some programs may appeal to only a relatively small cadre of employees. For those who need them, however, EAP and child-care assistance are highly appreciated. These are important in both maintaining and retaining employees. All employees not only appreciate but have come to expect physical safety and security in all organizational facilities and reasonable parking accommodations.

Succession planning is critical to the success of any organization. Many in healthcare plan only for the succession of the top few executives and then only when an employee is leaving. Employees appreciate the chance to have input into their careers and welcome the assistance that is often provided by HR. Some relatively large organizations are able to provide opportunities for career development. Promising employees are identified and offered positions on task forces, committees, or other temporary teams. In very large organizations, career ladders and parallel path progressions are possible.

Employee Separation

This category includes all activities involved in separating employees from an organization regardless of the reasons for separation. Some paperwork and filing always accompany any separation. When an employee is discharged for cause, all disciplinary actions must be documented. Activities after discharge may involve external agencies. Employees who are laid off must be reported to the state, so that they may receive unemployment compensation. Outplacement or access to similar services may be offered. Individuals who retire often appreciate counseling and planning assistance. Administrative work related to a pension plan is required to begin the flow of financial benefits. Occasionally, HR coordinates or arranges retirement celebrations. Every voluntary separation should include an exit interview. Most separations from an organization involve cessation of benefits. An interview or some other contact with HR is required to complete the necessary paperwork. When selected benefits are to be continued (for example, health benefits under COBRA legislation), HR usually completes alternative paperwork to ensure that services continue to be provided without interruption.

▶ Where Department Managers and Human Resources Personnel Meet

This section initially identifies the points at which a department manager can expect to come into regular contact with employees from HR or with the programs and activities that HR coordinates. A department manager will benefit by learning how to optimally utilize the services offered by HR to the fullest extent possible.

A typical department manager can expect to have frequent contact and considerable involvement in activities involving employment, employee relations, and labor relations (if there are unions present). Depending on the nature of a manager's supervisory responsibilities, periods of active involvement with training and development may be the norm. A manager should expect to have some involvement with activities involving compensation, benefits, safety, employee health, and payroll. The degree of involvement will depend on how such services are organized and provided as well as on the rate of turnover of departmental employees. The same manager should expect minimal involvement with HR personnel related to security, parking, child care, risk management, and other HR concerns. Contact with these services usually occurs when individual employees enter or leave a department's workforce.

The background, education, and experience of most department managers in healthcare organizations ordinarily stem from their basic education or their technical or professional specialties. A few have some general business knowledge, but the majority are not overly familiar with HR processes and requirements. Some basic HR knowledge and involvement with HR are necessary for individuals who want to supervise and coordinate their department's employees in an effective manner.

Employment

A successful manager must remain involved in recruitment and employment processes as a normal part of departmental activities. The intensity of this activity will depend on the turnover rate in the department and on how much employment activity is necessary.

When a manager finds it necessary to acquire a new employee, the initial step is to create or update (as necessary) a job description. A personnel requisition must usually be secured from higher management before HR can be contacted.

In some instances, a manager may be able to submit a personnel requisition directly to HR if the need is for a direct replacement of a departing employee. The requirement for such approval depends on the personnel practices of the organization. If the requisition seeks an additional employee, however, it usually requires thorough justification and subsequent approval by one or more managers in higher positions in the organization. This requirement intensifies when budgets are tight.

When a personnel requisition is received by HR, it is typically assigned to an employment recruiter who identifies an appropriate number of candidates. A department manager's next involvement usually occurs when HR sends the manager a file containing several applications or résumés of applicants who meet the stated minimum requirements of the job. The manager then reviews these documents and advises the HR recruiter which ones should be called for interviews.

An HR recruiter will conduct screening interviews. As long as the candidates remain appropriate after being reviewed by others for compliance with EEOC, the Americans with Disabilities Act (ADA), and other legal requirements and with organizational hiring guidelines, HR will arrange interviews for them with the department manager. Following the interviews, the manager compiles a list that ranks the candidates. This list is sent to the HR recruiter, who contacts the selected candidates. Depending on the size of an organization, the recruiter or a senior administrator or executive negotiates with the candidate and reaches an agreement on starting pay and other relevant details. One of these people extends a formal job offer and sets the desired starting date for the new employee.

For a variety of reasons that will become evident, formal offers of employment should originate only from HR. The responsibilities of most managers focus on providing services or producing products or information, but HR personnel are people professionals. Some senior executives may extend offers of employment should that be the norm for a given organization. Direct supervisors should not negotiate salaries with candidates because of the potential for ill feelings (if a particular salary request is not granted) after the job has been accepted. An offer is ordinarily made contingent upon positive reference checks and having the applicant pass a pre-employment physical examination. Once an applicant has been completely cleared and begins to work, it is a department manager's responsibility to ensure that the new employee is oriented to the department and properly started on the job in all other respects.

Benefits

A department manager should have no active role in administering employee benefits. However, the department manager is ordinarily an individual employee's primary source of information about the organization as well as the job (or is at least perceived as such by most employees). For this reason, managers can expect to receive regular questions about benefits from their employees. This suggests that a manager should become familiar with or have a reasonable working knowledge of commonly used benefits such as paid time off (vacation, sick time, personal time, and holidays). Answers to routine questions will save time and allow HR personnel to concentrate on questions concerning more serious or complex problems. When large numbers of managers reply to all questions related to benefits with "I don't know, go ask HR," HR appears to be lax in sharing information. This impression does not support HR in the short term. Over a longer period, an organization will suffer.

Most managers will benefit by having two levels of knowledge about HR. The first is knowing how the organization's benefits structure personally affects a manager. This knowledge will enable a supervisor to answer many common questions that employees might ask. The second is knowing from whom in HR employees should seek answers to more complex questions.

Compensation

A department manager must be familiar with an organization's compensation structure because it affects the pay of all departmental employees. This includes knowing about relevant wage scales, what they mean, where departmental employees are relative to the scales, and the relative position of each employee. Information about relative positions is needed to answer questions that are related to others who perform similar tasks and have similar lengths of employment but who might be paid at different rates. A manager should have sufficient knowledge of the compensation structure to recognize when inequities have crept into the department's pay rates and to raise questions about these inequities to HR.

The best information about how a job is performed resides with the person who does the job and the manager who directs that individual in doing the job. The department manager and an individual employee on the job are the primary repositories of knowledge of how a particular job is or should be performed. A manager must be able to apply this knowledge when creating, reviewing, or revising job descriptions. An accurate, up-to-date job description is an absolute necessity when determining the pay grade and salary range for any particular job. Thus, this essential component of compensation administration is largely the responsibility of a departmental manager. Human resources ordinarily participates in writing and updating job descriptions but cannot create quality job descriptions without departmental input.

Employee Relations

Each time a problem arises concerning an employee, the potential exists for a department manager to interact with HR. This involvement can come about because of complaints about employees. These may be made by employees or by persons from outside. They may be informal or formal, such as grievances. Complaints may be filed with agencies such as Human Rights or the EEOC. They may originate as lawsuits or disciplinary actions. They may be brought by a department manager or other person.

One employee-related activity that requires a manager's direct interaction with HR on a regular and recurring basis is compiling and filing performance appraisals. Human resources will ordinarily administer the appraisal system, keep the system up to date, provide training in the system's use, and follow up on appraisal completion. A manager's role is to perform the appraisals of employees who are directly supervised according to the guidelines established by HR and in accordance with timetables established by the organization.

Personnel Records

Human resources maintains the organization's personnel records. Department managers have a few regular areas or points of contact with personnel records. Much of the information that is filed comes to HR from department managers. Performance appraisals and disciplinary actions are among the most common of these items.

Managers occasionally have a need to review some fact or element of a subordinate's personnel record. Such requests often pertain to the work record and qualifications of someone who wishes to transfer into the department. Organizations create their own guidelines regarding access to personnel records. In general, information contained in personnel records is highly confidential and should not be available to any supervisor without a valid reason for access. Requested information should be provided by an employee from HR. Personnel records should be kept in a secure location, with access restricted to as few people as possible. Competent legal counsel should determine the parameters governing the long-term storage and retention of personnel records.

▶ Human Resources and the Organization

It is no secret that in many work organizations there is a degree of strain, at times even some animosity, between HR and managers of other departments. This is true of employees in health care as well as in other organizations or professions. Often these differences simply slow down the normal flow of business. Occasionally, however, the differences develop into overt antagonism that can significantly interfere with the efficient conduct of business.

"Line managers and staff human resource professionals spend a great deal of time talking at each other and often past each other and privately questioning each other's views about what goals and values are important" (Leskin, 1986). Why do such differences between HR and department managers exist? An examination of the differences between line management and HR may help to develop an understanding of why there is sometimes a credibility gap between the two.

Background and Qualifications

The backgrounds of HR practitioners are often varied. Some, a relative few but increasing in numbers over the past 15 years, have received specific education in HR. Despite the increase of people with specialized education, there are individuals working in HR who are educated in a number of different academic backgrounds, including business, psychology, sociology, organizational behavior, industrial relations, and education. People who started their careers in clinical or technical specialties have assumed management positions throughout healthcare organizations, but they are not commonly encountered in HR.

Supervisors and department managers in healthcare organizations tend to be educated in specific technical or professional occupations, invariably the operational areas they manage. On average, an HR practitioner's education has been liberal and nonspecifically focused. In terms of scientific training, personnel from HR are likely to have been educated in a so-called soft science such as those already mentioned. In contrast, other supervisors and managers in healthcare organizations are likely to have training in so-called hard sciences such as biology, chemistry, or physics. The educational focus of persons with hard science training tends to be narrower than their colleagues with softer science training. The particular educational backgrounds are relatively unimportant; they are simply different. However, people's initial education often sets a tone for their later outlook on organizational values and influences how they embrace concepts and facts or how they view theory and practice.

Staff Managers

Line managers frequently have to supervise and coordinate a variety of people who bring a mix of values into their jobs. Some of these people will require close, nearly constant supervision, while some are capable of independent work. A manager's working group may include individuals with an extremely broad mix of skills and educational backgrounds, often from within a single discipline. Consider, for example, a nursing manager who may supervise a group including nurse practitioners who have training at the masters level, as well as a variety of other nursing personnel with training that ranges from a bachelor's degree (registered nurses) to an associate's degree (some registered nurses, licensed practical nurses), to nursing assistants who may have attended certificate programs, and to persons with a high school education (clerical personnel). Such a diversity of educational preparation often poses managerial challenges. Human resources departments, in contrast, are usually considerably smaller than most line departments; they tend to be relatively cohesive groups composed of people who share similar values and have a common occupational outlook.

Management Style and Approach

The supervisor of a line department will ordinarily tend to manage with a downward orientation. Many decisions and supervisory interventions are accomplished on a one-to-one basis. The downward orientation clearly marks the subordinates of such a manager as being subordinates in the overall scheme of operations. A manager may sometimes have to perform the duties of a practitioner, but depending on department size and workload, such instances tend to be relatively minor components of a manager's responsibilities.

With the exception of clerical support staff, HR employees (HR practitioners) are more likely to view themselves as colleagues who are comparable with each other rather than as part of a hierarchical structure. With the exception of the largest healthcare organizations (multisite systems, teaching hospitals, and the like), in most healthcare settings the chief HR officer is likely to have some practitioner duties in addition to supervisory responsibilities. Because of this mix of duties, people throughout the HR department regard these managers and practitioners as organizational equals.

Expectations

The positional goals and expectations placed on line managers are usually relatively clear and easy to define. Line managers are expected to perform their assigned job duties to ensure consistency of quality and output. They are simultaneously expected to adhere to policies and procedures of the organization. Furthermore, they are expected to remain faithful to the mission, vision, goals, and objectives of the organization.

The expectations of an HR department may not be nearly as clear or recognizable as those placed on line departments. The expectations associated with HR will influence the manner in which line departments regard HR. Human resources may be perceived as being expected to control the affairs of other departments, retain the status quo, avoid making waves, or innovate. These perceptions will influence whether line departments regard HR with apprehension, indifference, contempt, or caution, or embrace HR as a helpful or useful organizational ally. As long as the expectations of HR and the line departments differ noticeably from each other, there is likely to be a degree of tension among them.

Orientation and Training

In regard to matching an appropriate person with each task to be performed, line management tends to hold the belief that selection is the most important factor. Put differently, many line managers feel that selecting the right person for a job is the most important factor related to accomplishing the task. Human resources practitioners, in contrast, often tend to believe that development is the most important factor. With proper development, any of several people have the potential to perform a given job. This sometimes leads to sharp differences between line management and HR in the area of recruiting. Human resources may supply several candidates, all having the potential to execute a particular job as expected if they are properly developed. However, none of the candidates may appear to have the exact qualifications or experiences or be precisely the right person for the job. This perception develops because line managers, knowingly or otherwise, often hold out for an ideal fit between candidate and position.

Participation

Line managers frequently exhibit a tendency to believe that the notion of employee participation in decision-making is no more than a theoretical abstraction, one that complicates matters by slowing things down and generally failing to contribute to departmental success. Human resources practitioners have a different view of employee participation in decision-making. Human resources proponents generally feel that when participation is properly implemented, it can generate improved organizational performance and increased employee satisfaction.

Employee Empowerment

The highest priority for line managers in a healthcare organization is taking care of patients and delivering services. As a result, they are often hesitant to delegate important tasks. More frequently, they adopt an approach reflecting the belief that managers or supervisors have the ultimate responsibility to provide needed services. In the extreme, they (the managers) will often provide the required services themselves. The philosophy and priorities of HR are different. The highest HR priority is performing a particular job or supplying a needed service. They often advocate employee empowerment as a vehicle for individual growth and development. This approach is taken because of their belief that in order to grow, people must have the freedom to fail.

Control

Line managers frequently act according to the belief that exercising control protects a department's staff and enhances an organization's ability to deliver care, programs, and services in a timely and cost-efficient manner. The human resources view, however, suggests that a controlling manager stifles creativity, discourages employee participation, and impedes employee growth and development.

Staff Performance

Line managers, especially in departments having a considerable mix of staff skills, qualifications, and educational levels, will ordinarily have to integrate or cope with varying levels of individual performance. As a consequence, managers must occasionally provide counseling, criticism, disciplinary action, and termination. Such people problems can consume a considerable portion of a line manager's time. In contrast, an HR manager usually supervises professionals and a few support personnel having comparable skills. As a result, their people problems are fewer, and they are far less likely to have to take corrective actions.

Reward Assumptions

Line managers often tend to believe that compensation is the most effective means of influencing performance and that their staff members are primarily motivated by the promise of material rewards. Human resources practitioners tend to place organizational culture, supportive management, employee participation, and opportunities for personal development above monetary compensation as providing motivation for employees over the longer run.

Regarding Change

The belief system that line managers seem to hold is that effective change occurs slowly over time and that as a consequence, true organizational change is always slow and incremental. The HR view is generally that genuine organizational change is achievable and can occur over a short term if it is driven and supported by top management.

Outlook

The orientation of line managers ordinarily views success or failure as occurring in the short run. The typical HR view usually involves a longer-term perspective.

What Results in Practice

In summarizing the apparent differences between line management and HR, the following points are useful: Line managers believe that HR departments impede progress by frequently obstructing what an operational department manager wants or needs to do. Furthermore, they view HR as being largely obstructionist, commonly citing laws to support their positions on why particular actions cannot be taken. In contrast, HR personnel feel that line department managers regularly try to evade laws and policies and generally insist on making decisions and taking actions that have the potential to cause legal problems for the organization.

What Can Be Done

Many rank-and-file employees, along with some department managers, do not trust HR. This often exists to the extent that some employees never go to HR with their needs because they feel that doing so will endanger their employment. As a result, these employees never utilize the HR processes and services that are available to them. Many employees apparently do not perceive HR as a resource for them. Rather, they view HR as a department that relates primarily with their managers and thus mainly serves the corporate hierarchy.

Department managers and HR personnel can both improve their situations by giving each other the benefit of the doubt concerning their motives. Translated, this means that HR's mission in life is not to obstruct and frustrate department managers and that department managers should not pour their energies into finding ways around HR. Rather, each should try to use every instance of disagreement as an opportunity to know more about the other.

A top priority of HR should be communicating how HR can be an important resource for all employees. This must be demonstrated to rank-and-file employees as well as managers. If HR is not communicating this critical information, then department managers and administrative personnel should take steps to ensure that this does occur. The HR department should never forget why it exists. Human resources represents employees and is an advocate for them. Human resources must ensure that managers are aware of employee needs and are motivating them to perform; HR must continually propose and champion programs and services that appear to be most needed by the employees of the organization that they serve. Senior management must never allow HR to forget why it exists and that it is needed by all in the organization.

▶ Conclusion

The activities of HR are reviewed from different perspectives. Most HR departments provide three basic services: employment or recruitment, compensation and benefits administration, and employee relations. When unions are present, HR frequently coordinates labor relations. Human resources provides other services in some but not all healthcare settings and may also coordinate employee health and safety activities, training and development, security, child care, award and recognition programs, and EEO and AA responsibilities. The following activities are occasionally coordinated by HR: risk management, executive compensation administration, organizational development, EAPs, outplacement services, and payroll. Alternatively, some of these latter activities may be outsourced.

Viewed from a different organizing perspective, HR activities may be grouped in an alternative manner. The groupings include employee acquisition, employee support or maintenance, employee retention, and employee separation. Line managers throughout an organization and personnel from HR interact most commonly on issues involving a small number of basic concepts or areas. These include employment, benefits, compensation, employee relations, and personnel records.

Despite these similarities, readers must remember that all HR departments or operations are not the same. Furthermore, the education and experiences of most line managers and HR managers are different. As a result, the expectations of people in these two groups are often different.

🔍 CASE STUDY: Resolution

Concerning the nurse recruiting situation at Community General Hospital, one might question the degree to which nursing director Jane Cassidy and employment manager Carrie Smith are actually working together. Carrie seems to be putting forth a fair amount of effort to locate candidates. However, she is deliberately vague about hours and shifts. Although she is appropriately sensitive about scaring off good candidates before they can be interviewed, she creates extra work for nursing staff and herself by not being open about hours and shifts and other scheduling requirements. When talking to new graduates, her hesitation in discussing the nursing department's rotation practices is unfounded because many new nurses seeking hospital employment expect to rotate shifts.

Jane might be considered luckier than many other nursing directors because of the availability of a group of nurses who prefer working steady nights. She has the good fortune to have staffing problems that are concentrated on one shift instead of two shifts, as is often the case.

Before Carrie and Jane talk with their recent applicant, they should quickly review their scheduling situation and current practices. If Jane continually has to adhere rigidly to her scheduling policy and the candidate nurses refuse the job as a result, then the shortage situation will worsen. A method must be found to recruit and hire qualified nurses during a time of shortage, even if doing so requires some compromise among existing employees and the internal movement of personnel to lessen the impact of any remaining schedule restrictions.

The nursing department and HR's recruiting personnel should consider closer collaboration. A key component of any new collaboration should include assembling a group of persons from both departments to review all of the nursing department's scheduling practices and searching for creative alternatives to replace the apparently rigid practices now used when scheduling nurses. The policies and practices governing nurse scheduling must be revised to reflect the reality of the nursing marketplace. Jane and Carrie must both be involved in this effort. With creative scheduling practices in place, no acceptable reason should exist to reject a qualified nurse applicant during a time of shortage. Considering the fact that quiet exceptions already exist, creative scheduling is already being practiced. This should ease the difficulty of the task.

SPOTLIGHT ON CUSTOMER SERVICE

Human Resource Activities, Managers, and Customer Service

In a manner similar to that of healthcare providers, human resource professionals often speak of practicing their craft. Over time, they improve their proficiency. This increases the efficiency with which they work while simultaneously increasing their value to the organizations that employ them.

Most managers become more proficient as their careers progress. They benefit from repetition. However, improved proficiency may be overlooked as managers focus on attaining their next promotions. This is due to changes in the nature of the tasks and responsibilities associated with their new positions.

Human resources provides services to an organization. When talking among themselves, managers often grumble about having to "support" human resources because that department generates no revenue. Such a view may be myopic to an extreme.

Human resource employees spend considerable portions of their working hours explaining regulations and other statutory requirements to employees. Many human resource employees become excellent teachers.

"That is nice," whisper managers, "but they (human resources) still do not contribute to the organization's bottom line."

The contribution to an organization's bottom line is indirect. One obvious reason should be teaching employees about the importance of customer service. Satisfied customers not only return to purchase additional services but also help to increase their organization's goodwill. When viewed from the opposite direction, dissatisfied customers rarely return. This reduces, rather than increases, the organization's revenue.

Modified from Leskin, B. D. (1986). Two different worlds. *Personnel Administrator, 31*(12), 58–63.

Questions for Review and Discussion

1. Outline a long-term approach that you would recommend for narrowing a credibility gap that might exist between an organization's HR department and its department managers.

2. Advance an argument either for or against having the employee health and safety clinic located within an HR department.

3. Describe the objectives and activities of risk management. Is risk management essential in a contemporary healthcare organization? Why, or why not?

4. Why is it a common practice to outsource an organization's EAP?

5. List several elements of a hypothetical organizational development program. Explain how and why such a program differs from management development.

6. Why is it preferable for a department manager to respond directly to the majority of employees' HR-related questions, rather than simply telling employees to "go ask human resources"?

7. What are screening interviews? Where and why are they ordinarily conducted?

8. Provide several reasons why a department manager should be familiar with the organization's compensation scales even though the manager is not expected to make specific salary quotations or negotiate salaries with prospective employees.

9. List three or four differing academic backgrounds that might be found among HR practitioners. What are the advantages or disadvantages of each in equipping an individual to provide HR services?

10. Describe the components of a typical outplacement service package. Explain why such services are almost always provided by an external vendor.

Reference

Leskin, B. D. (1986). Two different worlds. *Personnel Administrator, 31*(12), 58–63.

Resources
Books

Bucknall, H., & Ohtaki, R. (2004). *Human resource management.* New York, NY: John Wiley.

Fallon, L. F., & Zgodzinski, E. J. (2005). *Essentials of public health management.* Sudbury, MA: Jones and Bartlett Publishers.

Fisher, C. (2005). *Human resource management.* Boston, MA: Houghton Mifflin.

McConnell, C. R. (2019). *The effective health care supervisor* (9th ed.). Burlington, MA: Jones & Bartlett Learning.

Mello, J. A. (2005). *Strategic human resource management* (2nd ed.). Mason, OH: Thomson South-Western.

Niles, N. J. (2012). *Basic concepts of health care human resource management.* Burlington, MA: Jones & Bartlett Learning.

Society for Human Resource Management. (2005). *SHRM human resource outsourcing survey report: A study by the society for human resource management.* Alexandria, VA: Society for Human Resource Management.

Sutherland, J., & Canwell, D. (2004). *Key concepts in human resource management.* New York, NY: Palgrave Macmillan.

Periodicals

Bowman, B., & Stilson, M. E. (2005). Meeting the nursing shortage: A nursing camp for prospective nursing students. *Journal of Emergency Nursing, 31*(5), 512–514.

Graham, M. M., & Kells, C. M. (2005). The girls in the boys' club: Reflections from Canadian women in cardiology. *Canadian Journal of Cardiology, 21*(13), 1163–1164.

Lega, F., & DePietro, C. (2005). Converging patterns in hospital organization: Beyond the professional bureaucracy. *Health Policy, 74*(3), 261–281.

Luzzi, L., Spencer, A. J., Jones, K., & Teuser, D. (2005). Job satisfaction of registered dental practitioners. *Australian Dental Journal, 50*(3), 179–185.

Mathew, M. (2005). Nursing home staffing. *American Journal of Nursing, 105*(12), 15–16.

Matthias, R. E., & Benjamin, A. E. (2005). "Intent to stay" among paid home care workers in California. *Home Health Care Service Quarterly, 24*(3), 39–57.

Mulcahy, C., & Betts, L. (2005). Transforming culture: An exploration of unit culture and nursing retention within a neonatal unit. *Journal of Nursing Management, 13*(6), 519–523.

Parent, F., Fromageot, A., Coppieters, Y., Lejeune, C., Lemenu, D., Garant, M., ... De Ketele, J. M. (2005). Analysis of adequacy levels for human resources improvement within primary health care framework in Africa. *Health Research Policy and Systems, 2*(1), 3–8.

Prottas, D. J., & Nummelin, M. R. (2018). Theory X/Y in the health care setting: Employee perceptions, attitudes, and behaviors. *Health Care Manager, 37*(2), 109–117.

CHAPTER 5

The Manager–Employee Relationship

CHAPTER OBJECTIVES

After studying this chapter, readers will be able to:

- Recognize that groups composing the majority of healthcare organization departments are typically heterogeneous.
- Appreciate the value and importance of employee participation and input.
- Compare and contrast production-centered management and people-centered management, recognizing that most healthcare activities require people-centered management.
- Understand the importance of having a department manager remain visible and be available to the staff.
- Explain the value of a true open-door policy.
- Describe a manager's essential downward (toward the employees) orientation as opposed to an upward (toward higher management) orientation.
- Appreciate the importance of establishing and maintaining a solid one-to-one relationship with each employee and the need to know each as a whole person.
- Understand the department manager's key role in employee retention.

▶ Chapter Summary

This chapter advances the belief that in addition to many other responsibilities, every manager is also a coordinator of human resources (HR). Furthermore, this essential coordination is played out within a one-to-one relationship that the manager should have with each employee. However, work groups are composed of individuals, most of whom are different from one another in a number of ways, so that a manager's relationship with each employee may likewise be different in some respect from all other such relationships. Healthcare activities must ordinarily be more people focused than production focused. Managers must lead by example, remaining visible and available to employees while encouraging them and

🔍 CASE STUDY: "She Knows It All, Just Ask Her"

Two or three months ago, occupational therapist Alice Walters said to Kelly Miller, her manager and the director of rehabilitation services, "Kelly, it's obvious to me that we're not approaching the departmental budget sensibly. All we do is carry last year's actual expenditures forward, tack on some amount for an inflation factor and pile on some other guesses. We should be budgeting from a zero base, building up every line item and making each one justify itself every year."

Kelly replied something about simply following the budgeting instructions issued by the finance department and doing it the way they were told to do it.

Within a few days of the budget question, Alice approached Kelly with another question. "Shouldn't we change the way we approach performance evaluations? Surely most smart managers know that it's better to evaluate employees on their anniversary dates than it is to evaluate them all at the same time as we do it."

Kelly responded as before. As a manager, she was simply complying with the policies and practices of the organization. They discussed the matter for another 5 minutes. Although Kelly was not willing to take on higher management and work to change the evaluation system, she conceded that Alice had brought up a number of good points. To Kelly, it seemed as if Alice were picturing an idealized evaluation system in textbook-like terms. It was flawless but only in theory.

In the following weeks, Alice said more and more to Kelly about how both the organization and the department should be managed. It had taken Alice only a matter of days to get beyond generalized techniques such as budgeting and evaluation and to start offering specific advice on the management of rehabilitation services.

Kelly soon realized she could expect Alice to offer some critique related to most of her actions in running the department and many of executive management's policies in managing the organization. Kelly was disappointed with this annoying change in her relationship with an otherwise good employee. Kelly had always seen Alice as a better-than-average performer as a therapist, somewhat opinionated but not to a harmful extent. Recently, however, she had come to regard Alice as a sort of abrasive conscience, a critical presence who monitored her every move.

The worsening situation came to a head one day when Alice tried to intercede in a squabble between two employees. When Alice entered the situation, she proceeded to criticize Kelly's handling of the matter in the presence of the other employees. Kelly immediately took Alice into her office for a one-on-one discussion. She first told Alice that although she was free to offer suggestions, opinions, and criticisms regarding management, she was never again to do so in the presence of others. Kelly then said, "Lately, it seems that you have a lot to say about management in general and about how I run this department in particular. Why this sudden interest?"

Alice responded, "Last month I finished my first course in the management program at Community College, Introduction to Management Theory. Now I'm in the second course, Supervisory Practice. The concepts are not difficult. When I see things that aren't being done right, I feel that I have an obligation to speak up."

Kelly ended the discussion by again telling Alice that she expected all such commentary to be offered in private and never again in front of others. Overall, the conversation did not go well. On one or two occasions, Kelly felt that Alice's remarks were edging toward insubordination. Because of the uneasy feelings left after the discussion, Kelly requested a meeting with Carl Mason, the organization's director of human resources.

After describing her relationship with Alice in some detail, with a gesture of helplessness Kelly said, "She knows everything, I guess. Just ask her, she'll tell you. On the strength of a course or two of textbook management, she suddenly has all the answers. What can I do with her?"

Consider how Kelly Miller might address the problem presented by Alice Walters. Can Kelly do anything to curb the intrusions of an apparent know-it-all employee? If you were in Kelly's position, how could you encourage Alice to modify her apparently superior attitude? What suggestions would you offer to Kelly as she attempts to move her relationship with Alice to a more productive level?

depending on their participation and input. A healthcare manager must cultivate a genuine open-door attitude toward employees and must exhibit the essential downward orientation that says, "Although a member of management, the department manager's primary concern must be for the organization's clientele and the employees who provide services." A manager's task is to ensure that all employees are valued for what they can contribute.

▶ Every Supervisor a Manager of Human Resources

Some managers, particularly those who cling to old-fashioned and inappropriately narrow views of management, regard many employee-related concerns as something called "employee relations" rather than management. Their concepts of management may be described as production centered. They are concerned first, foremost, and always with getting the work done.

In organizations where HR practitioners are utilized to the maximum possible extent or nearly so, some managers have come to rely on them so heavily that, by default, they have transferred the primary responsibility for addressing all people-related issues to the HR department. Regardless of HR's strength and relative position in an organization, individual managers should retain responsibility for day-to-day employee concerns and remain involved with employee problems. However, HR should always be available for advice and assistance. By definition, this is an important role for HR. Many issues involving employees should not automatically default to HR. Most recurring, common, people-related tasks should be part of a manager's job and should not be referred to HR.

In the minds of some people, HR is an unnecessarily high-tone title encompassing activities that were formerly associated with a department called "personnel." However, "personnel" literally means *people*. In some modern organizations, the department that many refer to as HR is known by other names such as "people systems" or "employee affairs" or "employee services." In providing the people systems, literally the processes and procedures for serving all employees, HR simply provides a framework within which relations with employees should be conducted.

▶ The Heterogeneous Work Group

Workers in healthcare organizations bring with them an extremely broad range of educational backgrounds and levels of sophistication. Within a single group of direct reporting employees, a manager may have employees who require regular or even constant supervision (virtual hand-holding). In contrast, they may supervise employees, perhaps health professionals, who have been trained to act independently, make most of their own decisions, and determine most of their own behavior. These persons often require only the most general of direction.

Consider some examples appearing in many hospital organizations. Food service personnel can vary from entry-level employees who are hired without specialized skills or training to therapeutic dietitians who possess master's degrees. A manager in such a setting may be responsible for several levels of staff, each having different needs. Diagnostic imaging (radiology) employees may range from entry-level clerks and transporters to highly skilled special-procedures technologists and even physicians with whom a department supervisor must maintain working relationships even though they do not report directly to the manager. The manager in this venue may be responsible for as many levels of staff as a food service manager while also relating to physicians who can be either medical staff members or employees of the organization.

Other possible scenarios involve patient billing and housekeeping. In either activity, a single manager may be responsible for a number of personnel, all of whom are at the same level of education and sophistication (depending on how the activity is organized). In a modestly sized nursing unit, a nurse manager may have several levels of staff, such as nursing assistants and unit clerks, licensed practical nurses (LPNs), registered nurses (RNs), and nurse clinicians. In addition to multiple levels of education and sophistication, a heterogeneous work group can present its manager with another potentially troublesome condition—namely, differences among employees regarding their work ethic. For instance, significant differences in work ethic sometimes appear between newer employees and more established (experienced) employees or between older (in years) members of a group and younger workers. Although peoples' attitudes toward work and employment have shifted over the course of several generations, not all problems related to work ethic can be attributed simply to younger or newer workers having less experience.

Variations in work ethic suggest that within a single unit or group, a manager may have some employees who would never willingly miss a day's work or never intentionally shirk a responsibility, and some employees who think nothing of missing work on a whim and allowing responsibilities to go unfulfilled. In addition to striving to bring out the best in each employee, a department manager must be a visible example of a continually positive work ethic.

▶ Employee Participation and Input

An anonymous person—more likely several such anonymous people—claimed that, "When all is said and done, there's much more said than done." In few circumstances does this hold truer than concerning employee participation. Most managers claim they believe in employee participation and remain open to input from their employees; however, for the majority, their behavior contradicts their words. Managers repeat words they believe ought to be said or are politically correct because that is what "experts" are saying about contemporary management, especially in best-selling management books. Although such managers may repeat phrases and buzzwords from "Management 101," and say what they believe they are expected to say, on a day-to-day basis they continue to function as they have for years.

Some managers speak of their belief in participation, but in practice they only superficially tolerate it. Rather than participative, their style is consultative. A consultative manager is usually honest, conscientious, and completely well intended. However, such a person can rarely relinquish enough control to allow employees to participate or realize their full potential. For managers who behave in this fashion, any experience or process that involves sharing authority or control with employees smacks of abrogating responsibility and is perceived as weakness. Too often, this residual streak of authoritarianism remaining in modern management stifles employee participation.

Management has evolved for decades and will continue to do so. At the start of the 1900s, management, for all practical purposes, was largely authoritarian. In most settings, the boss was the only person in charge and was to be obeyed without question. During the same era, the top manager was likely to be the owner or principal stockholder of the organization. The human relations movement in management, a 20th-century phenomenon, began to take hold in the 1930s. It expanded steadily throughout the 1940s and 1950s. Today, many managers have been educated specifically for management. Like their supervisors and others who preceded them, however, they have acquired much of their managerial perspective from role models they observed and worked for. It is not surprising to find residual authoritarianism among many who manage today; their role models have been at least partly authoritarian. Authoritarianism in management is progressively weakening, but it is far from gone.

Department managers should always make it clear to employees that their ideas are valued and their input is not only welcome but also needed. Employee participation should be valued and promoted. Even consultative managers who reserve the right of final decision are well advised to solicit employee input, consider it carefully, and occasionally use employee ideas. In the end, such an approach or strategy usually pays dividends for both individuals and organizations.

When it comes to sources of knowledge about how to perform work better, faster, or more economically, the person who knows the inner workings of a job best is one who performs the duties day in and day out. Successful department managers remember this fact; the most successful managers are those who have learned how to tap into this source of knowledge.

▶ The People-Centered Manager

Depending on the particular work environment and kinds of work performed, most managers will tend to be either production centered or people centered. Because of the nature of some tasks, such as many found in manufacturing, a manager is required to be production centered. In production-centered situations, the work is ordinarily highly repetitive, many units of output are similar, output can be scheduled with some accuracy, and jobs can be defined in considerable detail. In a production-centered situation, employees are ordinarily assigned to specific work-stations. Other than keeping up with the pace of an assembly line or a sequence of related activities, they have little control over how they complete their jobs. In an assembly environment, the speed of the line determines the rate of output. If a particular employee does not keep pace, then another employee is substituted at that workstation. In a production-centered situation, a manager's priority concerns are usually keeping supplies and services entering the process and thus keeping the output flowing. In a production-centered environment, processes control the people and a manager's primary focus is on output.

In a people-centered environment, the willingness of employees to work main-tains output rather than the pace at which the work arrives or the manner of sup-plying the processes. In people-centered situations, the work is often irregular and varied. Rarely are two units of output identical. For this reason, scheduling output with true accuracy is very difficult. Jobs cannot be rigidly defined because demand on workers can be highly variable. In people-centered environments, employees control the processes. A manager's primary focus is on people, the producers, rather than on machines or conveyor lines or automatic processes.

Most situations found in a healthcare organization require people-centered management. In a healthcare organization, people primarily control the processes. Thus, people must be the primary focus of a successful manager. The following sections discuss some of the principal requirements of an effective people-centered manager of healthcare workers.

EXHIBIT 5-1 compares and contrasts several dimensions of production-centered management and people-centered management. Based on the characteristics

EXHIBIT 5-1 Comparison of Production-Centered and People-Centered Management

	Production Centered	**People Centered**
Nature of work	Repetitive	Variable
Nature of the output	Homogeneous	Heterogeneous
Pace controlled by	The process	Employees
Character of labor	More manual	More intellectual
Manager's primary focus	The process	Employees
Arrival of work	More predictable	Less predictable
Completion of work	Predictable intervals	Irregular intervals

encountered in the majority of healthcare delivery settings, it is evident that a manager using a people-centered approach to supervision best handles most situations that exist in healthcare settings.

▶ Visibility and Availability: Reality and Perception

A healthcare department supervisor must be generally visible to employees and must be both perceived as available and actually available. The matter of perception is stressed because, as far as employees are concerned, much of a manager's state of being visible and available is psychological. Although employees may never articulate the thought, seeing a manager around in a department and knowing that the manager can be accessed should the need arise provides most people with a level of comfort. Many employees are able to work independently for prolonged stretches; some even prefer to do so. On those occasions when a manager's judgment or expertise is required, however, the employees should know how to reach the manager in a reasonably short time. Even though only a few employees may be affected, a manager's presence in and around a work group will tend to limit inappropriate behaviors.

Consider the case of a manager who looked forward to moving from her small, glass-encased cubicle in the corner of the department to new and larger quarters some distance away from her staff. Formerly, all employees in the department could see that the manager was available. After the move, it was impossible to know her availability without leaving the department and traveling via a lengthy corridor. Within weeks following the move, complaints about the manager had noticeably increased. "Now she's hard to find when we need her." "She pays more attention to higher management than to us." "She no longer cares about us and our needs. Just look how she couldn't wait to get away from us." Her formerly noncomplaining employees uttered these phrases. Over the weeks and months that followed, staff absenteeism and tardiness increased, productivity decreased, and interpersonal problems among staff members increased. Absentee management may be appropriate in some retail business situations, but it is rarely appropriate when managing a department of people in an organizational setting.

Absence Impedes Communication

A manager often creates communication problems by not being reasonably accessible. When employees are forced either to wait to get answers or to take chances and act independently, time and material resources are wasted through delay and error. This may be especially troublesome in emergencies when time must be devoted to tracking down a missing manager.

Employees should perceive a department manager as the employees' direct conduit when communicating with other organizational elements. This is especially true for interactions with higher management. Employees may perceive a manager who is not readily visible or available as being uninterested and uncaring. This is true for supervisors who seem dedicated primarily to activities such as meetings, committee work, conferences, and the like that occur outside of a department. Such activities put strain on the relationship between supervisor and employees, and the employees begin to see such a supervisor as indifferent and impersonal. For many members of a working group, their department manager is a representative of the organization itself. This supervisor is the member of management that these employees know best and may be the only member of management with whom they have a speaking relationship. If employees perceive their supervisor as being cold, uncaring, and impersonal, then they are likely to perceive the entire organization in the same manner. In most instances, a first-line manager is a worker as well as a manager. These supervisory responsibilities provide an additional resource for a department. When a manager is unavailable, a potentially productive resource is lost.

A Genuine Open Door: Attitude and Actuality

Managers may occasionally use phrases often cynically described as coming from "Management 101." However, words alone are not sufficient; managers must back up the words with actions. Few managers have not said, "My door is always open." Unless the door is, in fact, usually open, employees quickly perceive reality. Few supervisors or managers are able to maintain a truly open-door policy. Supervisors are usually busy people, especially in times of shrinking managerial hierarchies and expanding responsibilities for individual managers. Contemporary managers must wrestle with problems, attend seemingly endless meetings, make and take telephone calls, and generally engage in many time-consuming activities. The effect of these responsibilities is that it is nearly impossible for a manager to sit behind a desk always available for any employee to drop in at any time.

Some managers are not easily accessible at any time because they are genuinely busy. Even though a manager has said, "My door is always open," the manager's attitude says, "The door may stand open, but I dislike interruptions and you should not consider entering without an appointment." The reality of an open-door policy depends largely on a manager's attitude. Even managers who are generally visible and available to their employees most of the time can discourage contact by projecting an attitude that discourages employees from approaching.

Easier for a First-Line Manager

An honest open-door policy, or a condition as near to that as practical, is easier for a first-line supervisor to maintain than it is for someone at a higher level of management. A first-line supervisor can usually address many problems and issues that enter via an open door in a direct manner. Persons in more senior managerial positions, however, usually must exert greater care when addressing issues brought directly to them by rank-and-file employees because of an espoused open-door policy. The actions of higher management must not subvert the authority of an employee's immediate supervisor. Thus, a higher manager's response must often consist of referring the matter down to the first-line supervisor or other source of assistance, such as the HR department or another intermediary.

A policy of easy access to first-line supervisors is often successful. First-line managers should remain appropriately visible and available and should strive to offer reasonably accessible open doors. They should maintain the open-door policy whenever possible. When other tasks require them to restrict access, they should have an alternative means for employees to schedule specific appointments. Barring emergencies, managers should always keep these appointments.

Show, Don't Tell

Surely many supervisors trap themselves with their own words by saying, "My door is always open" or something similar. It quickly becomes obvious that in many instances employees cannot have direct access to the manager, and employees immediately recognize the inconsistency between the manager's words and actions. A similar dilemma sometimes develops when supervisors claim to believe in participative management. Immediately following the very first instance in which a manager is unwilling or unable to allow employee participation, employees perceive the inconsistency between the supervisor's words and actions.

Contemporary supervisors are subject to the temptation to say the right things—that is, to repeat phrases that are well intentioned, trendy, and intended to convey the impression that employees always stand high among the manager's concerns; that is, to echo the platitudes of "Management 101." No matter how well intentioned a supervisor may be, however, it is not always possible for the supervisor to completely live up to words even though he or she may speak them with utmost sincerity. Such statements create inconsistencies that most employees eventually recognize. When inconsistencies between what one says and what one does become evident, contradictory perceptions result. The majority of employees see only that the leader has claimed to have one guiding belief but has acted contrary to that belief. When this occurs, a leader's credibility suffers.

Individual employees' perceptions of their manager's behavior may be correct, partly correct, or completely incorrect. The actual degree of correctness is irrelevant, but the perception itself is relevant, because to the perceiver, perception is reality. If an employee perceives a leader or supervisor to be untruthful for saying one thing and acting contrary to it, the perception becomes the truth.

It is rarely beneficial for supervisors to tell employees what kind of leaders they are. This invariably leads to negative perceptions at the first sign of contradictory behavior. Successful managers do not attempt to verbalize their supposed leadership style to employees. Subordinates are quite capable of deducing a leader's style from actions and behavior on the job. In other words, supervisors should show others their leadership styles and traits rather than talking about them.

▶ The Essential Downward Orientation

Strongly related to visibility and availability is the perception of whether a department manager or area supervisor is oriented upward or downward in the organizational structure. There is a strong and natural inclination for individual managers to be upwardly oriented—that is, spending more time being attentive to organizational superiors and executives than being focused on their subordinates. To a degree, some upward-facing behavior on the part of a supervisor is necessary; it is from above that the supervisor attains resources and receives praise and reward and gets noticed more readily when promotional opportunities arise.

Although the forces encouraging a supervisor to embrace an upward orientation can be relatively strong, it is essential to maintain a largely downward orientation toward members of the immediate work group and their needs. Downward is the direction in which the department supervisor must look most of the time; successfully leading subordinates is the primary reason for the existence of the supervisor's position. A first-line manager or supervisor is the leader of a group of people who perform the hands-on work of the organization. Employees depend on their leader for guidance; the supervisor is primarily the leader of the department's employees and is only secondarily a member of a greater organizational hierarchy called management.

A manager who is career minded and who wishes to advance is often inclined to seek the visibility obtained by maintaining an upward orientation. Although it may appear counterintuitive, supervisors who display an obvious interest in accomplishing the work of the department and who remain solidly oriented in a downward direction are most successful over time. Managers whose primary orientation is to their subordinates gain the most valuable experience for themselves and turn out the best work. They also build a reputation for caring for their subordinates. Simple visibility coupled with an ability to talk in a convincing manner has led to the promotion of many supervisors with limited people skills and capability. However, truly effective individuals in upper management are more likely to make promotions based on actual operating results rather than on superficial indicators. Quality leaders and managers require time to mature, and reputations require time to be established.

As with other elements of leadership, employees will readily perceive the fundamental orientation of their supervisor. A manager whom employees view as having an upward, self-serving orientation is likely to be seen as essentially separate from the working group and insulated from other employees by virtue of trying to identify with upper management. A downward-oriented supervisor is not only more readily accepted by subordinates but also more respected by employees as an advocate. Subordinates generally view such a person as a full-fledged team member for whom they will willingly produce.

▶ Essential Individual Relationships

A successful department manager must assiduously cultivate and maintain a one-to-one relationship with each employee. Doing so requires conscious effort. Effective avenues of communication are essential, but they are not formed automatically. Establishing and maintaining such a relationship with each employee should be a key concern of every department supervisor. This activity may receive higher-priority treatment than departmental productivity for brief periods. Maintaining a department's productive capacity is an ongoing priority. In labor-intensive working environments such as healthcare organizations, a department's productive capacity resides in its people.

Managers should treat each employee as a full-fledged, contributing member of a team. This is one of the most effective means of maintaining a labor-intensive department's productive capacity. This requires deliberate action to forge and maintain relationships between the supervisor and each employee. Managers should ensure that no one is excluded (except for the occasional individuals who exclude themselves; there are sometimes the few who want nothing more than to check their brains at the door for 8 hours a day as long as they are paid).

Most department managers are busy people, often having more demands placed on them than can reasonably be met on any given work day. This being the case, many supervisors tend to ignore employees who simply perform their job duties in an acceptable manner, never complaining or causing difficulties. Troublesome employees are invariably a minority, but they often consume inordinate amounts of a manager's time.

In any work group, consider who is noticed and who is not. Employees who perform at an outstanding level or who exceed the expectations of their positions are usually noticed. They often do not require much of a manager's time, although they surely do attract a supervisor's attention. Troublesome employees get a manager's attention and they consume the manager's time; these people consistently make mistakes, exhibit performance problems, violate work rules or policies, or do not meet the minimum expectations of their positions. The majority of employees, positioned between the outstanding performers and the troublesome ones, frequently go unnoticed and thus receive little or none of their manager's time and attention.

The 80–20 rule nicely summarizes this relationship: 20% or fewer of employees consume 80% or more of a supervisor's time. The majority of employees in the middle group who produce acceptable work day after day are neither outstanding nor problematic. These are the quiet ones who, for all practical purposes, are frequently ignored.

However, even the quiet ones should receive some attention from the supervisor if they are to maintain their output at an acceptable level and not become troublesome. Unless supervisors maintain relationships with these subordinates, their productivity may gradually deteriorate.

Other than addressing task-related matters, some supervisors convene face-to-face meetings with subordinates only on two occasions. One is to appraise performance, usually once each year, and the other is to address problems via counseling, disciplinary action, or other corrective processes. The invitation "Come into my office" raises considerable apprehension under such circumstances.

It is a good idea to meet with each employee periodically even in the absence of a pressing reason for doing so. The agenda can be conversation about the job or some discussion about the department's role or the organization and its future. Such meetings foster open environments and create opportunities for employees to ask questions and air perceived problems or complaints. These meetings can be instrumental to maintaining positive relationships with individuals. An occasional few minutes of ordinary social conversation totally unrelated to work can nurture essential relationships.

For managers, knowing each subordinate as a whole person, not simply as a producer of services or output, is important. Doing so not only ensures continued steady performance from an employee but also provides additional advantages for a supervisor. By knowing and understanding each employee, a supervisor will acquire knowledge other than that normally associated with individual capabilities. A manager will learn who occasionally needs more guidance or assistance; a supervisor will understand which subordinates are sufficiently motivated to take on additional tasks or learn new skills. Understanding employees allows a manager to evaluate potential candidates for promotion.

Regular communication with employees is a necessity for persons aspiring to be effective employee-centered managers. This means communication in a variety of settings and personnel combinations. Regular staff meetings should include the entire department. Project teams, work-improvement committees, and ad hoc working groups allow subordinates opportunities to experience and develop leadership skills. Against a backdrop of regular meetings and interactions, formal or semiformal one-on-one meetings such as appraisal interviews and counseling or disciplinary sessions become less threatening. Frequent informal or one-on-one conversations facilitate positive employee relations.

To elevate one's visibility and availability and to promote informal channels of communication with subordinates, supervisors should simply walk around and talk with their workers, practicing what has become known as "management by wandering around" (MBWA). Employees appreciate meeting on their own territory. This is an extremely effective employee relations practice.

A Team Is Composed of Individuals

The necessity for teamwork in the effective delivery of health care as well as in other endeavors is a topic of conversation in many locations. However, strong departmental teams do not survive without being attentive to the needs of individual employees. It is essential that a department manager strive to create a team environment in which all individuals feel that they are important elements of the group.

People who feel they are on the inside, that they are included, knowledgeable, and appreciated parts of the team, will be more satisfied and productive than if they feel they are left out. A supervisor's treatment of subordinates and the relationship with each employee are the most important factors in determining whether an individual worker feels included or excluded.

▶ The Cost of Ignored Employees

Regarding their employees, some managers have adopted an attitude that can be summarized by, "If this person doesn't work out, there's no problem—I can always hire another one." However, associated with such an approach are costs that are not always readily apparent. Employees who are ignored or taken for granted contribute to turnover. Costs associated with turnover are both obvious and hidden (direct and indirect).

Aspects of turnover that contribute to the overall cost of doing business include the diminishing efficiency of an individual who is preparing to leave. Each departing employee should be interviewed (in what is called an "exit interview") to gather information about the reasons for leaving. Such data can help to avoid problem situations in the future. The employee may be entitled to severance pay. Some departing employees may be eligible for unemployment compensation. The company may offer outplacement services. Such services, relatively costly, are uncommon at lower organizational levels, but companies generally provide them to senior managers and executives. In addition, clerical time is required to modify benefits and close out company records. While these costs are unavoidable and may be difficult to quantify accurately, they do represent real expense to any organization.

Other costs associated with losing an employee include the value of output that is lost while a position remains vacant. A new replacement employee is not as efficient in executing the duties of a position. The employee must take time to learn the new job. New employees require orientation and initial training. Until they have acquired proficiency, most people require additional supervision. The organization must supply new persons with equipment such as an identification badge, an employee handbook, and keys. The HR department frequently coordinates these activities, routinely processing paperwork and a myriad of forms.

Less obvious expenses related to employee acquisition include attending job fairs and developing and producing recruitment literature. The cost of a pre-employment physical and other testing is often allocated to the HR department. Recruiting for executive and senior managerial positions may involve travel and relocation fees. If an external source is involved, then an agency or finder's fee may be due.

Costs related to turnover are easily overlooked because so many of them are hidden. In summary, turnover is important to an organization because it is both costly and disruptive. Much turnover stems from how employees feel about their employment milieu, their supervisors, and how they are treated. Employees are more likely to remain if they feel valued as individuals and as producers and if they feel accepted as part of a group. Employees who remain loyal to their employers find acceptable amounts of challenge and interest in their work and see opportunities for personal growth and advancement.

Generous benefits and employee-friendly programs alone will not retain all employees. Among the strongest influences in determining whether particular employees will remain or depart are the relationships that employees have with their direct supervisors or department managers.

Consider that an individual's feelings of being accepted and valued, of being challenged and finding interest in the work, are entirely controllable by a manager. Depending on organizational policies, a manager may exert some influence on opportunities for growth and advancement. In the contemporary labor market, top performers, especially professional and technical employees, rarely encounter much difficulty finding new employment when they want it. For some occupations, such as those in nursing and a number of the other health professions, competing organizations are ready and willing to recruit good employees.

Two aspects of supervisor–employee relationships critically influence the likelihood of continued employment: how employees are treated and how employees are used. Treatment as individuals is equally important to all employees. Generally, fair and respectful treatment has a positive influence on all employees, while the opposite makes negative impressions. The effect of employee utilization varies with individual levels of enthusiasm and motivation. It is extremely important for employees to be used effectively, be continually challenged, have their ideas heard, be given responsibility, and have opportunities for growth. Top organizational performers find positive and encouraging responses from managers to be motivating. Managers strive to retain these people. Some of them will leave an organization for other opportunities to advance their careers. While organizationally challenging, such actions are preferable to premature departures because of dissatisfaction.

Individuals are unlikely to remain loyal or maintain their employment if they feel unwelcome, excluded, or otherwise believe they have few opportunities to excel or advance. Moreover, one of the most important factors in determining whether valued employees will choose to remain or depart is an individual relationship with their immediate superiors.

▶ Conclusion

Every supervisor has responsibilities in the realm of human resources. Department supervisors work as extensions of regular HR personnel. Healthcare workers and providers have broad and varied backgrounds. Their need for active supervision varies. Their individual work ethics vary.

The words and actions of supervisors and other managers must be consistent. Supervisors must support open-door policies with time that can be devoted to listening to employees. They must forward and act on solicited input. Persons making suggestions or providing input should receive feedback from the supervisor to whom the suggestion was initially made. Prudent supervisors listen to suggestions that subordinates offer.

The willingness of employees to work is crucial in a people-centered working environment. Successful supervisors are perceived as available. Not being present is detrimental to a supervisor's effectiveness. The perception of absence may be due to a closed door, physical separation from a working environment, or a reputation for not listening. The result is similar—ineffectiveness and decreased productivity.

Effective managers and supervisors have bidirectional orientations rather than simply being fixated on upper management and personal advancement. Supervisors who earn reputations for self-aggrandizing behavior have extreme difficulty overcoming them. In many cases, starting over in another organization is the only way to shed a poor reputation.

Most people appreciate some individual attention. Supervisors who take the time for one-on-one relationships are usually rewarded with positive employee attitudes and increases in productivity that far exceed the time invested in employee interactions. Though 20% of employees require 80% of supervisory time, effective managers are able to devote some time and attention to all subordinates. Understanding employees as persons usually facilitates earning their loyalty and respect.

🔎 *CASE STUDY: Resolution*

Returning to Kelly and Alice, to moderate a disruptive influence in the department (and contribute to her own peace of mind), Kelly should make a serious effort to curb Alice's know-it-all intrusions. Kelly could benefit by working with Alice in a one-to-one situation. Alice's superior attitude is based on book learning and some common sense. Kelly should put Alice into situations in which she is compelled to use the knowledge that she claims to have. This may require some thoughtful delegation on Kelly's part. However, people who must act on their claims of knowledge and expertise often learn how reality tempers abstract learning. If Alice is successful, then the organization may identify a potentially effective manager. If the situation is not critical, then Alice can have an opportunity to fail without incurring serious costs to the organization. Alice should learn and benefit from either outcome. Alice may discover that the gap between classroom and workstation is much greater than she may have imagined. Giving Alice a structured opportunity has a high probability of succeeding for all concerned. Kelly, Alice, and the organization will learn more about Alice and her true capabilities.

Kelly must directly address Alice's know-it-all attitude and behavior. Alice must understand how others in the department perceive her actions and attitude. However, Kelly must acknowledge Alice's initiative and willingness to learn. This requires some care and good judgment by Kelly. If Alice demonstrates that she is indeed knowledgeable, then Kelly could profit by using Alice as a sounding board for ideas and potential solutions to problems. Alice may have plenty to offer, but Kelly must learn to guide Alice so that the outcome is beneficial for the department and organization.

SPOTLIGHT ON CUSTOMER SERVICE

Customer Service and the Manager–Employee Relationship

Relationships between employees and first-line supervisors take on a variety of forms. An important factor is experience. People generally become more comfortable with their job duties as they perform them for longer periods of time.

While the experience factor is relevant for first-line supervisors, another aspect is also important. First-line supervisors are the interface between management and nonmanagement employees. Their job duties may be further complicated by the presence of a collective bargaining agreement (CBA). The net effect of these factors is to produce stress for all concerned.

Reducing stress should be a primary objective for all employees, as this contributes to productivity and is beneficial for any organization. Time is a prime antidote for insufficient experience. Acceptance may be the best course of action for accommodating a CBA. Because an organizational interface must exist somewhere, it is resistant to change.

Common goals and activities have the potential to reduce stress between managers and employees. Providing customer service should be an activity that is shared by all employees. In addition to providing good customer service, stress between workers and managers can be reduced. Few activities have that potential.

Regular communication with all employees, even if it means walking around and having brief conversations, promotes respect for supervisors by their subordinates.

Teams are composed of individuals. The weakest member limits a team's strength. Conscientious and caring supervision can augment a team's strength and utility to an organization. Ignored workers become unhappy employees. In time, they may leave.

Recruitment and replacement are costly. Avoiding these expenses by effective supervision contributes to an organization's financial vitality and success.

Questions for Review and Discussion

1. Why does this chapter advance the idea that every manager is, or should be, a manager of human resources?
2. Describe a healthcare organization or department that has a heterogeneous work group consisting of at least three levels of staff that differ in their educational backgrounds and job responsibilities.
3. Explain what the following statement means: The streak of authoritarianism remaining in modern management stifles participation.
4. Provide two or three examples each of activities that you believe could thrive under production-centered management or proceed most appropriately under people-centered management. Are these related to health care? Why or why not?
5. In your opinion, what is usually the major problem associated with a manager's claim to having an open-door policy? Why?
6. Why should it be necessary for a department manager to pay any particular attention to employees who steadily fulfill their responsibilities and cause no problems?

7. "This is a simple job we're filling. It is a no-brainer," the department manager said, "so just send me a warm body. If the first person doesn't work out, we can always get someone else, and we've lost nothing." Comment on this statement. Why do you feel as you do?

8. Why is a department manager's visibility and availability to employees considered to be important?

9. How does a department manager come to know which employees require what kinds of attention at what times?

10. If teamwork is so critically important in contemporary healthcare organizations, then why does this chapter place such strong emphasis on one-to-one relationships between supervisors and each of their employees?

Resources
Books

Borkowski, N. (2005). *Organizational behavior in health care*. Sudbury, MA: Jones and Bartlett Publishers.
Cranwell-Ward, J., & Abbey, A. (2005). *Organizational stress*. New York, NY: Palgrave Macmillan.
Furnham, A. (2005). *People business: Psychological reflections of management*. New York, NY: Palgrave Macmillan.
Kenton, B., & Yarnall, J. (2005). *HR: The business partner*. Burlington, MA: Butterworth-Heinemann.
Kulik, C. T. (2004). *Human resources for the non-HR manager*. Mahwah, NJ: Lawrence Erlbaum Associates.
MacLennon, N. (2005). *Coaching and mentoring*. London, UK: Ashgate.
McConnell, C. R. (2018). *Umiker's management skills for the new health care supervisor* (7th ed.). Burlington, MA: Jones & Bartlett Learning.
McConnell, C. R. (2019). *The effective health care supervisor* (9th ed.). Burlington, MA: Jones & Bartlett Learning.
Ulrich, D. (2005). *The HR value proposition*. Cambridge, MA: Harvard University Press.
VanDeVeer, R., Sinclair, G., & Menefee, M. L. (2005). *Human behavior in organizations*. Upper Saddle River, NJ: Prentice Hall.

Periodicals

Chang, E. (2005). Employees' overall perception of HRM effectiveness. *Human Relations, 58*(4), 523–544.
Hannes, L., Segers, J., van Dierendonck, D., & den Hartog, D. (2018). Managing people in organizations: Integrating the study of human resource management and leadership. *Human Resources Management Review, 28*(3), 249–324.
McConnell, C. R. (2018). Interpersonal competence in the management of people. *Health Care Manager, 37*(4), 358–367.
Parker-Oliver, D., Bronstein, L. R., & Kurzejeski, L. (2005). Examining variables related to successful collaboration on the hospice team. *Health Social Work, 30*(4), 279–286.
Sy, T., Cote, S., & Saavedra, R. (2005). The contagious leader: Impact of the leader's mood on the mood of group members, group affective tone, and group processes. *Journal of Applied Psychology, 90*(2), 295–305.
Varma, A. (2005). The workforce scorecard: Managing human capital to execute strategy. *Human Resource Management, 44*(3), 359–361.

CHAPTER 6

Position Descriptions

CHAPTER OBJECTIVES

After studying this chapter, readers will be able to:

- Understand the importance of a properly prepared position (job) description.
- Conduct a position analysis.
- Address the potential contributions of a position's incumbent.
- Describe the components of a position description.
- Create a position description.

▶ Chapter Summary

Position descriptions (or job descriptions—the terms are essentially inter-changeable) are the documents upon which the day-to-day tasks and activities of the employees of an organization are based. These important documents should support the mission, goals, and objectives of the organization. All job descriptions in an organization should use the same format and a common vocabulary. Well-written position descriptions include statements that clearly delineate duties and responsibilities and fully describe compensable factors such as the level of responsibility, the number of persons supervised, the resources controlled, and the experience and minimum level of education needed to perform the job successfully.

▶ Introduction

Lists of activities delineating a particular employee's tasks are called job descriptions or position descriptions. The term *job description* is older and evolved from the field of industrial psychology. *Position description* is a newer, more inclusive designation. The two terms remain interchangeable. With changes in the flow of work, position descriptions change. Fluidity of positions is especially pronounced in fields related to health. Managers must be aware of such changes and ensure that the descriptions of the activities that their employees perform remain current and accurate. This is

🔍 CASE STUDY: Creating a New Job Description

Julie Miller, the health officer of a large suburban health department, was planning for the future. The board had discussed creating a new position for someone to conduct training for employees of the health department. Registered sanitarians are the most common classification of employees in the health department; they are difficult not only to recruit but also to retain, so providing them with additional training and continuing education should help with retention.

Matt Jefferson has been employed as a registered sanitarian for the past 6 years. He recently completed a master of public health degree. He approached Julie to ask for the training position, briefly making his case that he was the best person to become the trainer. Julie told Matt that according to departmental rules, a search would have to be conducted to find the best candidate for the position. Matt replied that if the job description were written carefully, a sanitarian clearly would be the best candidate. After thanking Matt for his thoughts, Julie began to work on the position description, which she thought could be completed in half an hour. What comments or advice would you offer to Julie?

relatively easy for supervisors to address with an annual review of the descriptions of the positions they supervise. Human resources (HR) will ordinarily maintain a master file of all the organization's job descriptions.

A *job analysis* must precede the preparation of a position description. Position description formats may vary from one organization to another, but one general format is often found throughout a single organization. Health departments may sometimes use separate formats for exempt, nonexempt, and managerial positions. *Exempt* refers to the status of a position relative to the Fair Labor Standards Act (FLSA) of 1938 and its subsequent amendments, meaning exempt from the over-time provisions of FLSA. The FLSA established the length of a working week in the United States and requires employers to pay affected employees at a rate of one and one-half times their hourly wage for hours worked in excess of the specified work week. According to the FLSA, a position may be designated as exempt if it meets certain requirements addressing salary, level of responsibility, and the management or supervision of others. As long as a job meets the FLSA test as professional, admin-istrative, or executive, it is a "salaried" position exempt from the overtime require-ments of FLSA. Such positions typically include those of managers and supervisors, and any time these employees work in excess of 40 hours is assumed to be a part of their normal job duties. Employees who are paid by the hour are fully covered by FLSA regulations; they are referred to as being *nonexempt*.

A position description generally has three main parts: identifying information, a job summary, and a list of the principal duties performed. The process of generat-ing a position description begins with an analysis of the job or position.

Positions, not individuals, are classified. Occasionally, the temptation arises to write a position description for a specific individual, tailoring the requirements and experiences so that a preselected person becomes the best candidate in a job search. This should be avoided if that person leaves the position, the specifications may not readily change and finding a replacement may then become difficult. In all instances, a position description should be written for a job and not for a particular person.

▶ Position Analysis

A job description is the most obvious and visible output of a job analysis. Comprehensive and accurate job descriptions, developed as a result of job analysis, are used when selecting, training, evaluating, and compensating employees.

The basis of any employment decision is job analysis, a fundamental activity in human resource management. Accurate information about all positions is required to direct and efficiently control the activities and operations of any organization. Federal regulations and competition have both increased the importance of job analysis.

The human resources department does not produce revenue, yet HR consumes a portion of an organization's annual budget. Supervisors and managers must have current and accurate information about all positions to operate their departments, deliver services, and conduct programs in an efficient and timely manner. Smaller healthcare provider organizations and some health departments have sometimes omitted compiling complete sets of position descriptions; they rely on the professional nature of many employees' duties for guidance in supervising and evaluating professional employees.

Position descriptions provide more than just guidance for employees' workday; they are integral to an organization's efforts to be fair and equitable to all employees. Organizations providing healthcare services that do not have current position descriptions for all employees become vulnerable to accusations of discrimination in employment practices. One way to defend against charges of unfair employment practices is to conduct job analyses and prepare accurate job descriptions.

A job analysis involves extensive study of a specific position and yields information for a position description. The person conducting a job analysis gathers information about positions from several sources. These include interviews with people currently in the position, observing their performance of the job's duties or tasks, and examining worksheets or questionnaires completed by employees as well as information from sources such as the *Dictionary of Occupational Titles*.

Position analysts will compile their findings and review the resulting job analysis with the current position incumbent (unless, of course, the analysis applies to a new position as yet unfilled). Once agreement is reached with regard to a job description's accuracy, the preliminary document is given to an incumbent's supervisor for review. Supervisors may add, delete, or modify descriptions of duties, knowledge, skills, abilities, or other characteristics. Once approved, a final position description is prepared, signed, and dated. Copies are given to both the incumbent and supervisor. A copy is also filed for future reference in a master file ordinarily retained by HR.

Role of a Position Incumbent

Job incumbents have an important role in the process of generating accurate position descriptions. Position incumbents can assist in the process of analysis by taking time to think about their jobs. They should keep a diary of work-related activities or make notes about their job duties. These should include all activities that occur during one complete cycle of duties.

At the beginning of an analysis interview, incumbents should explain their concept of the job to the analyst. The analyst should try to help the incumbent focus on the facts. Job incumbents should avoid overstating or understating characteristics of a position, such as duties, required knowledge, skills, or abilities. Both analyst and job incumbent should remain focused and should minimize discussion of extraneous issues. Analysts are concerned only with the position. Personal performances, fairness of wages, complaints, and relationships with supervisors or coworkers are not relevant.

Senior managers determine the extent of a position's impact on an organization and the boundaries of a job. Position analysts do not determine consequences as part of their work; such decisions are made by senior managers. For example, salaries will not be reduced or a position eliminated because of the analysis process. An analyst may recommend title changes or other position realignments, but the final decisions are made by senior management.

Elements of a Position Description

A position description usually includes the following elements: the job identification information, a job summary, a section describing principal duties performed, and a job specification section.

Job Identification Information

Job identification information must include, at a minimum, the position title, the department location, and the last date on which the content of the position description was verified. Other data, such as the title of the supervisor, help to show how the position fits within a larger organization.

Job Summary

The job summary provides an overall rendering of the purpose, nature, and extent of the tasks performed by the person in the position. In a well-constructed system, the job summary should relate to the mission statement of the department in which the position is located and to the global mission of the organization.

Principal Duties Performed

This section presents job facts in an organized and orderly fashion. When preparing the principal duties performed section, a job is normally broken down into approximately five to eight different tasks or functions for the purpose of describing the position. The job tasks should be listed in order of decreasing frequency or occurrence. This means the task that requires the most time to complete or that is the most critical for a given position should be listed first. For each duty listed in this section, a description of the job's activities (i.e., what is done on the job), how the task is accomplished and why it is necessary, should be provided. This is a convenient method of organizing a position description. It quickly and effectively communicates a great deal of information about a position to a reader who is unfamiliar with the job or position.

An important precaution is in order: stick to the job's five to eight (or however many) principal functions; do not attempt to capture every task that may happen to arise. Many jobs in health care are complex and varied, involving many different tasks that may or may not occur regularly. Trying to capturing every task that may arise usually becomes an exercise in frustration, resulting in a long list that nevertheless still fails to capture everything the job incumbent may have to do some time or other. A reasonable job description that focuses on the job's principal duties in descending order of time consumed and overall captures 90% or more of everything the incumbent must do is a sound, manageable job description. It is for good reasons that many job descriptions' lists of duties conclude with a statement on the order of: "And all other incidental duties as directed by supervision."

Position descriptions should be written using sentences that are complete, clear, and brief, using action verbs and the present tense. In preparing a job summary, the purpose of the position must be clearly stated. This statement should be as brief as possible while still accomplishing its purpose. Words should be carefully selected to convey the maximum amount of specific meaning. General or vague terms should be avoided unless they are absolutely essential as a substitute for a long and detailed explanation.

The section describing principal duties performed follows the job summary and includes major job tasks, as previously outlined. Many organizations include a fourth section in their descriptions that covers job specifications.

Job Specification

The job specification section outlines the minimum specific skills, effort, and responsibilities required of an incumbent in the job. Job specifications provide the basis and justification for values that will be assigned to factors used in evaluating a position. Factors are elements created by a job analyst and subsequently used when comparing different positions within a single organization. Job specification statements must describe the extent to which a given factor is present and the degree of difficulty encountered in the position for that factor.

When writing job specifications, individual statements should be definite, direct, and to the point. Any unnecessary embellishments or complicated sentences should be avoided except where they materially add to an understanding of the details contained in the statement. Any specifications that apply only to occasional duties should be indicated accordingly so that the percentage of time or frequency with which the specification applies will not be overestimated.

Educational requirements for a position description must be supported by the analysis of actual duties. Higher educational requirements may legally be included if they are such that the skills or training can be acquired only through formal education or if it is only through formal education that an individual can acquire a particular license or certification that may be required to pursue the given occupation. Minimum levels of schooling must be used. For example, the formerly encountered requirement for a "high school diploma" for certain entry-level jobs has given way to the necessity for one to possess the ability to "read and write and understand simple instructions." Artificially high educational requirements have been judged to represent a form of discrimination. They are not only illegal but unethical. Skills must be supported by position analysis. These are factors that are linked to compensation. Other factors that must be compensated include the level of responsibility expected of an incumbent, the number of people supervised, the amount of funds managed, and the resources controlled.

Job specifications are then translated into position descriptions. These descriptions are for specific job categories, for example, Secretary 2, Nurse Aide 1, Sanitarian-in-Training, or Environmental Supervisor 1. The title suggests the major duties of a position. The number after it may indicate the level of the position in

TABLE 6-1 Position Description Components

Component	Explanation
Title	Specific title for the job
Status	Exempt or nonexempt
Summary of duties	Major tasks to be performed
Salary range	The minimum, midpoint, and maximum for the job
Knowledge required	Specific job training needed to perform the job; specific experience, both type and amount needed to perform the job
Skills required	Specific skills expected
Effort required	Both mental and physical; any heavy lifting
Responsibility	Consequences of an error
Working conditions	Hazards or other poor working conditions
General statement	Other duties as required

the organizational hierarchy. Higher numbers usually denote more senior or more responsible positions. Whereas job specifications may be recorded for individual incumbents, position descriptions are developed for general categories of jobs. Well-written position descriptions should contain the items listed in **TABLE 6-1**. An example of a completed job description in the described format appears in **APPENDIX 6-A** at the end of this chapter.

An Important Multiuse Instrument

A position description as represented in this chapter describes the major duties and responsibilities of an individual functioning in a specific position. This same instrument has a number of additional uses, including the following:

- Providing information for evaluating a job for the determination of status (exempt or nonexempt) and job grade and pay range
- Being used as a guide in recruiting and interviewing prospective employees
- Serving as a guide for new employee orientation and training
- Providing an outline for the conduct of performance appraisals
- Contributing to overall compliance with legal, regulatory, contractual, and accreditation requirements
- Providing an accurate rendering of a job's duties sometimes needed in addressing claims of discrimination

▶ **Conclusion**

Position descriptions are often treated as nonessentials, "frills" and unnecessary documentation stuck in files or binders and largely ignored. Largely ignored, that is, until a need arises and a new job must be graded and assigned a salary range or an existing job is altered such that job duties are changed. When such occurs, there is usually a flurry of activity to create or update a position description. Far better to maintain—either within an individual department or in human resources—a complete set of job descriptions that are regularly reviewed and updated and put to use as part of every manager's readily available resources.

🔍 *CASE STUDY: Resolution*

Returning to Julie, the health officer who began to write a job description for the new training position, a pause is in order. Job descriptions are not essays. They are based on an analysis of the new position. A thorough position analysis usually requires more than 30 minutes to complete.

Julie apparently intended to specify a master of public health degree as the minimum level of education for the job incumbent. While such a decision might appear to create a good opportunity for the sanitarian, formal schooling is not the only place where expertise in training can be obtained. An employee with several years of work experience who has had some leadership responsibilities should be able to become a successful trainer. Artificially high educational requirements are a form of discrimination. Julie should be reminded that job descriptions are written for positions, not individuals. To ignore this advice is to court problems when seeking a replacement for the proposed employee.

SPOTLIGHT ON CUSTOMER SERVICE

Customer Service and Position Descriptions

Data obtained from a convenience sample of 42 position descriptions from a number of different healthcare and public health organizations revealed that only one of the descriptions contained a reference to customer service. Holdings of the National Library of Medicine were checked. The search query stipulated the presence of two search terms, "customer service" and "position description." This approach identified 14 articles. One of the identified articles mentioned including customer service on position descriptions (Hill & Meyer, 1998).

If every position description in an organization included "provides good customer service," three criteria would be realized:

1. The single goal of addressing customer needs is clearly expressed in the program's name: customer service.
2. An organization requires only one customer service program.
3. Customer service is a priority activity that should be shared by all employees.

Modified from Hills, K., & Meyer, B. (1998). The worker of the future: A system outlines the competencies its employees will need. *Health Progress, 79*(2), 29–31.

Questions for Review and Discussion

1. What is the principal difference between "exempt" and "nonexempt" employees?
2. What are the main provisions of the Fair Labor Standards Act?
3. What is a job analysis?
4. Why is a job analysis important?
5. Briefly describe the main elements of a position or job description.
6. What, if anything, does a job incumbent contribute to a position description?
7. How is the education level required for a position established?
8. Describe several uses of a position description.
9. In addition to actual duties performed, what other information is contained in a properly prepared position description? Why is it included?
10. Why is the statement "Job descriptions are written for positions, not people" important?

Resources

Books

Cushway, B. (2006). *The handbook of model job descriptions*. London, UK: Kogan Page.

Farr, J. M., Ludden, L. L., & Shatkin, L. (2001). *Dictionary of occupational titles* (2nd ed.). Indianapolis, IN: JIST Works.

Mader-Clark, M. M. (2013). *The job description handbook* (3rd ed.) Berkeley, CA: NOLO.

McConnell, C. R. (2019). *The effective health care supervisor* (9th ed.). Burlington, MA: Jones & Bartlett Learning.

Noe, R., Hollenbeck, J., Gerhart, B., & Wright, P. (2017). *Human resource management* (10th ed.). New York, NY: McGraw-Hill.

Wilson, M. (2004). *Volunteer job descriptions and action plans*. Loveland, CO: Group Publishing.

Periodicals

Fooks, C. (2005). Health human resources planning in an interdisciplinary care environment: To dream the impossible dream? *Canadian Journal of Nursing Leadership, 18*(3), 26–29.

Hall, A. (2005). Dialing for jobs: How to make the most of a phone interview. *Biomedical Instrumentation and Technology, 39*(5), 377–378.

Kristof-Brown, A., Barrick, M. R., & Franke, M. (2002). Influences and outcomes of candidate impression management use in job interviews. *Journal of Management, 28*, 27–46.

Muskovitz, M. (April 18, 2011). The impact of job descriptions. *The National Law Review*, Western Springs, IL.

Smaglik, P. (2005). Seeking soft skills. *Nature, 438*(7069), 883–885.

Van Iddekinge, C. H., Raymark, P. H., Eidson, C. E., & Attenweiler, W. (2004). What do structured interviews really measure? The construct validity of behavior description interviews. *Human Performance, 17*, 71–93.

Van Iddekinge, C. H., Raymark, P. H., & Roth, P. L. (2005). Assessing personality with a structured employment interview: Construct-related validity and susceptibility to response inflation. *Journal of Applied Psychology, 90*(3), 536–552.

APPENDIX 6-A

Sample Position Description

Job Title: Community Practice Facility Controller

Unit or Section: Administration

Status: Exempt

Department: Finance

Salary Range: (intentionally left blank)

Basic Function: Plans, directs, and coordinates, on an efficient and economical basis, all facility accounting operational activities, including cost accounting, financial accounting, general accounting, information systems, and general office services

Scope: Work encompasses involvement in a broad range of accounting activities that are essential to the maintenance of facility operations and the dissemination of financial information to the board, senior managers, and owners

Summary of Duties

1. Coordinates all essential accounting operational functions in a timely and accurate manner, developing methods geared to providing management with information vital to decision-making processes.
2. Directs the development of methods and procedures necessary to ensure adequate financial controls within each of the facility's operational areas.
3. Performs analysis and appraisal of the facility's financial status.
4. Prepares recommendations with respect to future financial plans, forecasts, and policies.
5. Works closely with the chief executive officer (CEO) on confidential financial matters and expedites such matters to conclusion.
6. Directs this operation within the accounting parameters established by facility, third-party provider, state, federal, and generally accepted accounting principles (GAAP), rules and regulations.

7. Manages the organizational area in a manner that fully complements and interfaces with all other coordinating agencies or business partners.
8. Performs other duties and responsibilities as directed by the CEO.

Supervision Exercised:	Number of Employees:
Direct: General supervisors in operational areas	2–3
Indirect: Other facility supervisors, administrative and clerical personnel	15–20

Training and Education

Certified Public Accountant (CPA) required; graduation from an accredited program

Experience

Must have at least 5 years of experience in accounting with some supervisory responsibility

Responsibility

Budget of $3,500,000 per year
All required insurance for hospital
State and federal filings for tax and other financial purposes

Effort

Minimal physical effort required; no lifting
Mental effort requires ability to concentrate on numbers for long periods of time and to occasionally work under severe deadlines

Working Conditions

Well-lighted office; No exposure to hazards in the normal course of work
The earlier constitutes a general summary of duties. Additional duties may be required.

Approvals

Supervisor: _____ Date: _____

Department manager: _____ Date: _____

HR Department _____ Date: _____

Reviews

Person: Title: Date:

_____   _____   _____

_____   _____   _____

CHAPTER 7

Directions in Employee Relations

CHAPTER OBJECTIVES

After studying this chapter, readers will be able to:

- Understand the evolution of employee relations through three distinct philosophical eras: authoritarian, legalistic, and humanistic.
- Comprehend the emergence of scientific management and the development of other means of organizing and managing human enterprise.
- Understand fundamental assumptions about people that influence different approaches to management.
- Broadly describe the major theories of human motivation.
- Trace the growth of government concern for the social welfare of American workers.

▶ Chapter Summary

Since people began working in organized settings and some were placed in positions of authority supervising others, the subject of employee relations has been a workplace reality. Beginning as strict authoritarianism that was frequently exploitative, the primary drivers of employee relations have progressed from authoritarian management to legalistic management and finally to humanistic management. Authoritarian management continues to exist, but to a limited extent. Examples of legalistic management remain in significant numbers, but these are gradually but steadily diminishing as humanistic management continues to spread.

In healthcare organizations, the nature of a specific department or the personal style of senior managers usually sets the tone for the entire department or organization. Management style affects employee relations. The nature of a typical healthcare organization is people centered, as opposed to the production-centered character of many other kinds of organizations. Thus, a human resources practitioner or department manager who thrives in health care is one who understands that employees

🔍 CASE STUDY: "The Buck Stops Here"

Mary Johnson, a registered nurse and the new manager of the clinical staff at Community Health Center, was not happy with the way her job was going. Just a month into her new role, she already felt like walking away from the job.

Mary decided that the problem was resistance to change among staff members. She knew that a certain amount of resistance to a new manager was to be expected, but it seemed to her that everything she said or did was resented and resisted simply because it came from her. There was a great deal to do; her area of responsibility had coasted for years under an apathetic manager. The overall problem was so large that she hardly knew where to begin. With so much to be done, she had begun to fix everything that required change as rapidly as possible.

As Mary related to her friend Sally Drake, a nurse manager in another facility, "I resurrected the dress code and enforced it. You have no idea what was being tolerated in the way of appearance. I put a stop to personal phone calls and the use of food and drink and reading material within public view. I've started to enforce existing policies on absenteeism and tardiness. Sally, I can't tell you how long these people have been allowed to wander in and out whenever they felt like it."

She continued, "And what do I get? A nearly complete lack of support except for a couple of older employees who let me know they felt it was about time someone did something. I've told all the staff what was expected of them in no uncertain terms. I hold a staff meeting every week, and I'm trying hard to convince them of the need to improve the level of professionalism in the place, but it seems like every order or instruction I deliver just generates more bitterness and resistance."

Sally responded, "It sounds like you inherited a real mess. But are you sure you're not trying to do too much too quickly, giving orders and delivering mandates without trying to get people to accept your plan? Have you allowed them to give you their ideas and involved them in deciding what to do?"

Mary waved dismissively. "Oh, I know all about that involvement stuff. Get employees to help decide what to do and how to do it and all that modern management stuff from textbooks. I've never depended on employees to do my work for me, and as far as I'm concerned the buck stops here."

How would you describe Mary Johnson's management style? Identify what she appears to have been doing wrong. How would you advise her to proceed from here?

and providers are far more likely to be motivated by compassion and service than by economic considerations.

▶ Common Origins

From the beginnings of organized work activity when one person first directed the work of others, the subject of employee relations has evolved through three identifiable philosophies of management. In a sense, these philosophies represent periods of time, stages, or phases. Management experts hesitate to use the terms for the phases too freely because the eras they represent overlap significantly, and all coexist in varying degrees among contemporary organizations. The management philosophies governing employee relations are identified as authoritarian, legalistic, and humanistic.

Authoritarian schools of employee relations arose first, followed much later by both legalistic and humanistic styles of employee relations. It is still possible to identify organizations that continue to operate using an essentially authoritarian philosophy, although pure authoritarianism is infrequently found in American business and is steadily declining. There are many organizations in which a legalistic philosophy prevails. In a growing number of organizations, the humanistic philosophy is gradually replacing the others (Fallon & Zgodzinski, 2013).

Authoritarian Management

Authoritarian management encompasses the beginnings of organized enterprise, including master–slave relationships. Authoritarian management minimizes the importance of people. It operates on the assumption that people have to be pushed and continually told what to do in order to obtain the most output from them or the best possible results. Authoritarian management was the generally accepted form for centuries. It is conceptually simple. A boss gives orders and expects them to be carried out. A fundamental motivating force in authoritarian management is fear: do what you are told to do if you wish to remain employed.

This is not to suggest that authoritarian management is always harsh or cruel. Certainly, an authoritarian manager is autocratic, but a variety of autocratic styles exist. At one end of the spectrum is an exploitative autocrat. Exploitative autocrats are generally cruel leaders who literally exploit their followers for personal gain. When pondering the style of exploitative autocrats, think of them as coming from the "Attila the Hun School of Management." At the opposite end of the spectrum is a benevolent autocrat. Benevolent autocrats look after their followers and ensure that they are well cared for and protected. This benevolence continues only as long as the followers do exactly as they are told, without question. This can be referred to as the "Father Knows Best School of Management." Regardless of where on the spectrum they may be coming from, autocratic managers are unquestionably in charge. They establish the goals for their organizations, issue all of the directives, and give all of the orders. The only option followers have is to do as they are told or leave.

Authoritarian management is still practiced today. Many people now in the workforce have worked under strongly authoritarian managers. It is evident, however, that even though pockets of authoritarianism still exist, the philosophy and approach steadily diminished during the 1900s. The rate of change accelerated toward the end of the century.

For many years, authoritarian managers essentially acted as they wished. For a long while, employees had very few legal rights, so managers could manage as they pleased with little regard for resistance and little fear of encountering legal repercussions. But then legalism intruded.

Legalistic Management

The legalistic movement began in the 1930s with the passage of wage-and-hour laws and the enactment of labor laws. It blossomed significantly with passage of the Civil Rights Act of 1964. Since then, a steady stream of legislation has been addressing employment and employees. Many managers who were once strictly authoritarian have adjusted and changed, although their adaptation to accumulating legal restrictions has not always been made readily or willingly.

Managers began to treat employees differently because the law was now telling them what they could or could not do. This legalistic phase of employee relations has been shaped, defined, and bounded by legislation. Managers now interact with employees out of a strict regard for employee rights. These changes have not always been internalized. Rather, they are often grudgingly made because the law requires employers to act in a particular manner. Employee relations have been changed and restructured because managers wish to keep themselves and their employers out of legal trouble. The number of people simply complying with the law rather than undertaking actions because they want to do the right or proper thing is dwindling over time, helped along by turnover and changing attitudes.

Humanistic Management

Two significant areas of influence have contributed to the growth of humanistic management. One is the still-expanding structure of legislation that ushered in legalistic management and mandated humane treatment of employees. The other is found in the lasting effects of the human relations movement in management that has been growing and developing since the middle of the 1900s. The human relations movement recognized employees' rights before these became legally mandated. It fostered the belief that contented, well-treated employees who were dealt with fairly and equitably were generally better producers and more loyal than those who were not so well regarded.

A legalistic manager behaves in a particular manner because the law requires such behavior. Humanistic managers behave in a similar manner because of their belief that it is right and proper to do so. This is a fundamental difference between legalistic and humanistic management. Legalistic management may continue to be driven by pessimistic and somewhat authoritarian assumptions about people. In contrast, humanistic management holds the optimistic view that satisfied workers produce best. The progression from authoritarian to legalistic to humanistic management can be described in the parallel progression from pushing to directing and finally to leading people.

Residual Authoritarianism

If managers know why laws addressing employee rights are to be respected and obeyed, and if managers believe that satisfied employees are better producers, then why does managerial authoritarianism continue? The answer may lie in tradition. For centuries, autocratic management was the only management style. It became deeply ingrained in the population's overall view of management. Giving orders, bearing all responsibilities, making decisions, and placing or removing people as needed or desired was the norm. Management was authoritarianism by definition.

Most supervisors have traditionally learned about management by on-the-job observation. Although a growing number of managers now learn some of the basics of management in formal education programs, many still absorb most of what they actually use on the job through their management role models. A generation ago, the majority of managers learned by emulating their role models who were authoritarian in outlook and practice. Thus, a strain of authoritarianism is still present. It is weakening with each subsequent generation of managers but has nonetheless been passed down to contemporary managers. Human behavior often changes slowly, especially in a pursuit such as management, in which old beliefs and attitudes have solidified over hundreds of years.

▶ The Emergence of Scientific Management

Authoritarianism in employee relations was aided, prolonged, and intensified by the emergence of an approach that became known as scientific management. In the early years of the 1900s, a movement emerged based on the application of the scientific method of study to business management activities. The goal of scientific management was efficiency, defined largely by the amount of time required to perform any given task. Less time to accomplish the same work equated to increased efficiency because more tasks could be completed per unit of time. Frederick W. Taylor, Frank and Lillian Gilbreth, Henry L. Gantt, and Frank Bunker figured prominently in this movement. These pioneers of scientific management were largely responsible for defining the discipline of industrial engineering.

Scientific management seemed to intensify authoritarianism and sustain its existence in some business situations, especially manufacturing. It was extremely unpopular in other situations. Not all work activities can be reduced to a series of simple segments and repetitive activities. Scientific management focused on process and production while largely ignoring people. A November 1913 resolution of the American Federation of Labor referred to the Taylor system as a "diabolical scheme for the reduction of the human being to the condition of a mere machine" (Urwick, 1963).

Taylor and his colleagues used the term *scientific management* to describe their organized approach to analyzing work by the procedures that were used, employing standardizing methods and improving productivity. Scientific management made significant contributions to American manufacturing through the advent of assembly lines and other repetitive work processes. It strengthened the concept of production-centered management.

▶ The Development of Parallel Management Systems

Two systems or approaches to management developed in parallel during the early decades of the 1900s. One related to activities in which repetitive work was dominant, while the other related to activities in which varied work prevailed. These two different approaches were described by Rensis Likert (1961) as the *job organization system* and the *cooperative motivation system*.

In Likert's job organization system, repetitive work is dominant. Jobs are usually well organized with considerable structure to them so that extremely specific job descriptions are possible. The tasks of assembly line workers provide convenient examples. Tight controls are possible. Output can be scheduled with considerable accuracy. Inputs to the processes can likewise be accurately scheduled to feed into the system when and where they are needed. The overall speed of a process can be established and maintained at a predictable level. In a properly designed process using the job organization system, inefficiencies are held to a minimum and remain well under control. This approach to management is ordinarily advanced and well organized.

Management within the job organization system is production centered while being focused on the process and its output. It is the system that moves the people. More accurately stated, the people are carried along with the system. Picture an assembly line: the line runs at a set speed, and employees working along it keep up with its pace. If one person is not available to serve the line, another is plugged into that spot, and the line continues to move. The economic motivations of the workers keep the line moving. People come to work because they are paid to do so. This is the motivation that maintains the momentum in any variation of the job organization system. The success of the job organization system depends almost exclusively on economic motives. The work of Taylor and the other proponents of scientific management established and enabled the job organization system.

In Likert's cooperative motivation system, varied work prevails. Most jobs are loosely organized, with such a wide variety of possible activities and responsibilities that job descriptions are necessarily all-encompassing and decidedly nonspecific. In a healthcare setting, the position description for a registered nurse provides a convenient example. Tight controls are not possible. Output cannot be scheduled except in the most general terms. Some secondary inputs to the processes can be scheduled reasonably well, but the primary inputs enter the system with unpredictable frequency. In most situations, speed of a process cannot be maintained at a predictable level. An emergency department provides a good example in health care. People seeking treatment enter according to their own timing. Fixed schedules cannot be established or maintained. Further complicating the situation, the services that entrants may require are extraordinarily varied. While a systematic approach to management allows employees to be prepared for a variety of demands, this approach is not easily maintained. Hour-to-hour maintenance of such an environment requires judgment to be exercised regularly and decisions to be made in an impromptu fashion.

Management within the cooperative motivation system is necessarily people centered and focused on human elements. Both employees and the people seeking treatment or services provide examples from health care. People move the system. Again, consider a visit to an emergency department. Given the nature and timing of the problems encountered, the pace at which the department operates is determined by the workers; if one person is not available to work an assigned job, all of the personnel present have to adjust to perform the duties normally done by the missing person. Efficiency and output often suffer. Long waiting times are frequently the result. These can be eliminated by maintaining an extensive staff of specialists and providers in the emergency department at all times. Such an approach is economically untenable. In any variation of the cooperative motivation system, the employees keep the system moving. People come to work not only because they are paid to do so but also because they are willing to do so. The very operation of a cooperative motivation system depends on individual enthusiasm, motivation, and commitment to one's job and employer.

Management that is inclined toward authoritarianism is likely to encounter only token resistance within the job organization system. Within some environments, the same managerial approach (authoritarianism) may engender significant resentment and foment an adversarial relationship between workers and management. However, because many employees will be as production centered as management, they will expect, and to a limited degree accept, their situation of being a managerial focus that is secondary to output.

Management that is inclined toward authoritarianism is much more likely to fail in an environment where cooperative motivation often flourishes. Most

TABLE 7-1 Comparison of the Job Organization and Cooperative Motivation Systems

Characteristic	Job Organization	Cooperative Motivation
Dominant work	Repetitive	Variable
Job structure	Rigid	Loose
Controllability of system	Great	Minimal
Output predictability	Great	Minimal
Primary system driver	Economic	Personal values
Central focus of management	Production	People

healthcare situations fall under the cooperative motivation system, making them far more amenable to people-centered management than to production-centered management. With its focus on people, the humanistic philosophy of employee relations increases in importance.

To provide a summary, **TABLE 7-1** compares the characteristics of the job organization and cooperative motivation systems.

▶ Opposing Views of Employees

The work of Douglas McGregor contributed greatly to the human relations movement in management. In his classic paper, "The Human Side of Enterprise" (1957), McGregor provided a readily understandable continuum of assumptions about people in terms of their work activities in the form of his Theory X and Theory Y.

Within both Theory X and Theory Y, management is assumed to be responsible for organizing and applying the elements of productive enterprise. These include resources, initially money and then equipment, materials, and people. However, this is the full extent to which Theory X and Theory Y are alike.

Theory X assumes that employees are indifferent, passive, and resistant to organizational needs. Managers must actively and continuously intervene to direct the efforts of subordinates, motivate them, control their actions, and modify their behavior to fit the needs of an organization. This pessimistic view of people holds that employees must be persuaded to do what is needed, rewarded for doing their assigned tasks correctly, and punished for doing them incorrectly. In general, supervisors must constantly control their workers.

McGregor's Theory X has several underlying assumptions: People are indolent by nature and inclined to work as little as possible. Most people lack ambition, dislike responsibility, and prefer to be told what to do. When people become employees, they remain self-centered and generally indifferent to organizational needs. By nature, people are resistant to change. The average person is gullible, easily duped, and not particularly bright.

When applied, Theory X involves coercion, threats, punishment, close supervision, and tight controls on employee behavior. Conversely, Theory X also allows supervisors to be permissive, to satisfy people's demands, and to give employees what they want to get them to cooperate, accept direction, and produce as desired. Despite the approach taken, the unflattering assumptions about people remain the same. Furthermore, Theory X is inadequate for motivating employees because the human needs on which it relies are unimportant as motivators of human behavior.

The relationship between supervisors and employees is succinctly summarized in an overheard comment made by a worker to his supervisor. "Your job is to get as much work as you can out of me, and my job is to do as little as possible."

Theory Y is the direct opposite of Theory X. Theory Y assumes that people are not passive or resistant to organizational needs by nature. If they appear to be so, they have become this way through experience in organizations. The motivation, capacity, potential, and readiness to work toward organizational goals are innately present in all people. Managers are responsible for helping people to recognize and develop these characteristics. Supervisors must arrange conditions so that employees can best achieve their own goals by directing their personal efforts toward organizational objectives.

McGregor's work included a hierarchy of human needs that paralleled one described by A. H. Maslow in "A Theory of Human Motivation" (1943). Both McGregor and Maslow advanced the notion that humans were constantly trying to satisfy needs. As they satisfied needs at one level, other higher-order needs arose to take their place. The need hierarchies of McGregor and Maslow are similar. Physiological needs are the most fundamental. These include air, food, and water. Both McGregor and Maslow used the same terminology for this level. Next are safety needs. These encompass the need for protection from harm and for shelter. Both used identical names for these requirements.

After ensuring that physical safety has been established, McGregor called the next level of needs *social*, while Maslow labeled them *love needs*. By either name, these represent the need to belong, to be accepted, and to belong to groups.

Groups exist in a variety of situations, including work, family, religious, and social settings. McGregor summarized the next level of needs as *ego*, while Maslow called them *psychological*. These include the need for praise and reward, recognition, accomplishment, satisfaction in work, and the general need to feel good about oneself. At the ultimate level, McGregor identified a need for self-fulfillment. Maslow used the term *self-actualization*. These are essentially similar terms in that they represent the ultimate in need satisfaction that can be described as actions bringing individuals personal fulfillment and satisfaction. McGregor and Maslow both wrote that higher-order needs may be motivating only when all lower-order needs are satisfied. Thus, self-actualization is meaningless when people are hungry.

Inherent in the work of both McGregor and Maslow is the belief that a satisfied need ceases to be a motivator of behavior. In contemporary American society, physiological, safety, and social needs are met for a majority of people most of the time. When this is the case, individuals are then free to pursue fulfillment of psychological or ego needs. They are free to accomplish and achieve goals; acquire physical, intellectual, or technical competencies; acquire knowledge; and seek recognition or appreciation. Lower-order needs prevail only when a person has suffered some form of deprivation and gone backward through the hierarchy. For example, an individual who is out of work and running out of money must find employment to satisfy physiological and safety needs. Securing employment is far more important than social or psychological needs. McGregor and Maslow both made similar points. Capturing the essence of their insights, one may be able to live by bread alone, but only when no bread is readily available.

▶ Long-Term Trends in Organizational Management

Two long-term trends dominated management during the 1900s. First was scientific management, introduced more than 100 years ago. It had considerable influence on management practices. Even though it brought increases in productivity, scientific management had adverse effects on human aspects of organizational activities.

The other trend began shortly after the conclusion of World War I, when social scientists began taking a critical look at the negative aspects of scientific management. This was the beginning of the human relations movement in management. This trend, although burdened by social legislation, continues to replace scientific management.

The human relations movement made a number of significant advances beginning in the 1930s. Studies undertaken throughout the middle of the century showed that when workers' hostilities, resentments, suspicions, and fears were replaced by favorable attitudes, a substantial increase in production occurred (Likert, 1956). Experience with the human relations approach to management has led many experts to conclude that in most circumstances, people-centered management is more effective in inspiring productivity than is production-centered management. Furthermore, close supervision is associated with lower productivity when compared with more lenient supervision and giving people responsibility and some control over their work.

▶ Government Inspires a Major Shift

An important milestone was reached with passage of Title VII of the Civil Rights Act of 1964. This legislation has had a greater impact on society than most other recent legislation.

For a long time, the U.S. Congress had been urged by organized labor and other advocates to do more for working people. Since the 1960s, the federal government has shifted much of the social responsibility for workers to business and industry. Many laws affecting employment have benefited employees. People who are out of work can now receive unemployment compensation benefits. Applicants cannot be discriminated against when seeking employment. Furthermore, they cannot legally be discriminated against when seeking promotion or advancement in their jobs. People performing similar jobs must receive similar compensation. Employees are entitled to receive care and compensation if they are injured in the course of their employment. They are entitled to assistance and protection with difficult personal and family situations.

This growing structure of legislation has led to the legalistic philosophy of employee relations, under which managers have reacted by changing their behaviors to avoid legal trouble. To some extent, all of the laws affecting employment have added to the cost of doing business. For example, the Immigration Reform and Control Act (IRCA) adds effort, paperwork, filing, and occasional penalties to the cost of recruiting. The Family and Medical Leave Act (FMLA) necessitates replacement costs and other expenses related to covering jobs during leaves. The Americans with Disabilities Act (ADA) requires direct expenditures for reasonable accommodations when required.

Whenever Congress creates new programs, its members must consider how they will be funded. Three options exist to pay for new programs. Congress can discontinue an existing program, thus shifting funds for a new program. This action is usually politically sensitive and unpopular. Congress can raise taxes to cover the new program. This course of action is largely unpopular and often politically sensitive. Finally, Congress can find someone else to pay for the new programs. Therefore, businesses and other organizations are often put in the position of having to pay for the implementation of new programs enacted by Congress.

Congress has accomplished much through legislation affecting employment and has improved the well-being of millions of workers. However, the expenses added to the cost of doing business have raised the cost of goods and services for everyone. Members of the public in general and consumers in particular are paying for these improvements just as surely as they would through tax increases.

▶ Where We Are Now, and Where We Are Heading

Employees in the American workforce have changed dramatically over the years. More and more workers know about their rights under today's laws or are at least aware that they have well-defined rights. Employee knowledge has forced management into a legalistic posture. This trend has been enhanced by labor unions and other external advocacy agencies and groups.

Authoritarianism remains but is steadily diminishing. In general, authoritarianism is less common in healthcare organizations than in other industries. Legalism remains fairly strong and is common in many contemporary organizations, including healthcare organizations. Managers interact with their employees in a particular manner primarily because the law says that they must. However, legalism is slowly but steadily diminishing as the humanistic philosophy of employee relations grows in acceptance. Many people are slow to adjust when faced with societal change. Although a law can mandate behavioral changes, legislation in and of itself cannot change someone's attitudes and beliefs. The legislators who frame legislation are undoubtedly aware that much early compliance comes as a result of obedience to the law, not because people wish to change their ways. They do know that acceptance grows over time and that people who simply obey the law at first will eventually behave in the desired way as the new way comes to be seen as the right way.

Some humanistic managers have always existed. Their considerate and people-focused style is owing to their fundamental values as individuals, not necessarily because of a conscious belief in humanistic management. Upon casual observation or limited exposure, the legalistic and humanistic approaches to employee relations appear to be very much the same. Often, the difference between the two is that of management motivation. In a legalistic environment, managers provide fair and humane treatment because it is required by law and they wish to protect themselves and their organizations from legal troubles. In a humanistic environment, managers provide fair and humane treatment because they believe that doing so is the proper way to conduct themselves, manage others, and treat people.

▶ Conclusion

Authoritarian management remains alive in some contemporary organizations. It is often an organizational remnant or residue of earlier exposure to past role models. The approach can be found in isolated departments or pervading entire organizations.

Authoritarianism has been largely supplanted by legalistic and humanistic approaches to management. These were developed during the middle decades of the 1900s. They evolved from scientific management. Major theoretical contributions to humanistic management were made by Abraham Maslow, Douglas McGregor, and Rensis Likert. The legalistic environment has emerged since the enactment of the Civil Rights Act in 1964. Legal changes continue to be enacted.

🔍 CASE STUDY: Resolution

Mary Johnson's management style is clearly authoritarian. She shares this trait with a diminishing number of contemporary managers. Mary is legalistic in that she is sufficiently aware of the laws governing employment to avoid doing anything that is blatantly illegal. It is clear that she delivers mandates and gives orders with the expectation that what she says will be heard and obeyed.

The resistance by her subordinates is understandable. A change in immediate supervision is always upsetting. Mary's entry is all the more difficult because she seems determined to resolve all apparent problems at once even if she has to force unilaterally determined changes on the staff. She takes these actions with the belief that she is right.

Mary's friend Sally was correct in suggesting that Mary was trying to accomplish too much in too short of a time. The number of rules and policies is unimportant. If they have been ignored for a long period of time, then for all practical purposes they do not exist. Mary is unilaterally determining rules and policies and then trying to force them upon the staff.

Mary has made some of the classic errors of an authoritarian manager. Foremost among these is thinking that involving employees, listening to their ideas, and honoring their input are signs of weakness. Furthermore, she thinks that if she does not make all of the decisions by herself, then she is abrogating her responsibility as a manager. Her concept of management is authoritarian. Bosses give orders, and employees obey them.

Mary must slow down and reassess her own approach to management. She must earn her employees' trust, but this is likely to require time. Mary must involve her employees. She should consult with them to define problems and establish priorities. Then, she should address one specific issue at a time.

SPOTLIGHT ON CUSTOMER SERVICE

Customer Service and Employee Relations

In recent years, the economic climate has driven organizations to become more efficient. Supervisors have pushed their workers to become more productive. Organizations that have not participated in these trends are likely to have their former employees participating in unemployment insurance. Most experts agree that these demands are not likely to disappear. More likely, these trends are defining a new reality.

Employee relations must shift to support the new reality. Supervisors must find new or different ways to motivate their workers without also generating feelings of persecution. Employees must learn to accept these demands. If they do not, they risk being unhappy or frustrated in their jobs for the remainder of their working lives.

Customer service will continue to be appreciated. Because of its importance, customer service may become expected. Thus, it may provide a logical starting point for transitioning workers and their organizations to the emerging new reality.

Modified from Fallon, L. F., & Zgodzinski, E. (2013). *Essentials of public health management* (3rd ed.). Burlington, MA: Jones & Bartlett Learning; Likert, R. (1956). Motivation and increased productivity. *Management Record, 18*(4), 128–131; Likert, R. (1961). *New patterns of management.* New York, NY: McGraw-Hill; Maslow, A. H. (1943). A theory of human motivation. *Psychological Review, 50,* 370–396; McGregor, D. M. (1957). The human side of enterprise. *Management Review, 46*(11), 22–28; Urwick, L. F. (1963). The development of industrial engineering. In H. B. Maynard (Ed.), *Industrial engineering handbook* (2nd ed., p. 5). New York, NY: McGraw-Hill.

Questions for Review and Discussion

1. Cite two or three commonly observable practices in present-day organizational management that indicate the presence of residual authoritarianism.
2. Identify and describe the fundamental difference between legalistic management and humanistic management. Describe several indicators that can be used to distinguish one from the other.
3. Present three or four reasons why authoritarian management still prevails in American managerial situations.
4. In your opinion, why has authoritarian management prevailed for so long?
5. If scientific management was the diabolical scheme that some considered it to be, why was it so widely adopted in the early part of the 1900s?
6. Reduce the parallel discussion of the job organization system and the cooperative motivation system to a single statement that reflects the greatest single difference between the two approaches.
7. Name at least three major pieces of legislation that supported the advancement of the human relations movement in management. Why were they effective in producing change?
8. In your opinion, what will be the primary force that moves organizational management from legalism to humanism in the future?
9. Using concepts related to employment and work, explain the implications of Douglas McGregor's version of the statement presented earlier in this chapter, "Man lives by bread alone, when there is no bread." How does this relate to employee motivation?
10. Identify one organizational setting outside of health care in which strict authoritarian management is not only prevalent but preferred. Why is this so, and why is it needed?

References

Fallon, L. F., & Zgodzinski, E. (2013). *Essentials of public health management* (3rd ed.). Burlington, MA: Jones & Bartlett Learning.

Likert, R. (1956). Motivation and increased productivity. *Management Record, 18*(4), 128–131.

Likert, R. (1961). *New patterns of management.* New York, NY: McGraw-Hill.

Maslow, A. H. (1943). A theory of human motivation. *Psychological Review, 50,* 370–396.

McGregor, D. M. (1957). The human side of enterprise. *Management Review, 46*(11), 22–28.

Urwick, L. F. (1963). The development of industrial engineering. In H. B. Maynard (Ed.), *Industrial engineering handbook* (2nd ed., p. 5). New York, NY: McGraw-Hill.

Resources
Books

Bogardus, A. M. (2004). *Human resources jumpstart.* Alameda, CA: Sybex.

Connolly, P. M., & Connolly, K. G. (2004). *Employee opinion questionnaires: 20 ready-to-use surveys that work.* New York, NY: John Wiley.

Cummings, S., Bridgman, T., Hassard, J., & Rowlinson, M. (2017). *A new history of management.* New York, NY: Cambridge University Press.

Drafke, M. (2005). *Human side of organizations.* Upper Saddle River, NJ: Prentice Hall.

Hyter, M., & Turnock, J. (2005). *The power of inclusion: Creating a culture of development to unlock the potential and productivity of your workforce.* New York, NY: John Wiley.

Niles, N. (2013). *Basic concepts of health care human resource management.* Burlington, MA: Jones & Bartlett Learning.

Ristow, A., Amos, T., & Ristow, L. (2004). *Human resource management* (2nd ed.). Lansdowne, South Africa: Juta Academic.

Winfield, L. (2005). *Straight talk about gays in the work place: Creating an inclusive, productive environment for everyone in your organization* (3rd ed.). Binghamton, NY: Haworth.

Periodicals

Barney, J. (2001). Is the resource-based view a useful perspective for strategic management research? Yes. *Academy of Management Review, 26,* 41–56.

Brooke, L., & Taylor, P. (2005). Older workers and employment: Managing age relations. *Ageing and Society, 25*(3), 415–429.

Grandey, A. A. (2000). Emotional regulation in the workplace: A new way to conceptualize emotional labor. *Journal of Occupational Health Psychology, 5,* 95–100.

Herod, A. (2002). Towards a more productive engagement: Industrial relations and economic geography meet. *Labour and Industry, 13*(2), 5–17.

Lawler, E. E. (2005). From human resource management to organizational effectiveness. *Human Resources Management, 44*(2), 165–169.

Naile, I., & Selesho, J. (2014). The role of leadership in employee motivation. *Mediterranean Journal of Social Sciences, 5*(5), 175–212.

Pelletier, B., Boles, M., & Lynch, W. (2004). Change in health risks and work productivity over time. *Journal of Occupational and Environmental Medicine, 46,* 746–754.

Thomas, G. (2005). Leadership: The undervalued element? *Royal College of Medicine Midwives, 8*(10), 424–425.

Wang, G. G., & Li, J. (2003). Measuring HPT interventions: Dilemma, challenge, and solutions. *Performance Improvement Quarterly, 42*(10), 17–23.

Wang, G. G., & Wang, J. (2005). Human resource development evaluation: Emerging market, barriers, and theory building. *Advances in Developing Human Resources, 7*(1), 22–36.

Wilk, S. L., & Moynihan, L. M. (2005). Display rule "regulators": The relationship between supervisors and worker emotional exhaustion. *Journal of Applied Psychology, 90*(5), 917–927.

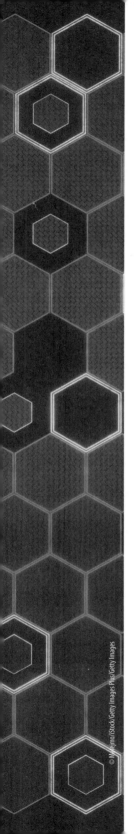

SECTION II

Services

The majority of departments or divisions in an organization produce products, coordinate programs, or deliver therapeutic remedies. Such outputs generate revenue. Rather than creating revenue, human resources departments provide important services to an organization. Section II introduces four important services of a typical HR department. Chapter 7 (Directions in Employee Relations) explores a variety of topics and different methods of delivering information. Chapter 8 (Compensation and Benefits) introduces the related concepts of pay and additional incentives. A relatively few benefits are required by law; the rest are provided at the discretion of senior managers or a governing board. Chapter 9 (Performance Appraisals) discusses methods for periodically evaluating employees. Chapter 10 (Succession Planning) reviews approaches used to replace organizational leaders.

CHAPTER 8

Compensation and Benefits

CHAPTER OBJECTIVES

After studying this chapter, readers will be able to:

- Describe the roles of human resources and department managers in matters of compensation.
- Understand the roles of human resources and department managers concerning benefits.
- Understand the basics of statutory benefits such as Workers' Compensation and short-term disability.
- Better understand a manager's role in the employment process and what occurs behind the scenes in human resources.
- Understand the role of human resources in performance appraisals.
- Be familiar with guidelines and precautions for managers who become involved in legal actions.
- Understand the involvement of human resources in external agency investigations and how these involve department managers.

▶ Chapter Summary

Compensation and benefits are the two significant human resources (HR) activities. Employees expect their compensation to be fair, and they expect HR to remain up-to-date concerning information related to compensation. Managers should be familiar with compensation scales that apply to their employees. Exchanging pay scale information with professional colleagues in different organizations is essentially illegal.

Next after their pay, most employees are vitally interested in their benefits. Benefits fall into two broad categories: those that are mandated by law, and those that are voluntarily offered by the employer. Organizational policies surrounding benefits have been changing. Currently, many organizations are changing from defined

🔍 *CASE STUDY: First Impressions Can Be Wrong*

Ben Baldwin, chief executive officer (CEO) of the Westside Health Consortium, summoned Rob Jameson, vice president for Human Resources, and Pat Collier, chief financial officer, to his office.

He told them, "Rob, I agree with your suggestion to change the structure of our benefits package. Pat has supplied financial data to support your suggestion. The costs of benefits continue to rise, with no end in sight. I am asking both of you to work together to develop options for a new plan to replace our existing approach that gives all employees the same benefits. I know that individual and family needs change with time. Westside must institute changes to control costs as well as to attract and retain skilled employees."

What steps should Rob and Pat take? What suggestions would you offer to them? Why? Should Ben provide additional guidance? If so, what information should he provide? Why?

benefit to defined contribution pension plans, and organizations that for years have offered the same benefits to all are adopting flexible or "cafeteria" plans that allow a range of employee choices. Statutory benefits include Workers' Compensation, unemployment compensation and insurance, and disability insurance. Government agencies investigating claims may involve an organization's employees, and inquiries from external agencies should be referred to HR.

▶ Introduction

Not all of the activities of HR are visible to department managers. Many of the activities discussed in this chapter are hidden in the sense that they occur within HR and elsewhere and are rarely the responsibility of a department manager. Compensation and benefits are matters of concern for most employees. This chapter is intended to provide a basic understanding of compensation and benefits.

▶ Compensation

One of HR's primary responsibilities is to maintain an organization's compensation structure. Human resources ordinarily endeavors to remain current and competitive with compensation levels in the healthcare industry and the local labor market. On a predetermined basis, usually annually, HR ordinarily makes recommendations for changes in compensation. Depending on organizational policy, these recommendations may be reviewed by an organization's board of directors before being implemented.

Annual compensation recommendations often include suggestions related to the timing of changes and the rationale for the suggested distribution of increases. Recommendations usually include the basis for the changes being proposed. These are typically related to prevailing industry or area compensation practices. Proposed wage increases may include all employees, perhaps as cost-of-living adjustments; they may be restricted to employees in specific professional groups; or they may have the effect of revising the organization's pay scales.

Knowing the Compensation System

Supervisors and department managers are usually the first persons to receive questions regarding compensation and benefits from their employees. To respond adequately to such inquiries, a manager should know how pay increases are related to performance and the general level of performance required for receiving merit-based increases. One must also know the differences between merit pay increases and increases provided through pay-scale changes. A manager should know when merit increases or scale increases can usually be expected to occur and how and when other types of pay increases, such as probationary increases, are granted.

A manager should be familiar with current pay scales for all positions in the department and should maintain current pay scale data for quick reference. When pay scales are changed, HR usually supplies up-to-date published scales to department managers. Current pay-scale information is needed when addressing particular employee questions, but the dissemination of this information should be selective and based on an individual's legitimate need to know.

Strategic planning figures prominently in compensation administration. Organizations must make decisions about the nature and extent of the compensation and benefits that they will offer their employees. Will they decide to pay employees at the regional median, similar to others in their region? Some consciously decide to pay less than the prevailing wage; they know they will be saving some money but will be accepting a higher than normal degree of employee turnover as a consequence of their decision. Others decide to pay at a rate or level greater than that of other organizations, accepting the higher wage costs in exchange for more highly skilled or reliable employees and a lower than usual level of employee turnover.

Organizations must make similar deliberate decisions concerning benefits. Will their benefits package be similar to or different from the packages of other organizations? A common question reflects the nature of the local pool of prospective job applicants and the extent to which they will have to compete for employees.

Yet another strategic decision reflects the nature of benefits that will be offered. For many years, the majority of organizations offered all employees a similar package of benefits that typically differed only in reflection of years of service in determining vacation entitlement. Today, many organizations are making strategic decisions to allow individuals to select benefits from a menu of options. Such an approach is referred to as a flexible benefits plan or a cafeteria benefits plan, under which employees are allotted a certain amount of benefits credits to distribute as they see fit among available benefits. Most employees welcome the ability to select options that best fit their individual circumstances, and organizations are able to better control or contain their benefit expenses.

Historically, benefits were offered to provide incentives for individuals to choose one organization over another. After employment began, benefits provided incentives to continue employment. Thus, companies were able to attract and retain desired employees. Funding for benefits reflects a financial commitment by employers. The ability to pay for benefits must be periodically reviewed as budgets are developed, as new employees are hired, and as collective bargaining agreements are negotiated.

Organizations maintain a mix of employees compensated at differing wage levels. The variety and extent of benefits that are offered broadly reflect the wage mix of an organization. Phrased differently, benefits are generally proportionate to wages. Some benefits are mandated; Workers' Compensation and unemployment insurance are common examples. All benefits other than those required by law are provided at the discretion of the employer.

Individual employees have the right to know the minimum and maximum rates for their pay scales as well as their own actual rates of pay. However, individual employees are not entitled to know other employees' pay scales or any other individual employee's rate of pay. Department managers have the responsibility to safeguard this aspect of employee privacy. A manager can exercise no control over those occasional employees who voluntarily share their pay information with one another, although this practice should be discouraged.

When Compensation Challenges Arise

A department manager is often the initial target when employees challenge the compensation system. Some individuals challenge the equity of their own rates of pay; they compare their pay with that of others who hold similar positions. The perceived similarity may be based on occupation, job title, or other means of comparison. A typical claim is that they are underpaid for performing the same or comparable work. Their information is often secondhand, inaccurate, or outdated.

A department manager should acknowledge several responsibilities related to possible pay inequities. First, a manager should know enough about the pay level for each person in the department to recognize pay inequities within the group when or even before they surface. In a relatively small group, substantial pay inequities are uncommon. A manager who has a small group of employees should be well aware of how these people stack up against each other in terms of pay. In a larger department, the cumulative effects of several years of hiring at differing levels as well as merit and probationary and annual pay increases may mask inequity until an employee raises the issue. When this occurs, the manager should do some preliminary research concerning the inequity. If warranted, the problem should be referred to HR for further analysis and a recommendation for change or correction.

A manager's other responsibility related to supposed pay inequities is to work with HR when the challenges involve claims of underpayment in comparison with what persons of comparable skills are supposedly receiving at other local facilities. Employees will sometimes approach the department manager with such challenges looking for the manager's support and advocacy. They want the manager to champion their cause and seek to have one or more pay scales increased and corresponding pay raises granted for individuals. Such claims must be addressed with care; in some instances, individuals have offered "proof" of higher wages paid by local competition by producing actual paycheck stubs bearing hourly rates clearly more generous than what their home organization is paying. However, investigation often reveals that these more generous payments are the rates paid to per diem employees who receive a higher amount per hour for limited hours because they receive no benefits.

Although conscientious and caring managers are probably inclined to be advocates for their employees, claims of pay inequity relative to other organizations should always be referred to HR. This action should be taken before agreeing to take on any employee's cause. Assessing such claims of inequity requires detailed information about wages paid in the immediate area. As previously noted, there are legal and practical restrictions on how such information may be obtained. It is no longer legal to do as many HR departments once did and simply survey the wage rates in one's local area. In the early 1990s, the U.S. Department of Justice put a stop to the direct sharing of wage and salary information. As part of a consent decree involving the settlement of a civil antitrust complaint, the Department of Justice laid down some rules for surveying rates of pay:

- Surveys must be designed, conducted, and published without the involvement of participating organizations (accomplished, for example, by a hospital association or other neutral third party).
- Surveys can include only historical or current pay information (that is, they cannot ask for intended increases).
- Surveys cannot request actual pay rates, only ranges and averages for specific job titles.
- Surveys must disseminate data of 10 or more organizations if current information is involved, or 5 or more if the data are more than 3 months old.
- No one organization's data may represent more than 25% of the weighted value of any statistic (this way, the data from one large facility cannot dominate the results).
- Data must be presented in such a manner that no individual participating organization can be identified.

Managers should never give in to the temptation to conduct a personal wage survey by calling on contacts or colleagues throughout the community to determine what other organizations are paying for the specific kinds of skills in question. Since the early 1990s, the free exchange of wage information has been regarded as price fixing under antitrust regulations. The Justice Department eventually decided that not-for-profit healthcare organizations should be held to the same standards as other industries. Therefore, department managers who solicit or exchange wage information with colleagues at other institutions are technically engaging in an illegal activity. Rather than attempting to verify the validity of employees' claims of wage inequity relative to other organizations, a concerned manager should take the issue to HR for investigation.

Wage surveys are permitted, but only when conducted according to established guidelines. They must be done by third-party organizations, such as membership associations of hospitals or other providers. They must include a sufficient number of organizations surveyed and present the results in such a way that no participating institutions can be readily identified. Generally, five or six organizations are enough for an appropriate survey as long as none can be readily identified (perhaps because of institution size or unique character).

Interviewing Prospective Employees

The department manager is expected to be conversant with all pay scales used in the department. Thus, in most organizations, a manager may cite the appropriate pay range for a job during an interview. However, a manager should not make a specific financial offer during an interview. Having made a decision to offer a position to a particular applicant, the manager should collaborate with the HR recruiter to determine the starting pay to be offered. The official offer will flow from HR to the applicant.

There are several reasons for making formal offers only through HR. First, all offers of employment are conditional pending successful reference checks, passing a pre-employment physical examination, and passing any drug or substance screening tests used by the hiring organization. Second, it is the responsibility of the HR department to protect an organization's compensation system against inequities. This can best be accomplished if all offers emanate from a single office. Third, some organizational policies for determining starting pay offers may state, for example, that people with a given amount of experience may be offered a starting pay at a specified percentage of the pay grade. This is also most easily controlled if all offers emanate from a single point.

A department manager should have a voice in recommending starting pay if there is any flexibility to do so. This input should be made in conjunction with HR, given that HR always extends the formal offer of employment.

▶ Benefits

A department manager should have basic benefits information available for employees. At a minimum, this should include information in the personnel policy and procedure manual and the employee handbook. No matter how strongly employees are urged to become familiar with their benefits, many of them show no interest in doing so until a specific need arises. When a specific need does arise, they do not read about the benefit. Rather, they choose to ask a person, usually their department manager or someone in HR. This is especially true concerning medical and dental insurance benefits, about which many employees remain nearly completely ignorant until a specific need emerges.

Department managers are not expected to be experts in the interpretation of employee benefits. However, managers should be sufficiently conversant with the benefits structure to answer simple questions and to know the appropriate person in HR to refer employees for inquiries about benefits. Some areas of employee benefits can become complex. For example, a large hospital may carry five or six different health insurance plans, each having hundreds of details. Questions about them are best addressed by a person who is qualified and knowledgeable about the different plans.

Flexible Benefits Plans

Flexible benefits plans proliferated through the 1980s and 1990s and remain popular today. They are frequently referred to as cafeteria plans, and their use recognizes that the majority of employees prefer to have some control over their benefits. The array of options available is often a consideration for an applicant in determining whether to accept a position with a particular employer.

The three benefits most preferred by the majority of employees, in order of their preference, are health insurance, a pension plan, and paid vacation. Despite the fact that these have formed the core of most organizational benefit plans, they are not of equal importance to everyone.

Employee benefits are available in many different forms and variations. Such variety is appropriate because not all employees want or need the same benefits. Even pension benefits, ultimately a concern for nearly everyone, are not a consistent choice for all employees at all times. Younger employees often pay less attention to pension plans than do older workers. Younger employees prefer cash or additional paid vacation time; older workers tend to prefer pension benefits. Choices were introduced into benefits programs as employers endeavored to stretch benefits budgets as much as possible while giving employees options for the benefits they perceived as most needed. Flexibility and choice will be increasingly important features of benefits programs in the future.

Flexible benefits plans have proven their appeal to many employees. An increasing number of employers are offering plans that are either entirely flexible or partly flexible around a small number of core benefits. Programs that allow an employee to waive medical coverage after establishing that coverage is provided by other means—for example, through a working spouse's medical insurance plan—and applying the value of that benefit elsewhere have been especially successful. Plans that permit buying or selling some vacation time by trading it off for other benefits are quite popular.

A logical progression beyond flexible benefits is the use of benefits vouchers. These provide employees with the equivalent of a set amount of money to apply outside of an organization as they choose. Stated differently, such a plan allows employees to spend an organization's contribution toward their benefits on whatever is most meaningful to them. Vouchers have proven to be especially advantageous to some employees during layoffs and downsizing. Many employer-furnished benefits end when employment is terminated, but benefits secured externally with vouchers are purchased for a fixed period of time and do not necessarily end when employment ceases.

Another emerging trend is the use of voluntary benefits. This approach allows employees to purchase specified insurance coverage and financial products for savings and retirement at their place of employment. Voluntary benefits have been used in work organizations for many years in the form of supplemental insurance programs. The concept appears to be spreading to include some products or options formerly regarded as core benefits.

Portable benefits are becoming more common in benefits administration. This concept has been advanced by many as the solution to maintaining benefits for workers in a mobile society. It recognizes that individuals may work for several different organizations during the course of a normal career and therefore may be best served by benefit products that can move with them. Defined benefit pension plans are being replaced by defined contribution plans. Because defined contribution plans limit liability exposure, they result in savings for employers. They also allow organizations that formerly offered defined benefit plans to escape the hassle of government reporting, avoid annual funding of plans, and get out from under the constantly increasing premiums charged by the Pension Benefit Guaranty Corporation (PBGC). Commonly defined contribution products include 401(k) plans for investments and savings and 403(b) plans for tax-deferred annuities. Individuals who have either plan can transfer the funds to subsequent employers.

The Health Insurance Portability and Accountability Act (HIPAA) addresses an aspect of benefits portability by providing for continuity of coverage when workers change employers.

Some experts have predicted that the ultimate development in benefits administration is to offer no benefits at all other than those required by law, such as those required by the Federal Insurance Contributions Act (FICA—that is, Social Security), Workers' Compensation coverage, and unemployment insurance. Employers will simply pay their employees the value of the organization's benefits contribution as a part of their salary and allow them to spend the money as they choose. This is in conflict with the direction and philosophy established by the government in employment legislation that encourages employers to assume greater social responsibility for their employees. Many workers in the lower tiers of the economy currently receive no benefits other than those required by law.

Statutory Benefits

Statutory benefits programs exist by virtue of legal requirements. These programs are usually administered by HR. Foremost among these are Workers' Compensation and unemployment compensation in all states. A number of states also have a legal requirement for short-term disability insurance. Human resources usually coordinates these programs, although there are implications for department managers.

Workers' Compensation laws are in effect in all 50 states, American Samoa, the District of Columbia, Guam, Puerto Rico, and the Virgin Islands. Including both medical benefits and compensation for lost income, billions of dollars in Workers' Compensation benefits are paid to American employees every year.

The medical benefits paid under Workers' Compensation laws generally equal full actual medical expenses. The amount of benefits paid for lost wages varies considerably from state to state. Nationwide, the most common benefit paid amounts to two-thirds of wages up to a specified maximum. Most states place limits on both maximum and minimum weekly benefits, the total number of weeks that benefits can be received, and the total dollar amount of benefit eligibility. Most states also provide lifetime payment for permanent disability. Some states pay additional amounts for dependents, rehabilitation services, and other benefits.

Department supervisors cannot exert much influence over Workers' Compensation costs, because managers are members of a group of people in an organization who have separate but not well-defined roles in controlling Workers' Compensation costs. The best approach to controlling such costs is to have an effective accident prevention program. Here, a manager's role is to be constantly aware of the requirements of the program and ensure that all employees observe those requirements. Specifically, it is up to managers to ensure that employees are thoroughly educated in safe work practices, including, in the healthcare setting, safe handling of needles and other sharp objects and safe lifting techniques. Puncture wounds have always been a concern in health care, and back strain resulting from improper lifting remains one of the most common on-the-job injuries experienced by healthcare personnel. Managers must enforce compliance with organizational safety procedures that have been mandated by governmental entities. They must also ensure that their employees are trained and appropriately use all required safety equipment as they perform their jobs.

When pursuing an effective accident prevention program, a manager is clearly responsible for encouraging a high level of consciousness about the need for safety among employees. Managers must discipline their employees for unsafe practices. Ignoring a safety procedure is no different from violating any other work rule or policy. Violators must be appropriately counseled. Continued violations must be handled through the organization's progressive discipline procedure.

A department manager should assist HR in monitoring Workers' Compensation claims and challenging those that appear to be inappropriate. To monitor claims properly, a manager must be thorough and timely in providing all documentation that may have a bearing on a claim. This includes all necessary incident and accident reports. These should be provided as soon after the fact as possible, and they must be clear and detailed.

Questions sometimes arise about whether a particular injury did indeed occur during working time or on an organization's property. It may be necessary to determine whether Workers' Compensation is appropriate or the case should be processed as a short-term disability resulting from an off-the-job occurrence. Employees may report off-the-job accidents as occurring on the job, because Workers' Compensation benefits are more generous than short-term disability benefits and generally more generous than applying individual health insurance (which may in some instances cover the medical aspects of a situation but offer no help concerning lost income). After an injured employee's personal physician, the employee's supervisor is often the next most important person in determining whether a given occurrence legitimately falls under Workers' Compensation.

Unemployment Compensation

The Social Security Act of 1935 made the individual states responsible for their own unemployment compensation insurance programs. A federal tax was imposed on employers, but most of this tax could be offset by state taxes. All programs were to be controlled at the state level.

Unemployment insurance programs are in effect in all 50 states, the District of Columbia, and Puerto Rico. These programs are continually undergoing change. The majority of such changes result in increased benefits for employees and increased costs for employers.

Although differences exist throughout the country, employers are generally subject to experience rating. This means they are taxed according to their past records. An employer that decreases its unemployment claims by employees will also decrease its unemployment tax costs. Many business organizations and virtually all profit-making businesses are taxed directly using experience-based rates established by each state. In a number of states, not-for-profit organizations, including most healthcare organizations, pay for their unemployment on a dollar-for-dollar basis rather than paying a tax based on a percentage of payroll. This means that such organizations pay actual unemployment costs as they are incurred.

Because unemployment compensation is intended to make up for wages lost due to periods of unemployment beyond an employee's control, unemployment compensation is not ordinarily made available to people who voluntarily resign their employment or who are discharged for cause. Rather, unemployment compensation is intended primarily for employees who are laid off through no fault of their own or who otherwise find that their services are no longer required. Individuals who have been dismissed because of their apparent inability to meet the requirements of their positions generally qualify for unemployment compensation. In a few states, employees who are on strike can receive unemployment compensation after a specified waiting period, usually six or more weeks from the start of the strike.

To the extent that it is possible for a department manager to influence some forms of employee turnover, a supervisor can have an effect on an organization's unemployment compensation costs. Care and thoroughness in hiring will help limit the likelihood of acquiring an employee who may turn out to be unable to succeed on the job. It is not possible to refine the hiring process to the point where the right choices will always be made. Nevertheless, if a manager sticks to minimum education and experience requirements and does not rush a decision based on insufficient information or an insufficient number of candidates, it is often possible to minimize or avoid performance problems before they begin. This also minimizes potential unemployment costs.

A manager should scrupulously follow all organizational policies regarding hiring, orientation, disciplinary action, and applicable legal processes. Disciplinary actions, especially those taken in a series that could eventually result in termination, are especially important. All such actions must be thoroughly documented and should be taken strictly in accordance with policy and Equal Employment Opportunity guidelines. It is frequently necessary to use records of disciplinary actions to refute nonlegitimate claims for unemployment compensation. Because the primary purpose of disciplinary action is the correction of behavior, it is often necessary to produce documentation of a series of related actions to demonstrate that an employee had the opportunity to correct errant behavior but failed to do so.

A manager should remove a substandard performer during the probationary period if at all possible. An organization's probationary period may be too short to enable a definite decision concerning an individual's ability, especially in the case of a marginal employee. However, the probationary period is usually sufficient to give a manager a fairly clear indication of an employee's potential. Separation for reasons related to performance is usually easier to justify if it occurs during a probationary period. Because unemployment costs are related to the length of time an employee has worked for an organization, separation by the end of the probationary period serves to hold costs down.

Working in conjunction with HR, a manager should challenge all unemployment claims that appear inappropriate. Many people automatically file for unemployment regardless of why or how they left their positions. They have nothing to lose by trying to collect benefits. Many former employees will state their reasons for termination clearly in their favor. The former employer then has the responsibility to dispute such claims to avoid unemployment costs. If a claim goes undisputed, then a former employee, deserving or not, will automatically collect unemployment compensation. Thus, every effort should be made to dispute claims that appear inappropriate.

A manager should consider the use of temporary help when it will be needed for only a short period of time. Hiring a regular employee to cover a given need and then laying the person off when the need has passed increases unemployment costs. Using temporary help for particular tasks or for brief periods of time will avoid such costs. In most parts of the country, 26 weeks of work are required for an employee to become eligible for unemployment benefits. Thus, any need that is less than 6 months long and can be met by using temporary help will reduce an organization's unemployment costs.

Short-Term Disability

Unlike Workers' Compensation and unemployment compensation, which are statutory requirements throughout the country, short-term disability is not a universal legal requirement. But if one's state requires short-term disability coverage, this becomes another cost-control concern for the department manager.

The premium for disability insurance is linked to usage. Technically, this is called an experience rating. The claims actually paid in a given year are reflected in the subsequent year's premium rates. Therefore, most organizations pay dollar-for-dollar. They eventually pay the total actual costs for all claims plus administrative expenses.

The single action that can have the greatest impact on an organization's overall disability costs is a corporate decision to become self-insured. Such a policy is typically coupled with a comprehensive employee health and safety program. At the level of an individual department, a manager can pass along information to employees concerning personal health and safety in general and particular hazards or illnesses that are germane to an organization. Supervisors should urge employees to take advantage of annual physical examinations or health assessments and should always be prepared to refer employees to the employee health office when questions arise or problems become apparent. Finally, managers should scrupulously fulfill all departmental responsibilities related to disability procedures by ensuring that all necessary forms are completed and submitted in a timely fashion.

Legal Actions

From a department manager's perspective, involvement in a legal action may take the form of brief periods of extremely intense and demanding activity, interspersed with lengthy stretches characterized by little or no visible activity. A department manager who may become involved in a legal action against the organization must be patient. Attorneys' schedules, court calendars, and official waiting times all extend the time that is required to resolve legal actions. There is little point in allowing the suspense of a situation to impact the routines of employees when the timing of events lies well beyond their control.

Supervisors must accept the normal sequence of events. During long, quiet periods, nothing may seem to occur. Many activities such as motions, depositions of various individuals, and settlement conferences that do not involve a manager may be transpiring. Managers should simply accept the apparently slow pace of resolution. Managers should not be overly concerned about being called for deposition or trial testimony. Expert preparation and support will be provided.

Individuals who are named in a suit or summoned in a case must appear in court. Because there is no way to avoid such an appearance, worrying about doing so is a waste of time and energy. Resigning one's employment will not remove the legal obligation. When completing any form, a manager should offer only what is necessary and always do so objectively and without personal bias or name-calling. The manager should complete all forms, being attentive to dates and signatures. Managers should remain sensitive to the implications of a case in their day-to-day dealings with employees. Words as well as actions have the potential to create problems. In response to direct questioning, managers should not discuss an open case with others in the organization except for those few who are actively managing the organization's involvement. Smart managers avoid the temptation to make predictions concerning the eventual outcome.

External Agency Investigations

Human resources staff members often spend a considerable amount of time interacting with representatives of different government agencies. Following is an overview of the agencies commonly encountered by an organization.

Equal Employment Opportunity Commission and the State Division of Human Rights

The Equal Employment Opportunity Commission (EEOC) and the State Division of Human Rights (DHR) address allegations of employment discrimination. Filing a complaint with one is essentially filing with both of them. In many states, a complaint reaching EEOC first is automatically referred to DHR for initial processing. The initial point of contact for both agencies is usually human resources. HR typically gathers the requested information and responds formally to a complaint. The manager of a complaining employee's department will often be contacted for information to help in developing the organization's response. That manager is likely to be interviewed during investigation of the complaint.

Occupational Safety and Health Administration

Using no particular schedule or set frequency, the Occupational Safety and Health Administration (OSHA) may send representatives to perform routine surveys of safety practices or to investigate specific complaints or allegations of unsafe practices that have been received. Human resources is often an organization's point of contact. The initial contact may be a particular administrator, a risk manager, or a safety manager. Engineering may also be involved because many safety issues or violations involve the physical plant. The manager of a department where a potential unsafe practice is observed or alleged can expect to become involved.

State Employment Service

Human resources is heavily involved in every claim for unemployment compensation. Since an employee's level of compensation is based on income, information about earnings must be provided. Human resources must supply the reason for termination and must indicate whether the claim will be protested. A protested claim usually results in a hearing before an administrative law judge. A hearing usually involves the former employee's immediate supervisor as well as an HR representative.

Immigration and Customs Enforcement

Under the provisions of the Homeland Security Act of 2002, the Immigration and Naturalization Service (INS) was dismantled in 2003 and separated into three components: the U.S. Citizenship and Immigration Service (USCIS), Immigration and Customs Enforcement (ICE), and Customs and Border Protection (CBP). Completed Employee Eligibility Verification I-9 Forms verifying individuals' status as legally employable in the United States and retained in employees' personnel files are subject to inspection and audit by ICE. Forms may also be inspected by the Department of Labor (DOL) and certain immigration-related branches of the Department of Homeland Security other than ICE. Financial penalties are imposed for missing or incomplete I-9s. Also, there can be significant legal repercussions should illegal aliens be discovered in the workforce. Usually, the department manager will have no involvement in an I-9 audit, except perhaps as the channel for an I-9 related question from HR to an employee.

Department of Labor

The DOL monitors compliance with wage-and-hour laws. Since both states and the federal government have wage-and-hour laws, an organization may be visited by either state or federal DOL representatives. Their interest may be a routine audit of selected wage payment practices. Overtime payments are often the subjects of investigation. The DOL also investigates employment practices such as compliance with child labor laws. DOL investigators occasionally investigate irregularities in wage payments. The primary points of contact in such investigations are usually human resources and payroll departments. Department managers can become involved in providing information to determine whether an employee is properly classified as exempt or nonexempt, or whether time worked has been appropriately reported.

Few people look forward to an investigation by an external agency. However, such contacts are inevitable. Most human resources departments regard external agency inquiries as opportunities to review selected practices for possible violations and determine how these practices can be improved. Even though an external investigator may appear to be unnecessarily forceful, nothing is accomplished when HR personnel or others respond by being defensive or uncooperative.

A considerable part of the role of human resources regarding external agencies is knowing the law as well as an agency's guidelines and procedures. When internally investigating a specific complaint, HR should first determine whether it is valid. If it is, HR can recommend corrective action in addition to formulating the organization's response to an external agency. There is no gain in resisting a complaint if an organization appears to be in the wrong. However, HR professionals are usually well aware that an external investigator who is acting on an individual's complaint has heard only one side of the story. Unless the particular complaint to be addressed is a discrimination charge from EEOC or DHR that cannot be disposed of at an early stage, human resources is usually able to keep a department manager's involvement with external agency representatives to a minimum.

▶ Conclusion

Compensation and benefits are important aspects of employment for most people. Compensation information is coordinated by HR. Benefits policies are changing. Organizations are trying to reduce expenses associated with benefits. Flexible benefit plans have evolved as organizations try to provide meaningful and relevant benefits to employees with a wide range of ages and interests. Rather than simply paying for a standard benefits plan for all, organizations are allowing individuals to make their own decisions regarding benefits. Benefit programs are usually administered by an HR department. Workers' Compensation, unemployment compensation, and insurance and disability insurance are required by law. All other benefits are offered at the discretion of an employing organization.

🔍 *CASE STUDY: Resolution*

Returning to the initial case study, Ben should either provide a general dollar amount to offer to each Westside employee or instruct Pat to develop such an amount. Rob and Pat should contact other organizations in the area that compete for employees to ascertain what components their benefits packages include. They should consider obtaining the opinions of a sample of Westside employees as to the desirability of the benefits under consideration. Once the fundamental questions of dollar amount and plan elements are addressed, Rob and Pat can develop a plan for Ben to consider. Based on employees' years of service and relative position within the organization, the plan should define the dollar amounts Westside will provide for its employees and the options from which they can choose for their benefits. Because they are thorough, Rob and Pat should develop a range of options for Ben to review. Ultimately, Westside's board of directors will have to approve the proposed changes in benefits.

SPOTLIGHT ON CUSTOMER SERVICE

Customer Service, Compensation, and Benefits

Customer service, compensation, and benefits are fundamentally linked by virtue of the fact that an organization must earn revenues in order to be able to pay its employees. Customer service, if regularly practiced by all employees, usually improves an organization's chances of not only staying in business but also prospering and expanding. Conversely, ignoring customer service may be an attractive option to persons seeking shortcuts. Such individuals are probably surprised when layoff notices are distributed to employees or an organization fails.

The bottom line in this thought process is to think of customer service as a form of insurance. Providing good customer service on a regular basis is an inexpensive form of insurance premium.

Questions for Review and Discussion

1. What is meant by the term *statutory benefits*? Provide several examples.
2. Why should a department manager be thoroughly familiar with pay scales appropriate to department personnel but refrain from making specific pay offers to potential employees?
3. How should a supervisor reply to a male employee who complains that he is being paid less than another individual who is doing the same work?
4. How should a supervisor reply to a female employee making the same complaint about a male colleague? Are the responses different? Why?
5. Why should a department manager avoid comparing employee pay scales with those of other organizations?
6. An employee asks, "What is the difference between a defined benefit pension plan and a defined contribution plan?" How would you respond to such a question?
7. Why is interest in portable benefits in health care increasing?

8. In your opinion, what should be a department manager's primary role in attempting to control Workers' Compensation costs?
9. Managers disagree whether a particular instance of time lost due to injury or illness should be considered under Workers' Compensation (job related) or short-term disability (not job related). Knowing that an employer ultimately pays for both, why is this distinction important?
10. What role should a department manager have in controlling the cost of unemployment compensation?
11. How should managers react if representatives of an external regulatory organization arrive at their departments to audit their activities?

Resources
Books

Baker, A. J., Logue, D., & Rader, J. S. (2004). *Managing pension and retirement plans: A guide for employers, administrators, and other fiduciaries.* New York, NY: Oxford University Press.
Beam, B. T. (2004). *Employee benefits.* Chicago, IL: Dearborn Real Estate Education.
Beyer, L., & Beyer, D. (2015). *The compensation handbook* (6th ed.). New York, NY: McGraw-Hill.
Bowey, A. M., & Lupton, L. (2005). *Managing salary and wage systems* (3rd ed.). London, UK: Ashgate.
Boyett, J. H., & Boyett, J. T. (2004). *Skill-based pay design manual.* Lincoln, NE: iUniverse.
Bragg, S. (2005). *Payroll best practices.* New York, NY: John Wiley.
Ellison, R., & Jones, G. (2005). *Dealing with pensions: The practical impact of the Pensions Act 2004 on mergers, acquisitions and insolvencies.* London, UK: Spiramus.
Henderson, S. (2005). *Compensation management in a knowledge-based world* (10th ed.). Upper Saddle River, NJ: Prentice Hall.
Rosenbloom, J. S. (2011). *Handbook of employee benefits* (7th ed.). New York, NY: McGraw-Hill.
Society for Human Resource Management. (2018). *The evolution of employee benefits.* Alexandria, VA: SHRM.

Periodicals

Baird, M. (2004). Orientations to paid maternity leave: Understanding the Australian debate. *Journal of Industrial Relations, 46*(3), 259–274.
Clark, I. (2001). Strategic HRM and a budgetary control mechanism in the large corporation. *Critical Perspectives on Accounting, 12,* 797–815.
Gornick, M. E., & Blair, B. R. (2004). Employee assistance, work–life effectiveness, and health and productivity: A conceptual framework for integration. *Journal of Workplace Behavioral Health, 20*(1–2), 1–29.
Michie, J., & Sheehan, M. (2005). Business strategy, human resources, labour market flexibility and competitive advantage. *International Journal of Human Resources Management, 16*(3), 445–464.

CHAPTER 9

Performance Appraisals

CHAPTER OBJECTIVES

After studying this chapter, readers will be able to:

- Know the value of having an up-to-date performance appraisal process.
- Understand the primary objectives of performance appraisal.
- Recognize traditional approaches to performance appraisal.
- Appreciate common obstacles to performance appraisal.
- Avoid problems presented by appraisal instruments that require evaluators to render personality judgments.
- Understand that sound position descriptions are the essential starting point for an effective appraisal process.
- Know the kinds of standards and measurements that can be applied in appraising performance.
- Define the critical differences between the terms *standard* and *average* as they are used in performance appraisals.
- Be familiar with the two most common approaches to appraisal timing.
- Schedule and conduct a performance appraisal interview.
- Know when and how self-appraisal can be a constructive element of the performance appraisal process.
- Appreciate important legal implications of performance appraisal.
- Know the role of human resources in performance appraisal, including the times in the process when a department manager becomes involved.

▶ Chapter Summary

Performance appraisals are important to employees and their organizations. They provide structured opportunities for supervisors and employees to talk about progress and performance. Knowledgeable organizations use structured forms for all employees and use written procedures to provide guidance for the process.

Poor or obsolete forms hinder the appraisal process. Useful forms are objective, easy to understand and use, and relatively brief. They rate performance, not personal characteristics or attitudes. The best appraisal forms are aligned with position descriptions and ask for evaluations that can be supported by data.

🔍 CASE STUDY: An Appraisal Conversation

"This is stupid and a waste of time," lamented Stu Johnson. "I supervise these people every day and know their working habits well. Upper management pays me to get work done, not to write out appraisals every year."

"Ah, even ignoring the fact that regular appraisals are required by policy, your employees look forward to them," replied colleague Marcia Stannis.

"Humph. If they want to know how they are doing, all they have to do is walk into my office and ask me. I'll be glad to tell them."

"How often does that happen?" asked Marcia.

"Maybe once every year or so," replied Stu.

"Do you walk around the office?" asked Marcia.

"Sometimes, when I have time," was the reply.

"How often is sometimes?"

"Every few weeks," said Stu. "You know we've been busy this past year."

"Did you know that Julie completed her degree?" asked Marcia.

"No."

"Or that Jeff is applying for a promotion?" Marcia continued.

"Huh? When did he do that?"

"Last month. Remember Jim, the problem employee?"

"How could I forget him? He was so lazy," Stu recalled.

"He lost his lawsuit for wrongful dismissal."

"That seems appropriate."

How would you describe Stu's management style? In your opinion, was he as knowledgeable about his employees as he thought? Why? Why do you think Jim lost his lawsuit?

A written appraisal must be followed by a personal interview to discuss the evaluation and provide the opportunity for employee input. Self-appraisals or team evaluations are used as appropriate. Human resources (HR) should oversee employee appraisal programs.

▶ Performance Appraisal Defined

A performance appraisal is a regularly scheduled, structured event. It involves a periodic assessment of performance to ascertain how well a particular employee is performing relative to what is expected. Performance appraisal involves two documents, a position or job description and a performance appraisal form. A permanent record is usually created and retained in an employee's personnel file.

Different organizations may use different names for the performance appraisal process. The more common titles are performance evaluation, performance review, and performance assessment. A newer term is performance management. Performance management purports to encompass not only evaluation but also the overall development and improvement of an employee as a producer. When completed correctly, however, a performance appraisal includes everything that performance management claims to include.

The Need for Performance Appraisal

Performance appraisal is used to facilitate improvement in employee performance, provide feedback to employees concerning job performance, and collect information for decisions concerning compensation and other personnel transactions such as promotions and transfers.

The primary purpose of an appraisal is to improve employee performance in the individual's present job. A secondary purpose is to maintain the performance at an acceptable level. The process contributes to two developmental objectives for an employee. It delineates an employee's progress toward advancement and assuming greater responsibilities. It helps senior managers to identify employees who are capable of advancement. Performance appraisals periodically remind employees about what their employers expect from them. From the perspective of individual employees, performance appraisals should enable them to know how they are performing. It also helps them to know what is needed to improve their performance.

Performance appraisal in health care is mandated by organizations and agencies that accredit and regulate healthcare facilities. In some instances, mandated evaluation has led to the development of performance appraisal systems that are little more than a formality; most such evaluation systems have minimal value.

Conducting a Performance Appraisal

Many methods have been employed to assess employee performance. The most often used ones employ rating scales based on comparing an employee's performance with a scale that represents expectations. Other approaches are sometimes used. Under particular circumstances, each of the following has been effectively used.

Essay

A supervisor periodically describes employee performance at whatever length is considered necessary. After the contents are discussed with the employee, the essay is signed by both parties. The employee is given a copy, and a copy is placed in the personnel file.

Critical Incident

Any positive or negative event that occurs outside of the ordinary is written up and retained for the next formal performance discussion.

Employee Comparison

Employees in a group are compared with each other and rank ordered from the best performer to the poorest performer. A different variation has supervisors placing their employees into a three-part distribution. A predetermined percentage of employees are rated as above average, a similar percentage must be rated as below average, and the remaining employees are rated in the middle.

Checklist

In this approach, an evaluating manager must describe employee performance by choosing from among a number of prepared statements. A variation of this method asks supervisors to select, from a group of prepared statements, the one that best and another that least describes each employee.

Management by Objectives

This is a participative approach commonly used with higher-level technical or professional employees and managers. The individual is evaluated on achievement of or progress toward specific objectives developed by the individual with the manager's concurrence.

Although every appraisal system has shortcomings, a rating-scale approach is most useful and equitable when it is applied correctly. It is neither appropriate nor fair to appraise the work of employees by comparing the performance of one to another. The most useful comparison that can be made via appraisal is the evaluation of individual employee performance over time; in other words, the only comparison applied to an employee is with his or her own past performance. Successive evaluation periods provide the basis for meaningful long-term assessment. Evaluators and employees must have similar expectations of how their organization's system works. This approach does not rely on the specifics of any particular rating system.

Managers and Rating

Appraisals occur so infrequently it is difficult to consider performance appraisal as a regular part of a manager's job. Thus, managers often view the process as extraneous and intrusive. Appraisals become extra work. They require supervisors to make difficult judgments about subordinates. As a result, employee appraisals are often dreaded or disliked. Managers are often uneasy about criticizing employees, especially on a performance appraisal that results in a permanent record in an employee's file and that could affect the person's pay, job future, and career.

One common approach to addressing anxiety or fear associated with having to evaluate others' performance is to ignore the appraisal requirement. When that option is unavailable, supervisors often accomplish the task in a hurry and avoid making substantive evaluation decisions. Such an approach is essentially useless. In business in general as well as in health care, periodic appraisals are a necessity. The best way to address appraisal anxiety is with knowledge, preparation, and practice.

▶ Obstacles to Performance Appraisal

Other obstacles to performance appraisals exist in addition to managers' and employees' often-felt dislike of the process. If evaluation is not taken seriously by an organization, managers will view performance appraisal as little more than a paper-pushing activity that has little relevance. The length and complexity of forms can deter department managers. Appraisal results may be converted to scores when used to determine pay increases. When this occurs, a performance appraisal becomes a scorecard, and the process becomes competitive.

Ensuring that all managers apply appraisals in a consistent manner is a common problem. Person-to-person consistency is important, especially when evaluation scores determine the amount of pay increases. Differences do exist. Some managers rarely give outstanding ratings, while others consistently give employees high ratings. Some managers cluster their ratings and group most employees in a narrow band around the middle of the scale. Different supervisors emphasize different parts of the system. One may emphasize quality of output, while another stresses interpersonal relationships.

After mergers occur, managers often find they have many more employees than before. Some supervisors feel they do not have sufficient time to do justice to so many evaluations; initial appraisals may be thorough, while later ones are likely to be rushed as deadlines approach. Managers with large numbers of employees may not be equally familiar with all aspects of every employee's work. Older performance appraisal systems were often based on the rating of personality characteristics. Even though such systems have mostly changed, longtime managers often continue to render personality judgments when appraising performance.

Personality-Based Evaluations

Older systems of performance appraisal often relied heavily on assessing personality characteristics. This yielded evaluations that were highly subjective and that did not focus on how an employee performed relative to an objective standard. **EXHIBIT 9-1** contains examples taken from an old rating form. Supervisors checked the statement that best described the employee being evaluated. Comments have been added to demonstrate the weaknesses of personality-based appraisals.

Exhibit 9-1 is typical of a performance appraisal that relies on subjective evaluations. Managerial uneasiness with such appraisals is understandable. A subjective assessment is merely an opinion when expressed by someone who is not qualified in the particular area of judgment. Few managers are qualified to render meaningful decisions about personality. Using criteria similar to those listed in Exhibit 9-1, managers were required to make judgments they were not qualified to make and could not possibly defend but that nevertheless could affect people's employment.

Such appraisals were as unsettling to employees as they were to managers. Few employees will willingly or readily endorse negative assessments. These performance appraisals were common in environments where authoritarian management prevailed. In such a situation, an evaluator could freely use personal opinions, unsupported judgments, and personal biases on evaluations. Employees who wanted to keep their jobs had no recourse other than checking their anger and returning to work.

Performance Appraisals

The appropriate way to appraise performance is to base the evaluation on what an employee *does* rather than on what an employee *is* or *knows*. For decades, managers rated employees on job knowledge. In addition to being subjective, such an assessment provided little or no value. Job knowledge is immaterial. What really matters is how knowledge is applied or what results are achieved.

The correct approach to appraisal is to base an evaluation on how well employees are performing the jobs they are expected to do. Preparation for appraisal begins by considering the specific tasks that make up the job being performed.

EXHIBIT 9-1 Example of a Personality-Based Rating System

I. Attendance
   1. Punctuality
      __ Always on time
      __ Occasionally late
      __ Requires occasional reminding
      __ Often tardy; treats job as unimportant
      __ Always tardy

      Commentary: In old evaluation systems, attendance was often the only quantifiable item. Above, subjectivity has been introduced. *Occasionally* and *often* are undefined. *Treats job as unimportant* is a conclusion that cannot be verified. *Always* and *never* are very dangerous words; rarely are they absolutely true.
   2. Dependability
      __ Perfect since last rating
      __ Rarely absent
      __ Frequently absent, but for cause
      __ Poor record, requires counseling
      __ Unsatisfactory; work suffers

      Commentary: Each of these statements is completely subjective. Again there are words, such as *rarely* and *frequently*, that have no absolute meanings. Evaluating whether an employee's absences are for cause cannot be done factually without violating an employee's privacy. As long as the employee has called in according to policy, the manager must take each absence at face value.
II. Personal qualifications
   3. Appearance
      __ Neat and in good taste
      __ Neat but occasionally not in good taste
      __ Sometimes careless about appearance
      __ Untidy
      __ Unsuitable for job

      Commentary: All five items are highly subjective. What is "good taste" and who defines it? When does untidy become casual? This entire subsection is out of line. If used in an evaluation, appearance should be brought up only in reference to an understood dress code or set of professional standards of conduct.
   4. Personality
      __ Exceptionally pleasing, a decided asset
      __ Makes good impression, wears well
      __ Makes good first impression only; does not wear well
      __ Makes fair impression only
      __ Creates unfavorable impression

      Commentary: Each of the five statements contains imprecise terminology. The entire subsection is completely irrelevant to an employee performance appraisal.
III. Attitude toward job
   5. Interest
      __ Shows intense enthusiasm and interest in all work
      __ Shows interest; enthusiasm is not sustained
      __ Passive acceptance; rarely shows enthusiasm
      __ Shows little or no interest
      __ Dislikes work

Commentary: Although often attempted, no one can appropriately evaluate or discipline attitude. These imprecise statements are useless in appraising an employee. The final one is an unwarranted and insupportable conclusion.

6.   Cooperation
    __ Goes all out to cooperate with management and coworkers
    __ Promotes cooperation and goodwill
    __ Moderately successful in cooperating with others
    __ Cooperates reluctantly and sometimes causes dissension
    __ Uncooperative; often breeds trouble

Commentary: How do the first two statements differ? The rest of the statements cannot be successfully defended.

IV.   Job performance
7.   Accuracy
    __ Rarely makes mistakes
    __ Above average
    __ Average
    __ Below average
    __ Highly inaccurate

Commentary: These statements are subjective without a quantified definition of average.

8.   Neatness
    __ Takes pride in appearance of work; has sense of neatness
    __ Usually turns out neat work
    __ Apparently lacks sense of neatness; needs reminding
    __ Too often sacrifices neatness for quantity
    __ Majority of work must be done over

Commentary: All questions depend on a subjective definition of *neat*.

9.   Quantity
    __ Unusually high output; meets emergency demands well
    __ Consistently turns out more than average
    __ Finishes allotted amount
    __ Does just enough to get by
    __ Amount of work done is inadequate

Commentary: Quantity is undefined, rendering it subjective.

Solid Position Descriptions

A sound performance appraisal begins with a solid position description. A position description is usually written by a department manager with assistance from HR and ideally with input from the person or persons doing the job.

Up-to-date position descriptions are necessary for several reasons, an important one being their use in performance appraisal. To evaluate employees on what they actually do requires a clear picture of what is expected of each employee. The tasks to be performed and the results to be achieved provide a baseline against which to compare observed performance. These are often referred to as *competencies*. Criteria refer to the requirements of a job or position, while competencies refer to mastery of applied knowledge and skills that fulfill the requirements of a position description.

A primary shortcoming of many position descriptions is the extent of detail their writers attempt to capture. A long and detailed position description leads to excessive length and detail in a performance appraisal. Position descriptions should be concise. For most entry-level jobs or nonprofessional positions, five to eight items describing the most time-consuming job responsibilities in descending order of time devoted to them are adequate. These should be able to capture 90% or more of the job duties and time spent in a year. Excessive detail places a manager at risk of paying as much attention to minor concerns as to major job requirements.

EXHIBIT 9-2 presents a sample description for the position of nursing assistant. The duties listed encompass more than 90% of the tasks an employee performs on a typical day throughout a year. Greater detail is possible but not desirable. The supervisors who know the job and employees as they should be able to provide competent and complete appraisals.

A position description should be one of the first considerations when a new position is created. An existing position description should be reviewed and

EXHIBIT 9-2 Sample Position Description

Department: Nursing
Position: Nursing Assistant, General Medical/Surgical
Grade: N-3
Job Code: 607
Reports to: Unit Manager (will occasionally report to designated nurse in charge)
Principal Duties (listed in descending order of approximate percentage of time required):

1. Provides timely personal care of acceptable quality to patients in accordance with established policies, procedures, standards, and approved individualized care plans in a manner mindful of patient privacy, comfort, and safety.
2. Performs routine treatments and other patient care duties as assigned, competently completing all assigned treatments during the scheduled shift; assists RN or LPN with nursing care and treatments as needed.
3. Assists RN or LPN in gathering data for patient assessment, including vital signs and height, weight, intake and output, and other measurements as applicable; demonstrates ability to recognize and report abnormal vital signs; demonstrates proper ability to collect and accurately label specimens and samples.
4. Maintains positive interpersonal relationships with patients, visitors, and other staff while ensuring confidentiality of patient information and protection of patient privacy.
5. Maintains conscientious work habits consistent with the standards of the Nursing Department specifically: documenting clearly and completely, managing assignments with normal supervision, completing duties within the assigned shift, accepting reassignment to other units as necessary, and responding favorably to reasonable requests to remain beyond the shift when needed.
6. Operates equipment and performs work in a safe manner, demonstrating proper body mechanics in lifting, pulling, pushing, and carrying.
7. Maintains the clinical and educational standards of the department: maintains CPR certification and demonstrates effective performance during "code" procedures; participates in unit and department in-service education activities; remains current with all continuing education requirements.
8. Undertakes other assignments as directed by the unit manager or officially designated charge nurse.

updated when it becomes necessary to recruit for the position, when there are obvious changes in the job such as new methods or equipment, or every 2 years, whichever occurs first. Another good time to review position descriptions for currency is when preparing to conduct performance appraisals.

Once a position description is current, attention should turn to measuring performance against the task requirements or assessing whether an employee's results are acceptable. Objective measures can usually be applied to many elements of most jobs.

Sources of Standards and Measures

Measures of performance should address four key dimensions: productivity, quality, timeliness, and cost. Sources of performance standards include detailed time-study and methods analysis. Accurate standards can often be developed using this approach, but the processes are time consuming and costly. Such approaches are most suitable in the development of standards for high-volume, highly repetitive activities that are infrequently encountered in health care.

Predetermined motion-time systems yield highly accurate standards, but these are also both costly and time consuming and again most suitable for high-volume, repetitive activities.

Reasonably, reliable standards can be established through work sampling. This is time consuming but not nearly as costly as the methods described earlier. Nevertheless, work sampling requires special skills and a person who can be dedicated to developing standards. Work sampling is most applicable to moderately repetitive activities.

Benchmarks are indicators of productivity that have been developed through the collective experience of several organizations or published by interested groups such as associations of healthcare organizations or technical and professional societies. Benchmarks are inexpensive. They are often free to members of an association or available via a purchased subscription to a statistical reporting service. Benchmarks are readily applicable but usually not as accurate as the other sources described. Benchmarks can be misleading because users often have no clear knowledge of the method on which a benchmark is based. **EXHIBIT 9-3** provides examples of indicators for which standards may be established or benchmarks acquired. These relate to productivity or quantity, quality, time, and cost.

Ranges

Benchmarks or other data provide the basis for assessing individuals or teams of employees. Ranges are preferable to absolute standards. Attendance provides a simple example. Rather than setting a rigid standard of three absences in a 12-month period, an organization may establish an acceptable range of three to five absences in a 12-month period.

This allows supervisors to caution employees about problems before they become serious. It provides a simple system for appraising behavior. Having 3–5 absences in a 12-month period constitutes meeting the standard. Employees with six or more absences fail to meet the standard. Those with two or fewer absences exceed the standard.

EXHIBIT 9-3 Examples of Objective or Quantifiable Indicators

For Productivity (Quantity)

- Number of patients served per unit of time
- Number of items processed or produced per unit of time
- Number of cases handled per unit of time
- Percentage of employees participating
- Percentage of employees absent or tardy

For Quality

- Percentage of retakes (radiology) or test repeats (laboratory)
- Error rate
- Percentage of down time (equipment out of service)
- Number of citations upon inspection or survey
- Percentage of work rejected
- Percentage of orders, bills, or other documents without error

For Time

- Number or percentage of bills out within a specified number of days
- Number or percentage of deadlines missed
- Number of days to complete a task or project
- Time elapsed or turnaround time
- Number or percentage of requests answered within a specified number of days

For Cost

- Expense compared with previous period
- Percentage of variance from budget
- Cost per item, per order received, per bill processed, per patient contact
- Overtime cost compared with target
- Contract help cost compared with target

Using Objectives

Some employees may be evaluated on how well they meet objectives that were based on previous evaluations. Objectives are best established jointly by individual employees and their managers. A manager ensures that each objective is pertinent, while an employee agrees that each objective is fair and reasonable. Some appraisal processes, especially those involving technical, professional, or managerial employees, rely on such objectives. Some objectives arise from weaknesses revealed during an evaluation. Some objectives relate to personal development.

The appraisal approach based on management by objectives, largely applicable to managers and professionals, consists mainly of objectives negotiated between employees and their immediate superiors. An appropriate objective always includes a description or definition of *what* is to be achieved, *how much* will be accomplished, and *when* it will be done (a date for completion). Without all three components, an objective is incomplete and lacks legitimacy.

EXHIBIT 9-4 Examples of Poor Appraisal Scales

Experience with more modern appraisal systems has shown that a small number of gradations are most desirable. Having an odd number of gradations places "average" in the middle position. Some systems use five points. Many highly effective job description–based systems use only three points. These are more than sufficient to assess performance. Each task on a job description should have a corresponding scale to rate the standard or expectation of behavior. An employee can then fall into only one of three positions relative to the standard or expectation: failed to meet the standard, met the standard, or exceeded the standard. Such a three-point scale is especially appropriate when standards use ranges rather than absolute numbers.

Scale Points

A number of older appraisal systems require an evaluator to measure or judge each evaluation criterion using a scale composed of gradations and check-off boxes or blanks. **EXHIBIT 9-4** contains examples of actual scales from older systems used for appraisal. Many different evaluation scales have been employed. Most of them have similar weaknesses in that they require an evaluator to render a subjective judgment using an arbitrary scale that lacks definition.

Average Versus Standard

In many appraisal systems, *average* is used to describe a desired level of performance. For example, a scale may place doing an average job in the center position. However, organizations often use standards or standard performance to indicate a minimally acceptable output. All too often, these terms are incorrectly and inappropriately interchanged. *Average* and *standard* are not the same.

Equating *average* with *standard* suggests that half of all employees are below the minimum acceptable level of performance and should probably not be employed. A goal of every reasonable appraisal system should be bringing all employees to an acceptable minimum or higher level of performance. *Standard* becomes the floor beneath which performance should not be considered acceptable.

Thus, *standard* is conventionally used as the minimum acceptable level of performance. If that is the minimum and all other levels of output are above it, then the true average or mean of a group is also above standard. *Average* may be a convenient way to compare or group scores once evaluations have been quantified, but *average* should not be used to describe the expectations of a performance appraisal process.

Appraisal Timing

An employee's initial performance appraisal typically occurs at the end of the probationary employment period, in most instances at either 3 or 6 months of service. The probationary evaluation is undertaken to assess whether the employee has learned the job adequately, after which the individual enters the regular evaluation cycle. In the majority of organizations, employees are evaluated annually, although in some organizations the evaluation interval is 6 months.

There are two common approaches to an annual appraisal. All employees may be evaluated in the same brief time once each year, or employees may be evaluated on or near their employment anniversary dates. Each approach has advantages and disadvantages.

For some supervisors, completing all evaluations during one brief period improves the consistency in applying evaluation criteria. Completing all appraisals at the same time can support a pay-for-performance compensation system by allowing the accurate distribution of a predetermined amount of money because all appraisal scores are known at the same time. For some supervisors, all-at-once evaluation puts an unwelcome task behind them for the better part of a year (or half-year, given a twice-a-year cycle).

Critics of simultaneous appraisals note that the task usually consumes a major amount of a manager's time and forces other important matters to be temporarily ignored. The quality of appraisals can diminish as the evaluator works through the group; this risk rises as the number of employees increases.

Proponents of anniversary date appraisal ordinarily contend that the appraisal workload is distributed more or less evenly throughout the year, thereby avoiding a rush within a brief period. Some see appraisals approached this way are likely to be fairer because they are not rushed. Opponents of anniversary date appraisal often contend that the process requires constant monitoring by higher management and HR rather than oversight for only a limited period. Seen this way, the appraisal task is never caught up. Performance appraisals should be completed faithfully for every employee at the appointed time. However, managers and their employees should have established relationships; simply meeting once each year for an appraisal interview is not sufficient. A manager must maintain an ongoing relationship with each employee and be available to discuss work performance whenever circumstances warrant. Supervisors make a serious error when they accumulate issues—"save up stuff" (especially negatives)—specifically for performance appraisal.

▶ Describing the Appraisal Procedure

An organization's performance appraisal process will ordinarily be described in a personnel policy and procedure manual. This document will explain the features of the process and delineate responsibilities for different stages. This description should be available for reference by employees at any time. **EXHIBIT 9-5** presents a model policy and procedure for an appraisal process based on anniversary date approach.

▶ The Appraisal Interview

Most performance appraisal systems stipulate that each employee receive a personal interview. An appraisal interview is a requirement; a manager's appraisals are not considered complete until all employees have had an opportunity to discuss their appraisals in detail. Managers should be certain that each appraisal interview occurs on time. Few events within a workplace can raise apprehensions and uncertainties faster than appraisal interviews that are late.

EXHIBIT 9-5 Model Policy and Procedure: Performance Appraisal

It is the policy of the hospital to provide a formal performance appraisal for each employee at least once each year. The purposes of the appraisal program are to:

- Maintain or improve performance in the job an employee currently holds
- Assist in employee development by providing learning and growth opportunities for those wishing to advance
- Assist the hospital in identifying individuals with advancement potential

Performance appraisal applies to designated employees as follows:

1. Newly hired employees:
   - The first appraisal will occur at the end of the initial 3-month probationary period.
   - The second appraisal will occur 3 months following the probationary appraisal.
   - The following appraisal will occur 6 months later, or on approximately the employee's first anniversary of employment.
2. Employees promoted or transferred:
   - The initial appraisal conducted in an employee's new position will occur at either 3 months or 6 months depending on the learning period established for the particular position.
   - Following successful completion of the learning period, the employee will revert to the normal appraisal scheduled per (3), as follows.
3. All employees:
   - Once having successfully completed the first year of employment or the learning period following promotion or transfer, all employees will be subject to appraisal on approximately the anniversary of their employment.

General Provisions of the Performance Appraisal Program:

- Appraisals in addition to those indicated in the foregoing may be instituted by the department manager when either a significant deterioration or a marked improvement in performance is evident.
- Regular communication with employees concerning performance is essential. Continuing positive communication can assist in motivating and reinforcing outstanding performance, which is the objective of the appraisal process. Regular communication may also call attention to specific needs for improvement in performance, and immediately addressing areas of need will help prevent them from emerging as major problems at formal appraisal time.
- An appropriate performance appraisal should:
  1. Provide an employee with guidance in growing and developing as a performer.
  2. Provide a manager with a means for personalizing management guidance to individual employees.
  3. Provide an employee with direction consistent with that appropriate for pursuing the objectives of the department and organization.
  4. Provide a manager with a means to assess an employee's performance and place a value on the effectiveness of this performance.
  5. Result in a more effective workforce, as individuals tend to perform more appropriately when they know what is expected of them and they are able to gauge their performance against periodic measurement.

(continues)

EXHIBIT 9-5 Model Policy and Procedure: Performance Appraisal *(continued)*

The following procedure applies to the performance appraisal process:

4. Approximately 30 days in advance of an employee's scheduled appraisal date, human resources will send the department manager an appraisal form for the employee with the heading information completed.

5. The employee's job description provides the basis for the appraisal. Before attempting the appraisal, a manager should ascertain that the job description is complete and accurate. If necessary, the job description should be updated at this time, before the appraisal is begun.

6. In addressing the appraisal, for exempt (salaried) professional, technical, and supervisory employees, the manager should assess performance primarily against the actual accomplishment of duties and responsibilities as delineated in the job description. Nonexempt (hourly) employees should be assessed primarily on the timely and accurate completion of assigned duties.

7. As appropriate, and provided that plans and objectives were delineated when the previous appraisal was discussed, consideration should also be given to employee growth and development and improvements in performance that might have occurred since the previous appraisal.

8. Objective, quantifiable measures of performance should be applied wherever possible. For example, the hospital's standards for attendance and punctuality may be applied, as may the output standards available in some departments. For duties for which no objective measure of performance is available, managers should be able to reasonably describe a normal expectation and indicate why, in their judgment, the employee did or did not meet or exceed the expectation.

9. Once completed, each appraisal must be submitted for review and approval by the next highest level of management.

10. When higher management approval of an appraisal has been secured, the manager may schedule the employee for an appraisal conference. Every effort should be made to accomplish this conference no more than 5 working days before or after the employee's anniversary date.

11. The manager is urged to follow good interviewing practices in conducting the appraisal conference by providing adequate time, privacy, reasonable comfort, and freedom from interruptions.

12. As appropriate (primarily for technical, professional, and supervisory employees), the manager and employee will jointly determine goals, objectives, and development plans to be pursued during the period preceding the next appraisal. As necessary, they should achieve agreement on interim dates on which to examine progress between appraisals.

13. At the completion of the appraisal conference, the employee should be asked to sign the appraisal document to acknowledge having discussed it and received a copy. If necessary, the employee may be reminded that signing the appraisal is simply acknowledgment and does not necessarily mean agreement with all that it says. The employee may add comments of disagreement or agreement in the appropriate space on the appraisal form.

14. Should employees refuse to sign their appraisal, a manager should so note the fact on the form. If, in the manager's judgment, the employee is in strong disagreement with the appraisal and may appeal or take other action, the manager should have another party witness the refusal to sign and so indicate on the form.

15. Following the conference, the completed appraisal is distributed as follows:
    - Original to Human Resources
    - Copy to employee
    - Copy retained by manager

Managers should schedule sufficient time for each meeting. Although an appraisal interview may seem routine to a manager, it is one of the most important annual events for many employees, so it should never seem rushed. Privacy and freedom from interruptions are important considerations. Employees should have several days' advance notice so they can be prepared.

If an appraisal involves objectives as well as ratings, then supervisors should review the objectives well beforehand and be prepared to discuss them. The manager should come to the interview with ideas or suggestions concerning objectives for the next cycle. If improvement or correction is needed, manager and employee should agree on appropriate steps to achieve both.

As with any other kind of interview, from a manager's perspective, the most important parts of an appraisal interview occur while the evaluator is listening, not speaking. Whenever delivering praise or criticism, the manager should be certain to address specifics; generalizations are not useful and should be avoided. Before concluding an interview, supervisors should ask employees to sign the appraisal form to acknowledge receipt. This does not indicate agreement with the findings or conclusions. If an employee declines to sign the form, this should be noted before the form is filed. Also, it is important to supply signed copies of all evaluation documents to employees.

Employees occasionally report to more than one supervisor. This occurs with overlapping shift assignments or split-shift responsibilities. When this occurs, the primary input must come from the manager who provides the most direct supervision. This is supplemented with input from other involved supervisors. The manager who provides the majority of direct supervision should be the one who conducts the appraisal interview.

Neither the written performance appraisal nor the appraisal interview should contain surprises for an employee. Employees should have a clear idea of their standing with their manager at all times; it is a manager's responsibility to ensure this is the case.

▶ Self-Appraisal

Self-appraisal can be a productive component of a performance appraisal system. However, self-appraisal is not appropriate for everyone. Some employees are intimidated by it. Others are apprehensive, fearing the possible consequences of rating themselves too high or too low. Self-appraisal is most appropriate for higher-level technical employees, professionals, supervisors, and managers. While self-appraisal has some potential advantages, many hourly employees are suspicious of the process and management's intent when using it.

While some people rate themselves higher or lower than may be appropriate, research has repeatedly shown that the majority of employees rate themselves no higher, and frequently lower, than their supervisors rate them. When it is used, an employee should complete a self-appraisal while a manager completes an evaluation. These tasks should be completed separately; that is, neither appraisal should be permitted to bias the other.

The forms should be similar and should address the same major job description criteria. The forms should be exchanged for the first time during an appraisal interview. The items on both appraisals should be compared one at a time. Both participants should note items on which they differ appreciably. Areas of divergence highlight an important aspect of self-appraisal and focus discussion where it is most likely to be needed. For example, if a manager evaluates an employee on 12 criteria and the employee does a self-appraisal using the same criteria and they find their two assessments are close to each other for 9 or 10 criteria, they know their ensuing discussion should focus on the two or three areas where their evaluations differ the most.

Self-appraisal is not appropriate for every situation. However, when appraising employees who are required to exercise some degree of independent discretion and judgment, self-appraisal can be a constructive adjunct to a performance appraisal system. Self-appraisal draws employees more deeply into the appraisal process and transforms it into more of a participative activity.

▶ Team Appraisals

Organizations have been assembling and using teams during recent decades. Teams present evaluation challenges to managers. Individual evaluations rendered in a team environment can be troublesome because they tend to undermine teamwork and cooperation by stressing individual competitiveness. They can encourage competitive individuals to circumvent team requirements for individual gain and to fail to nurture an open, problem-solving environment. Individual performance appraisals do not support team building because they lack a means of identifying the effects of individuals on the group or the group on individuals. Individual appraisals can impede effective team building.

Teams can be appraised as groups. However, a glaring weakness lies in the inevitable differences that exist among individuals. Different people perform in different ways. A properly managed team should be able to use the different strengths of all its members. Likewise, it should be clear to any group that functions well that a team is no place for either single stars or individual slackers.

As with individual performance appraisals, team evaluations require criteria and standards. These must be constructed specifically in terms of team performance. In many organizations, group or team appraisals supplement rather than replace individual performance appraisals. Thus, although the emphasis on groups and team performance continues to increase, most reward and recognition systems remain focused on individuals. This reinforces the need to appraise both team and individual performances.

▶ The Appraisal Form

A significant shortcoming of many performance appraisal systems lies in a tendency to try to address far too much detail. A lengthy, detailed appraisal form creates extraneous work for appraisers and rapidly fills personnel files with paper. Some organizations have tried to compensate for this by filing only a summary document. All too often, such an approach also requires a key for interpretation. Once filed, an appraisal should be a self-contained record that can be understood on its own if it is referenced in the future.

No single appraisal form is right for all situations. The most useful forms are those that have a minimum of fill-in spaces and a maximum of open writing space. Two or three pages should be sufficient for most performance appraisal forms. Following an appraisal interview and obtaining signatures from both supervisor and employee, three copies should be made of each performance appraisal. The original should be sent to HR and added to an employee's personnel file, a copy is given to the employee, and a copy is retained by the evaluator.

EXHIBITS 9-6 and **9-7** provide examples of actual performance appraisal forms. Exhibit 9-6 is generic, an open format that can conceivably be used along with many different job descriptions. The rating scale is simple and has three options. The numbers attached to these three levels of performance are simply a convenience for converting the appraisal results into an overall score for organizational use. Exhibit 9-7 contains an outline that is completed by adding specific information from a position description. It uses a three-point scale with the standard or expected level of performance in the middle. This exhibit allows individual components to be weighted. Exhibit 9-7 demonstrates how position descriptions and appraisal forms can be combined into a single document.

EXHIBIT 9-6 Generic Performance Appraisal Form

Employee Name: _____ ID No. _____

Department: _____ Hire Date: _____

Job Title/Grade: _____ Job Date: _____

Job Description Requirement Rating

No. Task and Expectation (Standard)   Not met   Met   Exceeded

_____

_____

_____

_____

_____

Scoring: Number Not Met: ___ × 0 = _____

Number Met: ___ × 2   = _____

Number Exceeded ___ × 4   = _____

Total   = _____

Average   = _____

Average less than 2.0 means improvement needed

Average of 2.0 means standard performance

Average greater than 2.0 means exceptional performance

Manager's comments:

Employee's comments:

Date of discussion:

Employee signature:

Manager signature:

EXHIBIT 9-7   Position-Specific Performance Appraisal Form

Job Title/Grade: _____ Job Date: _____

Department: _____ Hire Date: _____

Incumbent name: _____ ID No. _____

Summary: (obtain from position description)

Requirements: (obtain from position description)

I. First task (a):	Weight (c)	Rating Score (d)
Element (b) _ (c) _ _ (d) _		
a. Element one		1 2 3
b. Element two		1 2 3
c. Element three		1 2 3

Comments:

2. Second task (e):	Weight (c)	Rating Score (d)
Element (b) _ (c) _ _ (d) _		
a. Element one		1 2 3
b. Element two		1 2 3
c. Element three		1 2 3
d. Comments:		

Manager:

Employee:

HR:

3.   from position description with three specific elements; number of tasks is not fixed

4.   elements defined according to position description

5.   established by supervisor, manager, or HR per organizational policy

6.   weight × sum of total scores for all three elements

7.   handled in same manner as the first task

▶ Legal Implications of Performance Appraisal

Performance appraisal has become a regulatory necessity in health care. The Joint Commission (TJC) looks for appraisals in the personnel files during its periodic surveys, as do many state health departments. Performance appraisals are surely completed for employee development, but they must also be completed and signed and filed to avoid being cited for deficiencies when surveyed.

Although there are legal risks associated with completing and retaining performance appraisals, on balance the legal risks of not doing so are greater. When an employee is terminated for reasons related to job performance or is chosen for lay-off and the action is contested, performance appraisal documents in the personnel file become a central concern. Appraisals should support management's decisions. Decisions that cannot be substantiated by documentation are highly likely to be considered the result of discrimination or other personal bias.

Performance appraisals frequently figure prominently in wrongful discharge litigation. When there is a chance that a discharge was based wholly or in part on substandard performance, a wrongful discharge claim may be filed, and information will be sought in the appraisal records in personnel files. Thus, many wrongful discharge lawsuits are an outgrowth of inadequate performance appraisals. Consider: An employee is designated for layoff based on substandard work performance. The employee files a wrongful discharge complaint, and an investigation ensues. The individual's personnel file is examined, and what the investigator finds is several performance appraisals in which the employee has been rated at least satisfactory. This not uncommon scenario has played out in many organizations. Such "no-fault" appraisals are common, resulting when managers take what is apparently the easy way through an unwelcome task, rating everyone's performance at least nominally satisfactory so as to avoid coming to grips with issues of marginal performance. This is, in part, why appraisal is unpopular with many managers; they do not care to be critical on an instrument that can affect someone's employment in some way, so they look the other way and gloss over a few performance issues and create "no-fault" appraisals. But these kinds of appraisals can become troublesome when legal actions arise. Perhaps even more important, the manager who rates a substandard or marginal performer satisfactory is not doing the employee any favors; it is that manager's responsibility to address employee performance problems so as to provide every reasonable chance to enable the employee to improve and succeed.

The largest number of legal complaints centered on performance appraisal issues involves alleged violations of individual rights as specified under Title VII of the Civil Rights Act of 1964. Performance appraisal records may be examined closely if performance is used as a criterion in determining who will be included in a large layoff or planned reduction in force. This is emphasized if there appears to be a disparate impact on any group or class of employees, a common complaint arising from the layoff of older workers.

Although there is no way to avoid some subjective assessments in performance appraisals, these are best kept to a minimum. Always avoid potentially defamatory comments as well as insults, name-calling, and unsupported negative commentary. Whenever entering negative assessments, cite specifics that can be supported by data or otherwise proven.

An organization is not legally obligated to have a performance appraisal system. Once a system is put in place, however, an employer may be seen as having created an implied contract with employees to use the system as established and described. A performance appraisal system should be sufficiently formal to have published instructions for completing appraisals. These instructions, as well as any evidence that can be presented concerning the training of appraisers in the system's use, can be helpful in defending the appraisal system against charges of discrimination.

▶ The Role of Human Resources

The HR department is usually the custodian of an organization's performance appraisal system. The role of human resources in performance appraisal includes monitoring job descriptions and evaluation criteria to ensure that these are always up to date and currently applicable. Human resources typically designs an appraisal system. Ideally, design and modification should be a joint effort involving HR and managers of both line and support activities. Human resources should schedule the steps in the process, including establishing dates for forms to be sent out, appraisals to be written and discussed with employees, and completed documents sent back.

Human resources should provide forms, lists, and time schedules to department managers as needed. In a system under which employees are evaluated on anniversary dates, someone in HR should constantly monitor the system and send out forms and reminders as employees' anniversary dates occur. Human resources should monitor the incoming appraisals for completeness and consistency. Under some appraisal systems, appraisers are required to have their evaluations reviewed by the next level of management before they are discussed and submitted.

Human resources has a responsibility to hold classes for evaluators, providing both original and refresher appraisal training every year. Human resources usually responds to evaluators' questions about appraisal. It follows up to ensure that evaluations are completed within the proper time period. The HR department usually files completed evaluations in individual personnel files and addresses employee questions and grievances about the appraisal process.

Following up on appraisal completion is often stressful for line managers and HR staff. Managers may place a low priority on completing appraisals if they view the process as less than essential. They may complain about pressure and insufficient time to complete evaluations. In contrast, HR must follow higher management's mandate to keep the system moving. Timely appraisals are always important. Because they provide the reminders, many managers view appraisals as being an HR system at best and mere HR paperwork at worst.

▶ An Essential Process

Most employees perform at a satisfactory or better level. Individual results are seldom unacceptable. Despite this, some managers neglect to express appreciation of employee successes and instead focus on failures and weaknesses. Unfortunately, they take the good for granted. This tendency to focus on the unsatisfactory simply reinforces the reputation of performance appraisal as a negative process.

Human resources alone cannot guarantee a successful appraisal process; a few conscientious department managers working together also cannot do so. A critical element in the success of performance appraisal is the extent to which top management supports the process. Far too often, top management simply assigns supervisors to complete the process while failing to participate in any substantive manner. Lack of visible executive support increases the risk of appraisal becoming a meaningless routine. Many organizations, including those in health care, have performance appraisal systems. However, the existence of a system does not guarantee that performance appraisal is carried out in an effective manner.

▶ Conclusion

The importance of regular, structured employee appraisals cannot be overstated. Supervisors must be well trained and diligent about completing employee evaluations on time. Forms and procedures must be current. The personal interview that follows a written appraisal is often dreaded by employees. Successful managers use the interview as a positive experience to review and motivate their employees. Human resources supervises the appraisal process and collects and files completed appraisal forms.

🔍 CASE STUDY: Resolution

Returning to the conversation that Stu and Maria were having, Stu said, "I wonder what basis the court used for its decision?"

Marcia smiled. "The two latest annual appraisals that you completed."

"No."

"Yes," she said, heading out the door of Stu's office.

SPOTLIGHT ON CUSTOMER SERVICE

Customer Service and Performance Appraisals

Performance appraisals are not universally popular. More to the point, they are often dreaded by both supervisors and workers. Managers dislike them because they require both time and conversations with supervisees. Workers dislike them because they often involve hearing uncomfortable or unpleasant news. Despite their lack of popularity, performance appraisals are (or should be) completed every year for all employees in an organization. This should be an organizational policy for which no exceptions are allowed.

Because "Provides good customer service" is rarely included on position descriptions, it is not often included in annual performance appraisals. Two remedies are available for this problem. Both are relatively easy. The first is adding a line to existing appraisal checklists. The other is including customer service as a duty or responsibility on every position description used by an organization. Modifying an appraisal checklist has the advantage of requiring minimal effort and expense. Its disadvantage is providing a reminder about the importance of customer service only once each year. Modifying position descriptions requires considerable time and effort with associated expenses for labor. Offsetting these disadvantages, employees are frequently reminded about the importance of customer service. Candidates for employment and newly hired employees are exposed to the organization's commitment to customer service from the very beginning.

Questions for Review and Discussion

1. Explain the difference between *average* and *standard* as these terms are used in performance appraisal. Discuss how one is erroneously used.
2. Some management experts have recommended that performance appraisal be abolished. Provide three reasons why performance appraisals should be retained in modern healthcare organizations.
3. Consider an employee who always performs satisfactorily but has little or no opportunity to improve, and can go no higher in the organization and does

not aspire to do so. Why is it considered necessary to continue periodically appraising this employee's performance?

4. Why are employee performance appraisals often described as a manager's least favorite responsibility?
5. Why should all appraisal processes avoid addressing personality characteristics of employees?
6. Why is it appropriate to begin addressing an employee's performance with a review and update of the person's job description?
7. What are the three essential elements of an objective? Why are all three needed?
8. Why is it important to ensure that employee appraisals occur when they are scheduled to occur?
9. What is the primary shortcoming of team appraisal? How can this be avoided but still use a team appraisal?
10. Why is the HR department a reasonable place from which to coordinate an organization's performance appraisal process?
11. Managers do not always provide consistent appraisals. How can this problem be addressed?
12. How can past appraisals of performance influence the outcomes of employment-related legal actions?

Resources
Books

Delpo, A. (2005). *Performance appraisal handbook: Legal and practical rules for managers*. Berkeley, CA: NOLO.
Falcone, P. (2005). *2600 phrases for effective performance reviews: Ready-to-use words and phrases that really get results*. Chicago, IL: American Management Association.
Forster, N. (2005). *Maximum performance: A practical guide to leading and managing people at work*. London, UK: Edward Elgar.
McConnell, C. (2013). *The health care manager's human resources handbook* (2nd ed.). Burlington, MA: Jones & Bartlett Learning.
Paauwe, J. (2004). *HRM and performance: Achieving long term viability*. New York, NY: Oxford University Press.
Packard, P., & Slater, J. (2005). *Skills of appraisal*. London, UK: Ashgate.
Rothwell, W. J. (2005). *Effective succession planning: Ensuring leadership continuity and building talent from within* (3rd ed.). Chicago, IL: American Management Association.

Periodicals

Carmeli, A., & Schaubroeck, J. (2005). How leveraging human resource capital with its competitive distinctiveness enhances the performance of commercial and public organizations. *Human Resource Management, 44*(4), 391–412.
Cintron, R., & Flanikan, F. (2011). Performance appraisal: A supervision or leadership tool? *International Journal of Business and Social Science, 2*(17), 29–37.
Gerhart, B., Wright, P., McMahan, G., & Snell, S. (2000). Error in research on human resources and firm performance: How much error is there and how does it influence affect size estimates? *Personnel Psychology, 53*, 803–834.
Givan, R. K. (2005). Seeing stars: Human resources performance indicators in the National Health Service. *Personnel Review, 34*(6), 634–647.

Hitt, M. A., Bierman, K., Shimizu, L., & Kochhar, R. (2001). Direct and moderating effects of human capital on strategy and performance in professional service firms: A resource-based perspective. *Academy of Management Journal, 44,* 13–28.

Propper, C., & Wilson, D. (2003). The use and usefulness of performance measures in the public sector. *Oxford Review of Economic Policy, 19*(2), 250–267.

Robie, C., Johnson, K. M., Nilsen, D., & Hazucha, J. F. (2001). The right stuff: Understanding cultural differences in leadership performance. *Journal of Management Development, 20*(7), 639–650.

Wright, T. A., & Cropanzano, R. (1998). Emotional exhaustion as a predictor of job performance and voluntary turnover. *Journal of Applied Psychology, 83*(3), 486–493.

CHAPTER 10

Succession Planning

CHAPTER OBJECTIVES

After studying this chapter, readers will be able to:

- Understand the goals of succession planning.
- Appreciate the importance of creating succession plans.
- Understand the forces and factors that motivate healthcare organizations to create succession plans.
- Understand the process of effective succession planning.
- Recognize the importance of grooming successors.
- Understand why many healthcare organizations have not created succession plans.

▶ Chapter Summary

Succession planning is regarded by many as an organizational necessity for administrative positions and for a layer or two of executive management reporting to these top management positions. Succession planning need not be limited to just the positions in the upper reaches of the organizational hierarchy, but even in many organizations that have formal succession plans, it is approached just that way: What is to be done if the chief executive officer (CEO), chief financial officer (CFO), chief operating officer (COO), or other top brass suddenly drop off the organization chart? What will be involved in filling the gap created by an unanticipated departure?

This presentation of succession planning advances the belief that every management position, from CEO to the first-line supervisor, should be covered by some process for ensuring that a suddenly vacated management position will not go begging because there is no one ready to step into the breach. There will, however, be considerable differences in the depth and formality of a plan of succession depending on organizational level.

🔍 *CASE STUDY: Crash*

A private jet chartered to fly from New York City to Orlando, Florida, crashed in the ocean, killing all aboard. Among the passengers were the Memorial Hospital CEO, his three top managers, and the chair of the governing board. They were flying to Orlando to attend a national healthcare conference. The manager of human resources (HR) at Memorial Hospital was summoned to the phone to receive the devastating news. She gasped, turned pale, looked expressionlessly at her assistant, and uttered four words, "Now who's in charge?"

How would you handle the situation? How could this lack of continuity in leadership have been avoided?

▶ Introduction to Succession Planning

Succession planning is an important issue for nearly every organization. This chapter understandably focuses on the healthcare industry, but the points made are applicable to all organizations in virtually all settings. A considerable portion of this chapter addresses succession planning for the most senior executive position, CEO, with the understanding that most of what is pertinent to CEO succession is likewise applicable to other executive-level positions. It is perhaps appropriate, however, for an organization to first address succession plans for the CEOs before moving on to other executives.

Succession planning for middle managers is often described as *career planning*. Succession planning involves the preparation of a single, designated successor to a position, while career planning often involves preparing several candidates for a single position, which has the effect of creating a small pool of potential successors. This, of course, places multiple persons—perhaps as many as three or four—in a position of competition to determine who may be best suited to move up when the need arises.

In the context of the healthcare industry, succession planning is a structured human resources process intended to prepare the organization for a strong leadership transition. At the highest level, it involves identifying and preparing a successor for the CEO while the CEO is in place and there is no apparent reason to believe the position is about to be vacated. Succession planning is thus a proactive approach to ensuring continuity of leadership at the highest and most critical level of administration in an organization (Garman & Tyler, 2004).

▶ Preparing the Next Chief Executive Officer

Why Organizations Should Create Succession Plans

Demographic data reveal that the population of the United States is aging, a fact likely to lead to increasing numbers of retirements. The healthcare industry is not immune to such changing demographics. A substantial cohort of senior healthcare leaders will most likely retire over the coming several years. To maintain continuity of leadership, it is imperative to ensure that the next generation of senior leaders is adequately prepared to assume their roles. Changes in leadership at the top of any organization inevitably cause great stress and uncertainty among employees and members of their governing boards. In cases where a successor is not immediately apparent, uneasiness is intensified and may negatively affect organizational performance. Conversely, organizations with top-level succession plans are more likely to experience smoother leadership transitions. Given the pressure of impending retirements coupled with the potential loss of specific knowledge related to organizational experience (often referred to as institutional knowledge or memories), organizations must take appropriate steps to ensure leadership continuity by creating succession plans.

Organizations lacking succession plans are essentially leaving the development of their future leaders to chance instead of systematically identifying and preparing high-potential persons to carry on and provide the necessary leadership. Healthcare organizations in particular may benefit more from effective succession planning than other types of businesses; they are unusually complex and known to foster highly political environments. As a result, considerable time and effort may be required for outside persons to understand and learn how to navigate and lead in this unique environment. Many individuals have been drawn to the healthcare field because of its traditionally stable work environment, and smooth transition of a CEO can help to maintain both the look and feel of stability (Garman & Tyler, 2004).

Motivating Factors Behind the Creation of Succession Plans

In most instances, it is a CEO's responsibility to set succession plan development in motion and to direct the governing body until the plan is operational. A recent survey of more than 100 healthcare executives identified three factors that motivated their organizations to pursue succession planning. The first was either the presence of a governing board member or CEO having had previous succession planning experience. The second factor involved having a person within the organization initiate and coordinate the effort. The third factor was recognition of the benefits of succession planning to the organization (Hutton, 2003).

Many healthcare organizations do not have a key person such as a CEO or board member with previous succession planning experience. Managers who have had this experience, either with their current organizations or with others, are more likely to sponsor succession plans. Similarly, governing board members who come from organizations having succession plans in place are more likely to suggest or embrace such a plan. Furthermore, if governing board members have previously experienced the unexpected departure of a CEO, they are more likely to recognize the value of having a succession plan. Gaining knowledge from firsthand experience at replacing a CEO often comes sooner than most boards expect. The current reality is that many hospital CEOs remain in their positions for no longer than 5 years. Experts recommend that top management succession planning should begin 4 years before a CEO is expected to step down, so most hospitals should begin succession planning within a year of hiring a new CEO.

Human resources departments can and sometimes must step in and serve as the catalyst for effective succession planning. Ultimately, the HR department will have responsibility for managing the succession planning process. It is vital for a human resources director to earn and maintain the trust of the governing board and CEO. In some cases, an HR director or manager may have to broach the subject of succession planning with the CEO and hope that it is met with agreement. As with most projects, at least one person in an organization is needed to support and champion an initiative for it to become a reality. Succession planning is no different in this respect. The idea for creating a succession plan will usually receive more attention and have a better chance for acceptance if it is enthusiastically introduced and supported by the CEO or chairperson of the governing body.

Motivating the governing board by promoting the benefits of succession planning to an organization should not be difficult. Over the long term, succession planning will save organizations money. Executive search fees are eliminated when succession planning is practiced. The cost is high when an executive search firm is used to find a new CEO from outside. Fees for searches amount to 30% or more of a new CEO's first year's salary (Hutton, 2003). An organization maintains leadership continuity when an inside person is groomed for the position and promoted.

Grooming an internal person to take over has traditionally been considered a key element of for-profit sector succession planning (Rothwell, 2005). For-profit organizations that have hired external people to replace their CEOs have found maintaining financial stability more difficult than those for-profits that have groomed internal persons (Lucier, Schuyt, & Tse, 2012). More specifically, those that hire a CEO from the outside usually require 6–12 months before financial performance regains the level that existed prior to the replacement.

Five Principles of CEO Succession Planning

Each organization that develops a CEO succession plan will employ an approach unique to its particular organization. Key principles for succession planning have evolved among organizations that have gone through the succession planning process. Five key principles have emerged. Organizations should follow these principles when involved in CEO succession planning. It is important to remember that the governing board, the current CEO, the incoming successor, and the organization's human resources department all have critically important roles to ensure that any succession plan is successful.

1. CEO succession planning should be a board-driven, collaborative process. Furthermore, it should be one of the governing board's two or three most important tasks as it seeks to ensure a strong and viable organization. Selecting a successor must be a collaborative effort that includes the current CEO, but it is essential that the governing board have final accountability. The governing board and CEO should communicate openly about the process. Any agreements or promises the board makes must be communicated to the succeeding board leadership. If promises or agreements are made, the current and succeeding board should adhere to them (Caudron, 1999).

2. CEO succession planning must be a continuous process. A CEO can depart unexpectedly at any time. The untimely departure of the CEO from an organization without a succession plan creates an emergency with no short-term remedy. Up to 9 months may be required to recruit a successor from outside. At all times, a successor should be available, being groomed and ready to step in if needed.

3. Key leadership criteria and competencies must be defined for any potential successor. Potential successors with the appropriate skill sets and talents should be identified as early as possible in their careers. By identifying a specific potential successor for the CEO role, significant development assignments can be arranged to ensure that appropriate experiences are encountered. Building feedback loops into assignments will ensure that the successor is receiving the experiences necessary for professional developmental growth. Feedback can involve several approaches, including 360-degree feedback, standard reviews, informal discussions, and postassignment debriefings. This feedback should improve the governing board and current CEO's understanding of the successor's talents, aptitudes, and interests. It also increases the likelihood that the transition will be successful (Garman & Tyler, 2004).

4. The goal of CEO succession planning is to bring the right leader in at the right time. Specific goals and succession timelines should be created and monitored. Human resources departments play an important role in ensuring that planning is thorough and the assignment process is complete. It is important for the transition to occur as planned. For example, current CEOs should not delay the succession process in the interest of maintaining their current positions. A clear exit strategy should be developed for the outgoing CEO. It is important for organizations to construct and adhere to clearly written transition contracts (Gramam & Glawe, 2004).

5. Once the transition has taken place, a postsuccession assessment should be conducted to evaluate the results of the process. The human resources department should review the overall effectiveness of the program to generate understanding of what worked and what did not work.

When creating and implementing a succession plan, it is important to include a process that promotes diversity and multiculturalism. This helps to ensure that all potential successors are considered. A best successor rather than a clone of the past is more likely to be identified using this approach (Rothwell, 2005).

By following the foregoing principles, organizations are able to avoid some common mistakes and avert failure. One avoidable mistake is thinking that succession planning is a single event rather than a process. In other words, some organizations look at succession planning as a "big bang" theory of transition planning. They select an inside person as the heir apparent for a CEO. Without any work, 5 years later, suddenly a new CEO comes into being. Succession planning is much more than a series of mentoring talks or handing off responsibilities in one sweeping motion (Tyler, 2002).

Another common succession planning mistake is the failure of an organization to anticipate the concerns of key employees who may have been overlooked or feel like they have been ignored as potential successors. For the CEO position, it is best if only one specific inside successor is identified. Having multiple inside successors—picture several upper-level managers all with their sights on the top spot in the organization—can lead to a contest that can be destructive to the potential successors as well as the organization. In such situations, competing successors no longer behave as supportive team members. All are competitors in an environment that selects only one winner at the end. It is imperative that the selection process be conducted in a fair manner and that the actual selection of a new CEO is made by the governing body or board with input and assistance from the outgoing CEO and the HR department (Gramam & Glawe, 2004).

Grooming a Successor

Ideally, the succession planning process should begin to identify a successor at an early point in the potential successor's career to allow opportunities for orchestrating significant developmental assignments. An organization must ensure that the successor is provided with the types of developmental opportunities that foster insights and allow needed skills to be acquired and honed. The reward for such an undertaking is a new CEO who confidently and capably accepts new responsibilities. Developmental tasks should be sufficiently diverse to expose the successor to the entire organization and its departments and operations (Garman & Tyler, 2004). Grooming an inside person for the CEO position helps an organization ensure that institutional memories will be preserved. With inside successors, there is greater likelihood for the CEO to succeed and for the organization to maintain its current strategic vision and competitive position (Rothwell, 2005).

CEOs who have personally experienced being groomed for their current positions continue to be major supporters of this process. Testimonials from these individuals consistently attest to the benefit of having been groomed, reporting that existing relationships within their organizations had allowed them to "hit the ground running" (Hutton, 2003).

There are potential pitfalls involved in grooming an inside candidate as an heir apparent. Inside candidates may have connections to social networks and psychological ties within an organization that can complicate efforts to alter organizational culture if changes are needed. Some individuals being groomed for CEO positions may not have had appropriate experiences or may not have been tested in relevant ways. Persons from specific departmental areas within an organization may not be up to the task of leading the entire business. A significant shift in the nature of the industry or market could render the carefully groomed skills of some individuals irrelevant. There is always the possibility that the credibility of an outgoing CEO and existing management team is so sullied that only bringing in an entire new regime can sweep an organization clean (Ram, 2005).

When contemplating grooming a successor to a CEO, organizations may inventory their potential employees. This is often referred to as the process of assessing their inside bench strength. Those conducting the assessment may conclude that no suitable candidates have the necessary knowledge, skills, and abilities. Such organizations should consider hiring an outside person at least 18 months and up to 5 years in advance of the CEO's departure. This is where succession planning can become an economic issue because of the expense of maintaining two individuals with high salaries over an extended period of time, one for the current CEO and one for the replacement.

Why Organizations Do Not Create Executive Succession Plans

Succession planning for the CEO position should be considered a key goal of the governing board of every organization. Developing a succession plan requires time and thought but is not an overly daunting task. Surveys have revealed that few healthcare organizations have developed top-level succession plans. The reason given for this finding is that the task is invariably overridden by more immediate and pressing issues. Paradoxically, if a CEO departs unexpectedly, the most pressing issue for the governing board instantly becomes the planning for the next CEO (Tyler, 2002). Many governing boards do not address succession planning because of their lack of experience with the process and their lack of knowledge of its benefits. This lack of knowledge or experience was supported by survey results (Hutton, 2003).

Another reason for the low numbers of organizations having CEO succession plans is the unfounded belief that by implementing such a plan, the governing body or board is somehow hastening a CEO's departure. Some CEOs fear that they will lose power and become lame-duck leaders once a succession plan is adopted. This perception is strengthened if the succession plan names the next leader. This aspect converts a succession plan into an exercise in grooming. Some CEOs have said that they feel like they are planning their own funerals. Other CEOs have expressed the concern that if they talk about leadership change, their governing board will think they are planning to leave soon.

Governing boards may not want to talk about succession planning because they do not want to imply loss of confidence in their CEO. In any of these cases, CEOs and governing boards must understand that while succession planning and implementation can be uncomfortable, it should be considered an essential strategic goal that is important for the continued success of the organization. Leadership is critical for the long-term effectiveness of contemporary organizations (Hall, 2006).

Some organizations avoid succession planning because their governing boards believe that regardless of available inside talent, an outside person should be recruited to replace the CEO. Unfortunately, this philosophy is more common among healthcare organizations than it is among large corporate businesses. Relying on replacing an outgoing CEO with an outside person can be risky. The CEO is a prominent organizational position. The more visible a position is, the more difficult it is to find and recruit a suitable candidate. Cultural and political influences inside a healthcare organization can create problems and make it difficult for a person recruited from outside to fit in and to survive and thrive. Furthermore, too much reliance on recruiting an outside person can come at the expense of developing a new CEO from within. Although succession planning focuses primarily on developing inside talent, there can be situations when an organization finds itself looking for an outside person (Greenwald, 2001).

Many of the barriers to succession planning are composed of self-imposed fears and concerns. These can easily be overcome if a CEO or governing board seriously wants to develop a program (Hutton, 2003). By providing more and better knowledge about the practice of succession planning, human resources managers can mitigate most existing fears and concerns (Greenwald, 2001).

Case of a CEO Succession Plan

An appropriate succession plan clearly defines a successor's qualifications, establishes a time frame for the transition, and is tailored to an organization's unique needs. Organizations that have expended the time and effort to create and implement succession plans are in the best possible position during a leadership transition to maintain their momentum and direction because there is a seamless transition to a new CEO. Although some barriers to succession planning exist, many CEOs recognize that a significant measure of their success is how their organization fares after they leave. Embracing succession planning and grooming a successor can help to ensure that a gratifying and memorable legacy remains.

▶ Succession Planning Below Executive Level

It was stated earlier that succession planning for middle managers is frequently described as *career planning*. This may or may not be strictly true in all instances, although preparing someone against the eventuality of having to take a step upward in the management hierarchy is surely a part of career planning, along with engaging in continuing education and pursuing other avenues of self-development.

Middle management is, of course, that loosely defined layer of management between the executive level and the first-line supervisors, "loosely defined" because it can be more than just a single layer of management. Three levels may be precisely correct when, for example, a billing supervisor reports to the accounting manager, who in turn reports to the CFO; the accounting manager is clearly the middle manager. In some other function, however, for example, a large nursing department, there may be two or three or more management layers between the head nurse of a unit (the first-line supervisor) and the top nursing executive. These intervening layers are also rightly referred to as middle management.

It was suggested that in some instances multiple individuals may be prepared to ascend to a particular middle management position. The approach can be carried too far; it may be acceptable to have two promising underlings in a position of learning about the next position up the hierarchy, but too many people with their sights set on the next upward step can foster unhealthy competition.

Just the Middle Manager?

It is not only the middle manager that should be backed up with a potential successor. The backup—call it a succession plan—need not be as formal and far reaching as the succession plan for the CEO position. Whether a true, lone middle manager and a first-line supervisor in a hierarchy, or three or four middle management layers between the top and the first line, every position in which someone supervises the work of others should be backed up in such a manner that there will be a person to turn to in the event of a sudden vacancy. There need not be a formal plan anywhere near as detailed as that for the CEO position, but there should be some designated individual who has been sufficiently prepared to step up and ensure some measure of continuity.

First-Line Supervisor

Preparing for management succession should begin with the lowest level in the hierarchy, the first-line supervisor—that all-important manager who oversees the performance of the individuals who do the organization's hands-on work. And that which can be said about backing up the first-line supervisor's position can and should be applied to middle-management positions. Supervisory skills programs have for years advised anyone who would supervise others to identify and prepare one or two potential successors. Although this may be accomplished informally, preparing potential successors is succession planning at its most fundamental level.

▶ Why Prepare Potential Successors

The most obvious reason for having one or two people knowledgeable of at least the most important aspects of the supervisor's role is the need for coverage should the supervisor suddenly no longer be there. Bad things can happen: death, accident, illness, unanticipated termination, resignation without notice, any event that suddenly leaves the department with no leader. Such transitions, difficult enough when someone can take over at least partially, are an invitation to chaos when no one in the department knows what to do. Also, having a capable backup will allow the supervisor to remain relatively at ease while experiencing a short-term illness or going away on vacation.

Another important reason for identifying potential successors resides in consideration of the supervisor's future. A supervisor identifies potential successors by trying them out with delegated tasks. One important factor often examined when a supervisor is being considered for possible promotion is whether there is someone in the department capable of stepping up if this supervisor is promoted. A supervisor who has prepared no one, who has not expended the time and effort necessary to develop a potential successor, is less likely to be promoted. The lack of potential successors often tells higher management that this supervisor has not taken the time and effort to develop backup, and that this supervisor does not delegate well or at all.

Having a knowledgeable backup can be of considerable benefit to the supervisor. A backup can handle time reporting in the supervisor's place, can attend committee meetings and other gatherings when there is not enough of the supervisor to go around, and can generally keep this functioning when the supervisor is ill or on vacation.

▶ Preparing Potential Successors

One of the supervisor's most important activities is—or certainly should be—employee development. Much of employee development resides in expanding employee knowledge of how the department functions and in general preparing employees to grow and eventually move up if that is what they desire. This is pursued largely through proper delegation, which assists the supervisor in identifying employees' capabilities and encouraging them. Relative success at accomplishing delegated tasks tells the supervisor much about the growth potential of employees. And delegation possibilities are usually numerous, consisting of any of the supervisor's normal tasks except those describable as personnel management (hiring, firing, disciplining, promoting, demoting, and such). Trying out an employee with delegated tasks of increasing responsibility and using that employee to fill in for the supervisor when needed is in fact developing a potential successor.

▶ Potential Downside

There is a downside to almost everything; the best one can hope for is that the benefits of any action or activity greatly outweigh its shortcomings. There are some limited possibilities that may sometimes cause a supervisor to wonder whether the preparation of potential successors is a worthwhile activity. However, employee development is an important part of the supervisor's job, and surely the development of potential successors is employee development.

One possible downside of developing one or two potential successors is that one or two of the supervisor's more promising subordinates may leave for a greater opportunity elsewhere.

Employees who respond to growth opportunities usually have the desire to advance. If such an employee is eager to advance but the supervisor is going nowhere in the foreseeable future, the employee may seek placement in another organization or another department. When this occurs, the supervisor may feel that all he or she has done is prepare one of the department's better employees to leave for greener pastures.

There is another possible downside to the development of multiple successors—competition between two potential successors as they try to outdo each other in the eyes of the supervisor or actively try to undermine each other. This condition is not often encountered, but when it occurs, the supervisor needs to address the issues with the employees or perhaps reevaluate either or both as potential successors.

▶ An Essential Process

The development of one or more potential successors at the first-line supervisory level is an essential part of employee development. Unfortunately, employee development too often takes a back seat to the problems of the moment. Yet when the problems pile up and the supervisor feels forever pressed for time, this is when some practical, well-thought-out delegation can begin to reveal some employee capabilities that will soon contribute to reducing the pile of problems.

🔍 CASE Study: Resolution

Returning to the case study, given the magnitude of the leadership loss, a succession plan for the CEO alone would have been insufficient. The experience of Memorial Hospital demonstrates the need for identifying potential candidates for advancement to executive ranks in addition to having an ongoing formal succession plan for the CEO. Many organizations have policies that prohibit key executives and managers from traveling together. Lacking an identified successor, Memorial Hospital has few options. One choice is to engage the services of an executive search firm. A more drastic response may be a merger. While disruptive and unplanned, such a decision could provide experienced executive leadership.

SPOTLIGHT ON CUSTOMER SERVICE

Customer Service and Succession Planning

Succession planning is an organized and deliberate process that is designed to reduce problems related to the departure and replacement of key employees. Due to limitations of resources (time and money), most organizations limit their succession planning activities to the position of CEO. This assumes that an organization actually practices succession planning, though a great many organizations do not do so.

Some organizations create succession plans for many employees at differing levels. These activities are more likely to be career-path planning rather than succession planning. Participants are given assignments in a variety of departments. The benefit of widespread exposure is to develop career paths that will be mutually and maximally beneficial to employers and employees.

Customer service provides a stark contrast to succession and career-planning activities. Customer service is (or should be) an activity that is practiced by all employees. The beneficiaries are users or purchasers of an organization's products, programs, or services. Organizations do receive some benefits, primarily in the form of increased sales or participation rates due to satisfied customers. For employees, customer service involves giving, rather than receiving, specific benefits.

Modified from Caudron, S. (1999). The looming leadership crisis. *Workforce, 78*(9), 72–76; Garman, A. N., & Glawe, J. (2004). Succession planning. *Consulting Psychology Journal: Practice and Research, 56*(2), 119–128; Garman, A. N., & Tyler, J. L. (2004). *CEO succession planning in freestanding U.S. hospitals: Final report*. Chicago, IL: American College of Healthcare Executives; Greenwald, S. (2001). Why succession planning can't wait. *Workforce, 80*(12), 34–38; Hall, H. (2006). Planning successful successions. *Chronicle of Philanthropy, 18*(6), 47–49; Hutton, D. H. (2003). Succession planning—Dress rehearsal for the under-studies. *Trustee, 56*(6), 27–32; Lucier, C., Schuyt, R., & Tse, E. (2012). CEO succession: The world's most prominent temp workers. *Strategy+Business.com*. Retrieved from http://www.strategy-business.com/article/05204?gko=47020-1876-9227977; Ram, C. (2005). Ending the CEO succession crisis. *Harvard Business Review, 83*(2), 67–72; Rothwell, W. J. (2005). *Effective succession planning* (3rd ed.). Chicago, IL: AMACOM Books; Tyler, J. L. (2002). Succession planning: Charting a course for the future. *Trustee, 55*(6), 24–28.

Questions for Review and Discussion

1. Why is succession planning important?
2. Briefly describe the five principles of succession planning.
3. From the perspective of an organization, what are the advantages of succession planning?
4. What are the disadvantages of succession planning?
5. Succession planning is widely practiced in industry. It is fairly common among large hospitals and medical centers. In your opinion, why is this so?
6. Succession planning is very uncommon among public health organizations. What are some reasons for this? In your opinion, are these reasons valid?
7. Briefly describe the elements of a succession plan that is based on grooming an internal candidate as a successor.
8. What are the advantages and disadvantages of grooming an internal candidate as part of a succession plan?
9. What are the advantages and disadvantages of seeking an external candidate as part of a succession plan?

10.   Would grooming an internal candidate or seeking an external candidate be the most advantageous approach to succession planning in your own place of work (or proposed place of employment if you are a student)? Why?

11.   Why do organizations resist succession planning? In your opinion, are these reasons valid? Why?

References

Caudron, S. (1999). The looming leadership crisis. *Workforce, 78*(9), 72–76.

Garman, A. N., & Glawe, J. (2004). Succession planning. *Consulting Psychology Journal: Practice and Research, 56*(2), 119–128.

Garman, A. N., & Tyler, J. L. (2004). *CEO succession planning in freestanding U.S. hospitals: Final report.* Chicago, IL: American College of Healthcare Executives.

Greenwald, S. (2001). Why succession planning can't wait. *Workforce, 80*(12), 34–38.

Hall, H. (2006). Planning successful successions. *Chronicle of Philanthropy, 18*(6), 47–49.

Hutton, D. H. (2003). Succession planning—Dress rehearsal for the under-studies. *Trustee, 56*(6), 27–32.

Lucier, C., Schuyt, R., & Tse, E. (2012). CEO succession: The world's most prominent temp workers. *Strategy+Business.com.* Retrieved from http://www.strategy-business.com/article/05204?gko =47020-1876-9227977

Ram, C. (2005). Ending the CEO succession crisis. *Harvard Business Review, 83*(2), 67–72.

Rothwell, W. J. (2005). *Effective succession planning* (3rd ed.). Chicago, IL: AMACOM Books.

Tyler, J. L. (2002). Succession planning: Charting a course for the future. *Trustee, 55*(6), 24–28.

Resources

Books

Byham, W. C., Smith, A. B., & Paese, M. J. (2002). *Grow your own leaders: How to identify, develop, and retain leadership talent.* Upper Saddle River, NJ: Prentice Hall.

Carey, D. C., & Ogden, D. (2002). *CEO succession planning: A window on how boards can get it right when choosing a new chief executive.* New York, NY: Oxford University Press.

Rothwell, W. J. (2005). *Effective succession planning: Ensuring leadership continuity and building talent from within* (3rd ed.). Chicago, IL: AMACOM.

Rothwell, W. J., Jackson, R. D., Knight, S. C., & Lindholm, J. E. (2005). *Career planning and succession management: Developing your organization's talent—For today and tomorrow.* Westport, CT: Greenwood.

Weisman, C., & Goldblum, R. I. (2003). *Losing your executive director without losing your way: A nonprofit's guide to executive turnover.* New York, NY: Wiley.

Periodicals

Cantazarro, T. E. (2006). Succession planning. *Veterinary Clinics of North America: Small Animal Practice, 36*(2), 355–371.

Cohn, J. M., Khurana, R., & Reeves, L. (2005). Growing talent as if your business depended on it. *Harvard Business Review, 83*(10), 62–70, 155–157.

Dolan, T. C. (2005). Increasing succession planning: Executives at all levels have a responsibility to ensure leadership continuity. *Healthcare Executive, 20*(3), 6–14.

Frauenheim, E. (2006). Succession progression. *Workforce, 85*(1), 32–34.

Hadelman, J., & Spitaels-Genser, E. (2005). Succession planning: The art of transferring leadership. *Trustee, 58*(8), 4, 14–17.

McConnell, C. R. (2006). Succession planning: Valuable process or pointless exercise? *Health Care Management (Frederick), 25*(1), 91–98.

Oonan, P. R. (2005). Succession planning: Aligning strategic goals and leadership behaviors. *Nursing Leadership Forum, 9*(3), 92–97.

Sherrod, D. R. (2006). Succession planning. *Nursing Management, 37*(2), 64–67.

Szot, A. (2005). Systems look to future: Stand-alone hospitals lag in succession planning. *Modern Healthcare, 35*(25), 17–22.

CHAPTER 11

Employee Training

CHAPTER OBJECTIVES

After studying this chapter, readers will be able to:

- Appreciate the importance of training and development as continuing activities.
- Outline the essential role of department managers as teachers.
- Appreciate the importance of new-employee orientation.
- Understand applicable principles in addressing staff training and development needs.
- View cross-training as a means for improving employee capability and know-how to approach on-the-job training.
- Understand employee mentoring.
- Appreciate the importance of developing potential managers.
- See how human resources can help managers meet departmental training needs.

▶ Chapter Summary

Training is an essential activity leaders use to ensure that their organizations will have the best possible chance to survive and grow in the future. It helps ease an individual's transition into an organization and facilitates movement within the organization. Training takes many forms. New-employee orientation, mentoring, and on-the-job and off-site training are just some of the training approaches. Managers often provide training in formal or informal settings. Cross-training of employees with similar types of jobs provides organizational flexibility. Giving developmental opportunities to potential leaders facilitates succession planning.

▶ Introduction: The Role of Training and Development

Senior managers in most healthcare departments can be counted on to support and praise the value of continuing education. Unfortunately, many managers drop training and development when budgets get tight and expenses must be reduced. This is

🔍 *CASE STUDY: A Blue Monday*

"Monday mornings should not be so complicated"—at least that is what Sam, the health commissioner, thought. The new epidemiologist was scheduled to report for work that Monday at 10:00 A.M. A second new employee was scheduled to begin on Friday. "Two new people on two different days in the same week," thought Sam, with a feeling of defeat.

Sam had been reading about the importance of developing potential new managers. The usual departmental duties would not diminish. Because the previous Friday was a state holiday, the morning volume of e-mail was extra heavy. This had become more of a problem since a prankster had spread Sam's e-mail address to websites that specialized in body reshaping surgery or drugs to enhance performance. "Why couldn't both new employees start tomorrow?" mused Sam. What advice would you give to Sam?

partly because of the difficulty of pinpointing cost savings that can be attributed to continuing education. Most individuals in management believe or know intuitively that education ultimately saves money; however, it is more difficult to measure the results of education in terms of costs versus benefits than it is to measure cost savings in most other areas of organizational activity. As a result, money spent on education is often viewed as expending resources with few tangible results; the financial outlays can be clearly seen as money going out, but the benefits are largely hidden and slowly accruing.

As important as training and development are to every healthcare organization, in many instances, they receive minimal attention from top management. Simply reminding department managers that they have a responsibility for employee development is insufficient. Managers must be encouraged to view training and development as important because they keep valuable employees interested and challenged.

Factors that motivate employees are found primarily in the nature of work. Among the strongest motivating factors are the opportunity to do interesting and challenging work and the opportunity to learn and grow. Better-performing employees are usually so motivated. They are also the individuals who are most likely to leave in search of more interesting and challenging work and greater overall opportunities. One way for department managers to increase the chances of retaining their better employees is through visible support for training and development.

A department that places no emphasis on training and development may seem to be standing still. In reality, such a department is essentially going backward because the world continues to move ahead. With technologic, economic, legislative, financial, and social change constantly occurring, no department or organization can afford to stand still. A certain amount of forward progress is necessary simply to remain abreast of change. As contrary as it may sound, one must move ahead to stay even. Therefore, maintaining or improving the abilities of staff must be an ongoing effort. Continuing education is essential.

The Manager's Role in Employee Training

Under the blanket heading of training is an entire range of employee development activities, from providing new-employee orientation to assisting employees in moving up into management. Employee development should be one of the most important aspects of a manager's job.

Department managers are likely to possess greater depth and breadth of technical knowledge and expertise in the areas or activities they manage than is found anywhere else in the organization. Managers are mostly educated in the fields in which they work. In addition, they have the advantage of practical education acquired through experience. Therefore, managers are primary resources for information about their departments and the work they perform. Department managers are uniquely positioned to pass on their knowledge and expertise to others. Department managers have the responsibility for maintaining and improving the capability and competence of their staff.

The Manager as a Teacher

Because the department manager is usually well versed in the department's tasks and activities, the manager is best suited to provide some, although probably not all, of the teaching in the department's continuing education program. For some of the topics, the manager will clearly be the most qualified individual and the most readily available instructor, but chances are there will be a few topics that other individuals can better address. For example, a supervisor in health information management (formerly medical records) who is interested in cross-training several assistants in chart completion review might prefer to use the person regularly assigned to this task as the instructor. With proper encouragement and assistance, the person who knows best how to perform a given task can be the best resource for teaching that task to others. Regardless, however, even if the department manager does not do all the teaching, this manager nevertheless remains responsible for the department's continuing education program.

Teaching a class can loom as a formidable task to the manager who has not previously done so. But a manager who is hesitant to adopt the role of instructor can rest assured that just about everyone involved in teaching or any other form of public speaking has experienced similar qualms. It helps to regard one's early experiences in teaching as learning experiences in themselves, remembering that one is not a professional teacher and that the department's employees are familiar faces and not a group of unknown "students." The keys to building one's effectiveness as an instructor are preparation and practice. The more one teaches a given subject, the better it can be taught in the future. The more often one faces a group of learners, the less troublesome the feeling of uneasiness about teaching will become.

A manager who will be required to serve as a teacher is advised to acquire knowledge of adult learning principles. Pertinent information is available from a number of sources, including some of the resources listed at the end of this chapter. Most healthcare organizations of any appreciable size have internal resources available. Depending on organization size, human resources (HR) may have a training function that can assist managers, or a separate education department may be available. At the very least, it is usually possible to obtain information about adult instructional methods from nursing in-service education. From a manager's perspective, teaching should be accepted as an integral part of the management role. Teaching is also an essential part of delegation, as proper and effective delegation requires instructing the person who will undertake a delegated task. Unfortunately, in the pursuit of everyday business, such employee development activity is often overlooked.

External Requirements

The importance of continuing education and training is underscored by the extent to which different accreditation and regulatory agencies assess training activities during their periodic surveys. For example, The Joint Commission (TJC) publishes specific requirements for the continuing education of physicians, nurses, and certain other personnel. The accrediting organization checks via periodic surveys to see whether employee orientations are routinely scheduled and attended. Some states have requirements for all-employee orientations to address certain particular topics and offer annual refresher education on the most critical topics.

Another indicator of the importance placed externally on continuing education is the fact that many healthcare practitioners are required to provide evidence of completing a certain number of continuing education units each year to maintain their professional licensure.

▶ New-Employee Orientation

All healthcare department managers should have a new-employee orientation plan for their own departments. This is in addition to the separate orientation to the organization overall. Orientation plans are required by accreditation and regulatory agencies.

An organization usually provides a general new-employee orientation that addresses common matters. Ordinarily prepared by HR, a general orientation addresses such topics as the organization's structure and leadership, employee benefits, the performance appraisal process, the organization's dress code, employee parking, facility security, infection control, and universal precautions. Employee health and other benefits, the employee assistance program (EAP), employee work rules, and generally applicable policies are also typically included.

A department orientation should provide an introduction to the people in the department and program areas and to the physical space, equipment, processes, and any special department policies, as well as on-the-job guidance in getting started doing the work for which the new person was hired. It is highly inappropriate to simply allow new employees to begin working without the benefit of an orientation. Even experienced and well-educated new employees require some guidance concerning variations specific to a particular department or program, as well as need some time to ask questions about the new job.

As part of a new employee's orientation, it may help to appoint a mentor. A mentor is an experienced person who can provide guidance through the new person's first few days or weeks on the job. Mentoring offers valuable benefits; it provides a personally guided orientation for a newcomer, and it affords an opportunity for further development of an experienced employee.

Training to Correct Performance Problems

Training must (or at least should) be a high priority for every manager. Running a program or department and getting out the expected work is a supervisor's number-one priority; nevertheless, training is important as well, especially regarding new or revised work procedures and the correction of performance problems.

When assessing employee performance, supervisors continually compare observed performance with expectations. Managers may have to be teachers when helping employees correct performance problems. When an employee displays performance problems that command the manager's attention, it is always appropriate to consider whether reasonable efforts are being made to help the employee succeed. Many employees fail at their jobs because they were inappropriately trained, insufficiently oriented, or inadequately supported.

It may sometimes be necessary to impose a requirement for a particular kind of education or training as a condition of continued employment. For example, an individual whose telephone manners have elicited many complaints may be required to complete a program in telephone etiquette, or an individual whose job requires writing but who has experienced problems with grammar may be required to take a remedial English program.

▶ Determining Departmental Learning Needs

If a variety of learning needs seem to be present throughout a department, then it is helpful to conduct a needs analysis for basic remediation. One approach consists of making a simple chart for each job description in a department, with columns indicating the principal required skills and rows listing the employees whose work includes those activities. It becomes a matter of assessing all employees in terms of whether their skills are adequate to meet normal job expectations. Each assessment that falls short of normal expectations indicates a learning need. This approach helps managers focus training activities on areas of greatest need. In addition to managers' assessments, noticeable performance problems also indicate areas of need, as do tendencies toward repetitive errors or actions that generate chronic complaints by customers, coworkers, and others.

A manager's initial assessment of training needs must then be translated into training objectives. Learners must know initially where they are headed. Once a goal is determined, learners and managers can consider how to get there.

A learner's motivation is key to the eventual success of training. Managers must be prepared to help employees answer one particular question about what they are being asked to learn: "What's in it for me?" In correcting a severe performance problem, the answer may be as basic as, "You get to remain employed." There are numerous other possible responses, such as, "You get to learn something that may eventually help you to be promoted," "You get more variety in your work," or "You get to do something more challenging than what you've been doing."

Employee Training Within a Department

The following principles may assist the manager when addressing staff training and development needs. All employees who are expected to learn something deserve to know why they are learning, and all employees should be advised of specific goals and objectives. Employees learn better when they actually become involved in the process. The more hands-on or learn-while-doing components that can be incorporated, the more likely a training program is to be successful. Experienced trainers know that trainees are likely to retain a limited amount of what they simply hear, a greater amount of what they both hear and see (thus, the use of visual aids), and the greatest amount of what they simultaneously hear and see and do.

Employees will more quickly and more accurately absorb material that applies to their daily work rather than having to learn material that they see as irrelevant. Thus, in-department employee training should be practical and immediately applicable rather than theoretical.

Most employees will accept new ideas more readily if these ideas support their previously held beliefs. New material, techniques, and processes are best presented within the context of a department's mission. For example, "We're still here to serve members of the community, but now it can be done more quickly and at lower cost." Some employees learn best when allowed to pursue their own areas of interest or needs at their own rate. For these employees, managers must provide clear expectations, necessary information and materials, and general guidance. Many employees must be encouraged to find learning pleasant. For some employees, the possibility of education of any kind essentially means going back to school, which renders them resistant to training. These people must be shown what is in it for them.

Cross-Training for Efficiency

Department managers who supervise employees working in comparable positions in terms of job grade or pay scale have the opportunity to implement cross-training. For example, an office manager may have three clerical-level employees who are assigned in different capacities: a file clerk, a program secretary, and a data entry specialist. These three jobs reside in the same pay grade. As long as the three people simply do their own jobs, the department has limited flexibility. If one person is on vacation or is ill, no one is trained to assume the missing person's duties. If all three people are capable of doing all three jobs, the employees can be moved around as needed. Resources can be shifted as workloads or backlogs demand, and any of the three people can cover for any of the others as necessary.

This type of flexibility can be obtained by training the three employees in one another's jobs. This requires time and effort. Each of the people can train the other two in job particulars, with the supervisor providing general guidance. This training will ultimately repay the time and effort involved. A department gains considerable flexibility in addressing backlogs and covering for vacations and illnesses. The individuals gain greater interests and challenges associated with their work through increased task variety.

On-the-Job Training

On-the-job training is appropriate under many circumstances. For some learning needs, it may be the best available approach. Also, it is frequently the nearly ideal learning combination of hearing, seeing, and doing. Much on-the-job training is best accomplished under the direct supervision of a manager or under the direct guidance of an experienced employee. Employees receiving on-the-job training receive step-by-step instructions on how to accomplish a task while actually performing it. After employees perform the task a sufficient number of times under this direct guidance, the instructor may then reduce or eliminate the verbal guidance and simply watch until assured that the activity is being performed in a satisfactory manner. Thus assured, the instructor may further withdraw to a position of being readily available to answer questions.

On-the-job training is not simply allowing employees to learn by trial and error with only a rough idea of expected results. However, this is precisely what it becomes when managers decide that they are too busy to address training in a proper manner and simply turn new employees loose on the job.

Improper or inadequate on-the-job training can be dangerous or destructive. Employees may learn to perform their tasks in a highly inefficient or incorrect manner, creating inappropriate work habits that can conceivably become deeply ingrained and difficult to correct. It is far better for managers to ensure that sufficient time and attention are devoted at the start of the learning process so that on-the-job training can succeed as intended.

Another common but inadequate approach to training, or at least to satisfying annual in-service education requirements, is to give staff members files or folders of information to review. Often, accreditation agencies or state regulations require these documents to be reviewed. A reading package is circulated among the staff with instructions for each recipient to review the documents as required, check off to indicate that they have done so, and pass the material to the next person. This is the loosest and weakest approach to training. Short of questioning each recipient in detail, there is no way to ensure that the material has been read and absorbed.

Most people recall a certain portion of information they hear (approximately 10%), a somewhat greater portion of what they both see and hear (estimated to be 20%), and almost all of what they simultaneously see, hear, and do (often 90% or more). This suggests that the most effective job-related training should include a combination of lecture, demonstration, and hands-on practice.

Using multiple channels of sensory input increases the likelihood of learning. This is why personal reading alone can be the least effective way of learning, and why lecture alone is not a great deal better. When multiple senses are used simultaneously, the chances of learning increase. Repeating the same material after a lapse of time, and presenting it in varying forms, can be highly effective in ensuring that the material will be retained.

Effective Mentoring

Mentoring can be most effective if it is officially sanctioned. It need not take place within the context of a formal program, but it should be acknowledged as an actively used employee development technique rather than simply an ad hoc practice whereby people might happen to link up with each other. The extent of the formality required may be minimal. A new employee and an experienced employee or mentor are intentionally brought together by the manager, and all three parties agree on the objectives of the relationship, specifying what the new employee is expected to learn. The manager remains close enough to the process to be able to evaluate both the new employee and the mentor during and after the relationship period.

By officially addressing mentoring as a means of employee development, an organization sends a strong message to all employees concerning its commitment to their development. Although mentoring is one of the least costly development tools available, it can be extremely effective. Its visible use proclaims that the organization cares about the development of its people.

For a new employee, a mentor can be a valuable facilitator, sounding board, and source of advice and guidance. The mentor benefits as well. Mentoring can provide a sense of fulfillment and satisfaction, especially for a senior employee who is in need of additional challenges and who stands to benefit from more interesting work experiences. The process helps mentors further refine their skills and keep them sharp.

Employees most likely to realize significant benefits from a mentoring relationship are those who demonstrate a willingness to learn, are proactive in expressing this willingness, and are ambitious and enthusiastic. Effective mentors are able to assume full responsibility for their own growth and development. They are receptive to coaching and constructive feedback and have the ability to change behaviors based on positive experiences.

Experienced employees who are considered for mentoring responsibilities should be persons who are willing to serve voluntarily and give the undertaking the time and energy it requires. No mentor should ever be unilaterally assigned or forced to serve. Similarly, managers should not force new employees to work with any particular mentor. Both parties should have an option to change a mentoring relationship if either becomes dissatisfied. Potential mentors should possess sufficient knowledge and expertise in the new employee's areas of responsibility. They should have good interpersonal skills and patience, and they should be supportive, friendly, and effective listeners. Above all else, potential mentors should demonstrate interest in the development of others.

Developing Potential Managers

An essential part of every supervisor's responsibility is to help identify and develop new managers. This includes identifying and developing one or more potential successors. Many managers fall short of properly addressing the latter need.

The development of potential successors is closely associated with the practice of proper delegation. This is the primary means by which succession planning evolves. It is an area of concern or threat for some managers, especially people who are often insecure in their positions and fear competition from intelligent, up-and-coming subordinates. Many managers simply do not think beyond the present. They are ill prepared to imagine being moved up or out or becoming incapacitated and no longer able to function in their positions.

Development of a potential new manager may not occur within a department because it requires serious and progressively more responsible delegation. This takes time and planning on the part of management. Such development requires delegating tasks that involve increasingly more responsibility.

At the very least, the manager who has a potential successor under development usually has readily available coverage for vacations and illnesses as needed. No person is or should be considered absolutely indispensable, but the loss or absence of a group's leader when there is no ready backup person can create significant inefficiency and inconvenience.

A manager who entertains ambitions of advancing higher in the organization should take seriously the need to develop a potential successor. Higher management will often look closely at a manager's track record in delegating tasks and especially at whether that manager has one or more capable successors in the wings. Enlightened higher management may well conclude that a supervisor who has paid no attention to developing a potential successor shows little strength in delegation, a skill that becomes increasingly important as one moves up in an organization. Executives in an organizational hierarchy may be unwilling to promote a manager if doing so means having to conduct an external search for a successor or promoting an untried insider.

No manager wants to lose good employees; however, some are going to be lost regardless of a supervisor's actions. Managers who put time and effort into developing potential successors may see many of them eventually lost to other departments or other organizations as they take advantage of opportunities to advance their careers. But these employees are likely to be lost to the organization anyway if they are not given opportunities to develop. Some of them will be lost even sooner if they remain unchallenged in their jobs. Therefore, prudent managers should take full advantage of the talents that are available in their groups by delegating tasks to the better and more willing employees and helping them to develop.

Only rarely does a manager have anything to fear from a subordinate who is encouraged to develop and grow and learn some aspects of the manager's job. In fact, having one or two sharp, up-and-coming subordinates is often just what a manager needs to remain effective and to continue to grow.

▶ How Human Resources Can Help

It is customary for an organization's general new-employee orientation to be presented or at least coordinated by HR. As far as this orientation is concerned, ordinarily all a manager has to do is ensure that each new employee attends. However, some managers have to be reminded of the necessity for all new employees to attend the orientation. Some of these new employees may be filling positions that have been empty for some time, and the department may be behind in its work. Occasionally, a manager may decide that a new employee cannot be spared for the few hours required for orientation. There may be a tendency to regard orientation as just another nonessential HR thing that intrudes on a manager's ability to run a department. In most instances, however, a general orientation to the organization includes topics that are required by accreditation or regulation. Orientation then becomes partly a response to external requirements and partly a service performed to get new employees pointed in the proper direction.

Beyond ensuring that new employees attend general orientation, it is the manager's responsibility to become aware of training needs and ensure these needs are met. When addressing issues of employee training and development, a department manager should expect HR to work with supervisors to diagnose particular problems and determine the kinds of training or education that might be helpful, to provide certain kinds of needed training, to secure the involvement of other in-house training expertise, to identify external sources for specifically required training, to determine how these sources are accessed, and to guide employees in using an organization's tuition assistance program when appropriate.

Training needs should be addressed on a continuing basis, both to assess present circumstances to determine the skills and attitudes that must be adopted or improved to meet current needs, and to attempt to determine future needs based on trends that appear to be coming during the next 1 or 2 years. Information for evaluating training needs can be gathered in a variety of ways, including questionnaires completed by managers and employees, focus group discussions, individual interviews with managers and employees, and exit interviews at which departing employees are asked for their opinions concerning developmental needs. Subjects that are frequently mentioned merit consideration as potential program topics.

Human resources can contribute information relevant in determining training and development needs from direct contact with people on the job, both managers and rank-and-file employees; from reviewing performance appraisals, performance improvement records, and disciplinary actions; and from monitoring trends in public health.

When guiding training and development activities, HR may recommend involving both managers and employees in preparing training agendas and determining program content. It often starts with needs that employees appear to be the most strongly motivated to address. Human resources focuses on present jobs and needs first, then looks to the future, focusing primarily on behavior, in the belief that if skills are appropriately implanted or modified, then proper attitudes will follow. It will use on-the-job experiential learning to the maximum practical extent, supplemented with training from other sources.

When evaluating training efforts, HR will attempt to determine whether the needs assessments that were conducted were accurate, whether targeted skills have been learned and incorporated in new behaviors, and whether employee attitudes appear to have been modified. Human resources must assess what has been learned and how this audit of results can support the next cycle of training.

▶ Conclusion

Training and development should be ongoing and essentially continuous activities. Managers are central to training efforts, identifying needs and often serving as trainers. New employees must be properly and completely oriented to a healthcare department as well as their own specific program areas. Cross-training provides flexibility, especially in times of crisis. On-the-job training is important and often conducted by a mentor. Potential new managers rarely emerge without assistance. They must be nurtured and developed by providing opportunities for them to actually supervise others or guide programs. Human resources personnel may provide assistance in training and development.

🔍 CASE STUDY: Resolution

Returning to the harried health commissioner in the opening case study, Sam should seek volunteers to serve as mentors for the new employees. This will provide support for the new people and give Sam a chance to evaluate the leadership potential of two subordinates. Sam should decide to take the new employees to lunch on their third day of employment.

Although it would be efficient to provide one initial orientation session for both new employees, Sam should avoid the temptation. This would require the epidemiologist starting on Monday to either start without any training or to waste 4 working days. Either alternative sends a negative message to the new employee.

One year later, both new employees had become fully integrated into the health department. One of the mentors seized the opportunity to shine and was promoted 7 months later. Both mentors reported increased job satisfaction. Sam noticed the improvement in their job productivity. The epidemiologist volunteered to serve as a mentor in the future.

SPOTLIGHT ON CUSTOMER SERVICE

Customer Service and Employee Training

Providing employee training on the topic of customer service would seem to be an obvious priority for organizations interested in promoting the concept. With that commitment made, the next decision becomes how to provide the necessary training and what modality or approach to use. A common response is to hire a consultant to teach employees the fundamentals of customer service. Another less common approach includes using data from questionnaires completed by people who have received or purchased products, programs, or services (Thies, 1999). A third (Darby & Daniel, 1999) obtains input from senior managers.

Each approach has advantages and disadvantages. Purchasing a generic training package will reduce expenses, but at the cost of including situations that are unique to the organization. Gathering data from users via questionnaires should provide information focused on the unique needs of an organization. Obtaining such premium data would demand premium prices. Tapping into the ideas of senior managers would not be expensive but would include local biases.

The most pressing truths are the importance of customer service and ensuring that all employees are adequately trained.

Modified from Darby, D. N., & Daniel, K. (1999). Factors that influence nurses' customer orientation. *Journal of Nursing Management, 7*(5), 271–280; Thies, S. (1999). Customer service: Moving from slogan to point of differentiation. *Medical Group Management Journal, 46*(5), 34–38.

Questions for Review and Discussion

1. Why are training and development opportunities important to some employees but apparently not to others? To which employees do they appear most important?
2. Why is having training and development opportunities available to employees important even if many do not take advantage of them?
3. Why must in-service training or on-the-job education be continuing?
4. Why is education usually one of the first line items to be reduced or eliminated when it becomes necessary to cut budgets? Is such an action organizationally prudent? Why?
5. What activities could a department manager undertake to continue involving employees in education with little or no direct budgetary impact?
6. How you would implement a program of cross-training among three or four roughly comparable positions? Use actual or hypothetical positions as an example.
7. How do a department manager's skills as an instructor, teacher, or mentor relate to the ability to delegate tasks?
8. Why should a department manager who plans on remaining in place for as long as practical develop one or two capable employees as potential successors?
9. It is frequently claimed that it is difficult if not impossible to quantify the cost effectiveness of education. Do you believe this to be true? Why?
10. What are the advantages of using capable senior employees as mentors or trainers for newer employees?

References
Darby, D. N., & Daniel, K. (1999). Factors that influence nurses' customer orientation. *Journal of Nursing Management, 7*(5), 271–280.

Thies, S. (1999). Customer service: Moving from slogan to point of differentiation. *Medical Group Management Journal, 46*(5), 34–38.

Resources
Books
American Society for Healthcare Central Service Professionals (ASHCSP). (2005). *Training manual for health care central service technicians* (5th ed.). San Francisco, CA: Wiley.

Baume, S., Pink, D., & Baume, D. (2005). *Enhancing staff and educational development.* New York, NY: Taylor & Francis Group.

Bubb, S. (2004). *The insider's guide to early professional development.* New York, NY: Taylor & Francis Group.

Buckley, R., & Caple, J. (2004). *Theory and practice of training* (5th ed.). London, UK: Kogan Page.

Jacobs, R. L. (2003). *Structured on-the-job training* (2nd ed.). San Francisco, CA: Benett-Koehler Publishers.

Kahnweiler, W. M., & Kahnweiler, J. B. (2005). *Shaping your HR role: Succeeding in today's organizations.* Sudbury, MA: Jones and Bartlett Publishers.

McConnell, C. R. (2007). *The health care manager's human resources handbook.* Sudbury, MA: Jones and Bartlett Publishers.

Reddington, M., Withers, M., & Williamson, M. (2004). *Transforming HR: Creating value through people.* Sudbury, MA: Jones and Bartlett Publishers.

Roberts-Phelps, G. (2005). *Training event planning guide.* London, UK: Ashgate.

Silberman, M. L. (2005). *101 ways to make training active* (2nd ed.). San Francisco, CA: Wiley.

Stimson, N. (2002). *How to write and prepare training materials* (2nd ed.). London, UK: Kogan Page.

Wilcox, M., & Rush, S. (2004). *The CCL guide to leadership in action: How managers and organizations can improve the practice of leadership.* San Francisco, CA: Jossey-Bass.

Wilson, J. P. (2005). *Human resource development: Learning and training for individuals and organizations* (2nd ed.). London, UK: Kogan Page.

Periodicals
Hegeman, C. R. (2005). Turnover turnaround. *Health Progress, 86*(6), 25–30.

Helgeson, L. (2005). Human resources I.T. starting to deliver. *Health Data Management, 13*(11), 48–52.

Karsh, B., Booske, B. C., & Sainfort, F. (2005). Job and organizational determinants of nursing home employee commitment, job satisfaction and intent to turnover. *Ergonomics, 48*(10), 1260–1281.

Longman, S., & Gabriel, M. (2004). Staff perceptions of e-learning. *Canadian Nurse, 100*(1), 23–27.

Price, J. H., Akpanudo, S., Dake, J. A., & Telljohann, S. K. (2004). Continuing-education needs of public health educators: Their perspectives. *Journal of Public Health Management and Practice, 10*(2), 56–163.

Stengel, J. R., Dixon, A. L., & Allen, C. T. (2003). Listening begins at home. *Harvard Business Review, 81*(11), 106–117.

Sumrow, A. (2003). Motivation: A new look at an age-old topic. *Radiology Management, 25*(5), 44–47.

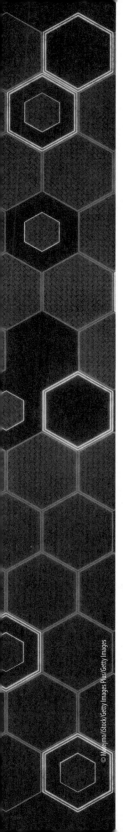

SECTION III

Recruitment

Identifying, locating, and recruiting new employees is a never-ending activity for human resources. Each of the two chapters making up Section III addresses a different aspect of this essential activity. The goal of the chapters in this section is employing individuals who will succeed in their jobs while aligning their activities with the mission and objectives of organizations. Chapter 12 (Department Managers and the Recruiting Process) introduces the responsibilities that managers are normally expected to assume in the process of attracting new employees. Chapter 13 (Conducting a Successful and Legal Selection Interview) provides guidance about interviewing. Guidelines, legal requirements, and pitfalls are presented and discussed.

CHAPTER 12

Department Managers and the Recruiting Process

CHAPTER OBJECTIVES

After studying this chapter, readers will be able to:

- Describe the steps in the recruiting process.
- Understand the essential partnership between department manager and human resources in recruiting employees.
- Be knowledgeable of the legal risks and hazards inherent in checking references or answering references requests.
- Understand the concepts of defamation and negligent hiring as they relate to recruiting.
- Understand a department manager's role in locating job candidates.
- Know the advantages and occasional disadvantages of promotion from within the organization.
- Be knowledgeable of special recruitment concerns, such as recruiting during periods of labor shortage.

▶ Chapter Summary

Every department manager should participate in recruiting actively partnered with the employment section of human resources (HR). This collaboration begins with determining and approving a staffing need, identifying the most appropriate recruiting channels, and agreeing on the contents of a position description (job description). The content of an existing job description must be revised and updated as necessary. The partners specify any special recruiting requirements that may be present, consider both internal and external candidates as they become

🔍 CASE STUDY: "Didn't Cut It? Hire Another"

Kathy Gray was hired by Meadows Nursing Home for the position of business manager. Hers would be a small department: two employees other than herself plus one open clerical position. Although she had considerable experience with business office operations, this was Kathy's first supervisory position.

One of the first tasks facing Kathy was hiring someone to fill the open clerical position. She asked the individual who handled HR matters for help in finding some candidates for her to interview. There was no HR department as such, just one person who also coordinated purchasing for the home. Kathy's manager, nursing home administrator Sam Weston, chose to sit in on the interviews, citing Kathy's newness to supervision as his reason. Because Kathy had never interviewed or hired before, Sam reasoned that he should assist her in the process.

Kathy and her boss jointly interviewed four candidates. Of these, two appeared to be reasonably qualified for the job. One of these was a young woman named Louise Bennett who worked in the home's food service department. The other was a young woman named Emily Smith whose total work experience consisted of working in a convenience store for a few months.

Following the interviews, Kathy expressed her desire to hire Louise Bennett from food service because she seemed to have the ability and exhibited a strong desire to better herself. She reasoned that selecting Ms. Bennett would show a commitment by the home to develop employees from within the organization. Sam disagreed, telling Kathy that she could do the hiring "the next time a job opened." Sam himself made the decision to hire the other candidate and personally communicated the offer to Emily Smith.

As the 30-day probationary period progressed, it became increasingly evident to Kathy that Emily was not shaping up in a satisfactory manner. Even after providing Emily a good orientation, providing her with reasonable guidance, and extending her every benefit of the doubt because she had been "the boss's choice," Kathy still had to conclude that the nursing home would be making a mistake by keeping Emily.

On the 28th day of Emily Smith's employment, Kathy Gray went to see Sam. She had kept Sam informed, so it was no surprise to him when Kathy said they should let Emily go and start over.

"Okay," Sam replied. "She didn't cut it? Let her go and hire another person."

Kathy hesitated, then finally said, "I don't believe I should be the one to let her go. I'm not the one who hired her."

"She's your employee," Sam said, "so you get rid of her."

What management errors were committed? Remembering that Emily Smith reported to Kathy even though Sam had hired her, do you believe that Sam dodged his responsibility by ordering Kathy to get rid of Emily? How might this whole situation have been handled in a more professional manner? What effect might the Emily Smith incident have on the future relationship between Kathy and Sam?

available, and conduct professional interviews to identify the most appropriate of available job candidates.

Because of contemporary legal concerns, including the risk of charges of defamation or negligent hiring, a department manager's involvement in checking references and responding to reference requests should be limited to providing information to the human resources department as needed. Of special interest to department managers is the importance of promoting from within the organization.

▶ Legal Concerns in Recruiting

A number of legal requirements exert considerable influence on the employment process. Especially pertinent are those having to do with opportunities for equal employment, especially Title VII of the Civil Rights Act of 1964.

An HR department is primarily concerned with much of the legislation reviewed in previous chapters; however, there are implications for department managers. Managers must be aware of many aspects of legislation and regulation when interviewing prospective employees.

▶ Partnerships with Human Resources

Obtaining employees is an area of activity in which a department manager and HR personnel ordinarily must work together closely. Although the process may vary somewhat from one organization to another, the following discussion represents a fairly standard recruiting relationship between HR and the other departments of an organization.

Initially, the department manager provides an approved personnel requisition to HR. The requisition may specify replacement for an employee who is resigning, retiring, or being discharged. Alternatively, it may request an employee to fill a position that did not previously exist. A department manager will have procedures to follow involving steps mandated by the organization before HR receives the requisition. The specific steps to be taken are usually related to the nature of the requisition.

If a request is for a new employee who represents an addition to a department's workforce, in the majority of organizations the department manager will be expected to go through a justification process to secure approval for the added position from higher management. This process may or may not involve input from HR. However, for a new or additional position, HR will be unable to recruit without approval from higher management. In some organizations, if the personnel requirement is for a direct replacement, a department manager may be empowered to initiate a requisition and submit it directly to HR.

Close attention may be brought to bear on staffing levels. In organizations experiencing financial difficulties or undergoing reengineering or a significant rearrangement of personnel, senior managers may elect to review all positions that become available to determine whether they must remain unfilled. In such an environment, higher management may reserve the right of review and approval for all staffing requests, even direct replacements.

Once a personnel requisition is approved, it travels from the department manager to HR. The HR department may or may not know a particular requisition is coming. Human resources will expect a requisition if it is to replace a retiring employee or person who has been discharged, because HR will have been involved in processing the retirement or the discharge. If the requisition is for an employee to fill a newly created position, then HR may not receive advance notification.

The next step involves the job description for the position in question. A department manager or direct supervisor usually has the responsibility to provide an accurate job description, either new or updated, as appropriate. If a requisition is for a direct replacement known in advance to HR, then the appropriate job description will usually be recovered from company files and reviewed. The direct supervisor of the position in question will typically be asked to examine the position description and determine whether it should be updated. If a request is for a newly created position, then HR will expect to receive a new job description along with or immediately following the requisition. The HR department is often able to assist in developing or updating a job description. However, most of the information necessary for doing so will be available to the position's direct supervisor rather than to HR.

An accurate job description is essential for getting the recruiting process properly started. Human resources will require an understanding of the major job duties of the open position so as to produce a job posting seeking internal applicants, if possible, and to advertise for external applicants. As soon as people begin to apply for the position and screening interviews are started, HR will require information from the job description to accurately describe the position to applicants.

At the time an approved personnel requisition is submitted, the department manager should have an accurate, up-to-date description of job duties and a checklist of the necessary experience and qualifications of individuals who are to be interviewed. This information is contained in a comprehensive and correctly written job description. A department manager should be prepared to review appropriate internal candidates as well as those from outside, interview the best prospects for the position in question, and have all applicants' references checked and academic credentials verified as necessary. These steps must be completed for all applicants. When the HR department receives a personnel requisition, its initial consideration is to determine whether the position is to be posted internally. Most organizations, especially large ones, maintain job-posting systems for use by existing employees. These provide opportunities for promotion or transfer to current employees. In some locations, internal posting and external advertising commence at the same time. Typically, an organization-wide posting system will provide a reasonable time period, typically a week, for internal candidates to apply before external candidates are considered. An exception occasionally arises when a position requires specialized training or a specific skill that is known to be missing among present employees. Such positions usually involve skilled technical or professional expertise. In such a situation, an external search is started immediately upon receipt of a requisition.

Regardless of the source of applicants, HR has the job of providing a department manager with a number of candidates who meet the stated minimum qualifications of the position. The number of candidates to be supplied varies. Salient factors involve normal departmental or organizational practices, considerations of equity and diversity, and the labor market from which candidates are to be sought. Conducting interviews can be costly. Some highly skilled professionals may be in such short supply or high demand that an organization may have only one or two qualified candidates. For most entry-level positions, however, HR should be able to provide five or six reasonably qualified candidates without consuming too much time conducting screening interviews.

When hiring entry-level personnel, a manager should be able to select one suitable employee from among five or six candidates who all meet the published minimum requirements for the position. Human resources and department managers do not always agree on the appropriate number of candidates. Managers may insist on interviewing an excessive number of candidates, searching for one who significantly exceeds the minimum requirements of the position, looking, in short, for the "ideal" candidate. Finding the ideal candidate will usually reduce or eliminate the need for training; however, the effort and expense involved in searching for an ideal candidate usually does little more than create extra work for the recruitment system. An ideal candidate rarely appears. If a position truly requires a highly qualified and experienced individual, an ideal candidate, then the minimum requirements submitted in a requisition should be adjusted to reflect this need.

When applicants are plentiful, HR may simply forward the résumés of people who appear to be minimally qualified. Such a determination is usually made by reviewing information appearing on paper and not by actually conducting screening interviews. Managers then review the applications and select candidates to interview. While some managers prefer to work in this manner, such an approach creates more work for them and tends to subvert the effectiveness of an established system, because these managers are actually conducting their own initial screening as well as interviewing candidates, and human resources is often inappropriately blamed when a poor selection decision is made.

Human resources' time spent finding and referring candidates and a department manager's time spent interviewing are normal organizational costs related to recruiting. Lost productivity as well as training and orientation activities must be included when calculating the true cost of recruitment. The latter are indirect costs, but they are nonetheless real. The extent to which the department and HR personnel are able to cooperate in recruitment will directly affect the efficiency of the process.

When meeting with candidates, department personnel should avoid discussing compensation except in the most general terms, such as perhaps describing the pay range for a position. Discussion or explanation of employee benefits should not be attempted by departmental personnel. Benefits information can rapidly become complicated, especially when an organization has a benefits structure that includes individual choices and when HR is the only department prepared to address or explain benefit options.

The interviewing manager should not extend an offer of employment during a departmental interview. This admonition is even more important when a candidate interviews well and the manager is becoming positively inclined toward the person. All offers of employment must be processed through HR. Formal offers must be extended conditionally and considered firm only upon completion of successful reference and background checks and receipt of medical clearance via a preemployment physical examination.

An occasional point of contention between a department manager and HR occurs in establishing a new employee's starting date once an offer has been made and accepted. Some managers often feel that new employees ought to be able to start work immediately unless working out a period of notice for other employers.

Human resources will ordinarily take all reasonable steps to have new employees begin work as soon as possible, but reference and background checks and preemployment physical examinations are absolutely essential and require time.

▶ Reference Checking and the Department Manager

Department managers who want to become personally involved in checking applicant references or personally answering reference requests should not be allowed to do so. A centralized function—specifically, HR—must handle all reference information, checking applicant references as well as answering reference requests from other employers. The HR personnel conducting the activity are familiar with applicable laws, can check all pertinent applicant references in a similar way, and can respond to all reference information requests in a consistent manner.

Exchanging reference information is another activity that sometimes generates friction between HR and department managers. On the surface, it would seem that allowing health professionals who manage others to exchange reference information with their counterparts in other organizations without HR intervention would be a logical approach. To paraphrase a manager who insisted on personally exchanging reference information about high-tech employees: "It requires my level of specialized knowledge to render judgments on an individual's capabilities." The reason why the manager should *not* become involved in exchanging reference information is revealed by the use of one word in that statement: *judgment.*

Judgments have no place in exchanging reference information. Reference responses must include nothing that is subjective in any way—no opinions, no judgments. Subjective statements can always be challenged because they cannot be rendered as absolute, objective truths. Only information that can be verified in a personnel record is completely safe to give out when answering a reference check. Furthermore, only information that is relevant to the request should be offered.

Reference requests are best answered by someone who has access to the appropriate personnel files. All reference requests should be answered impersonally and directly from the record. Time and again attorneys and advocates have advised, "For all practical purposes, information not contained in a file or record does not exist." Documentation to substantiate statements made in a reference conversation is imperative. Anything said in response to a reference request must be verifiable in a personnel file.

Organizations often become overwhelmed with fear of legal repercussions resulting from reference requests on both the receiving and sending sides, especially the sending side. Many have adopted the practice of either not answering at all or limiting their answers to the verification of job titles and dates of employment. Some organizations exhibit an obvious double-standard concerning references. When checking references of potential new hires, they try to obtain as much information as possible from prior employers. In contrast, when they respond to reference requests. They limit their responses to the minimum, verifying only dates, titles, and occasionally salaries.

There are opposing sides concerning the legal dangers involved in giving and receiving reference information, with one side receiving far more attention than the other. The more obvious apparent risk is being charged with defamation. Many employers fear being sued by an unsuccessful candidate who feels a job opportunity was lost because of comments received from a reference. This, of course, causes many former employers to limit their answers to reference-information seekers and to disclose as little information as possible.

The other potential legal hazard related to reference checking is negligent hiring. This can occur when an applicant's references are not checked prior to extending an offer to hire. A negligent hiring charge may arise when a hiring organization does not make a good-faith effort to check references on an incoming employee who later causes harm to people or property. Many people do not consider this to present as much risk as defamation, but it has the potential to inflict serious harm on an organization. Assume that an employer hires a new employee without checking references and that employee has a record of serious misdeeds known to the former employer. If that employee causes harm while working for the organization that failed to check references, then the organization is at risk of being charged with negligent hiring. A secondary danger exists for the person's past employer. If the past employer had relevant and documented knowledge of a serious problem (e.g., assault or theft) and did not reveal that information upon request, the former employer could be at risk for legal action brought by the new employer.

Charges of defamation are relatively common. Unsuccessful candidates often file charges of defamation, claiming they were not hired because of something said in a response to a reference request. A few such complaints go on to become legal cases that can require months or years to resolve. Such cases are time consuming and can be costly. For department managers who choose to unilaterally give out reference information, such actions can become extremely frustrating. Legal actions involving negligent hiring are not nearly as common as those involving defamation, but negligent hiring cases tend to be considerably more serious and decidedly more expensive. A final reason for restricting all reference contacts to HR is simply practical. Should a charge of defamation or negligent hiring become a full-scale legal battle, HR, not an individual department manager, assumes the responsibility for all legal issues and activities.

Organizations are usually fairly safe in answering reference requests with documented truth from the personnel record, as long as what is said is pertinent in assessing the person for the job being sought and as long as the information is not conveyed with malicious intent. Those who are responsible for answering reference requests should do so without attempting to interpret the record. They should supply information directly from a former employee's record. For example, concerning attendance, one might say, "Absent 9 times and tardy 12 times in 3 months," but should never say, "Frequently late or absent. The person can't be depended upon to be there when needed." The former is in the record and cannot readily be disputed. The latter is imprecise and renders a judgment. "Frequently" does not have a quantifiable definition, and the judgment about dependability is a personal opinion or interpretation. Judgments and opinions are subjective. An exception to this guideline can sometimes occur if a supervisor has rendered a judgment in writing; relaying the words of another can sometimes be considered an objective recitation of information that is already contained in the record. But one must remain cautious in doing so; if the judgment that is repeated is inflammatory or otherwise controversial, the effect might be to simply shift some of the emphasis for defamation charges to the individual rendering the original judgment.

Even if no HR department exists, as is the case in some very small organizations, reference requests should still be centrally addressed. The person responsible for maintaining the organization's personnel files should handle such requests.

A note documenting the information in a reference telephone call should be added to the personnel record. The date, information provided, name of the organization, contact information, and person receiving the information, and the name of the person supplying the information should be noted on a separate sheet and added to the permanent personnel file. Such information is usually sufficient to resolve most legal claims.

Regardless of precautions and guidelines about handling reference requests and information, there remains a tendency for some managers to exchange such information with peers and colleagues. In most geographic areas, many of the people in the organizations constituting the local healthcare community tend to be well acquainted with each other. Managers are ordinarily acquainted with their counterparts, as they often attend conferences together or belong to the same professional organizations. It is often natural for managers to speak with each other about employee capabilities, especially as employees change jobs and move from employer to employer within the community. A manager who engages in such conversations is essentially trading reference information. Although this practice is likely to continue, supervisors should nevertheless observe the essential rule: offer no judgments and convey nothing that cannot be verified in the personnel file.

The foregoing advice was disputed by a department manager who said in effect, "It's no one's business what I might say in a private conversation with a friend and colleague. We can discuss anything we wish and nobody can do anything about it." That manager was asked to consider the following: "If you find yourself in the witness chair in federal court, under oath, and you are asked specific questions about a particular conversation with your friend and colleague, how will you answer? How will your friend and colleague answer?" It is best to avoid the possibility altogether by leaving the giving and receiving of reference information to the HR department.

▶ The Manager's Role in Finding Candidates

A constant concern of HR is finding and retaining people with the skills and talents needed by the organization. This should be a continuing concern for each department manager as well.

Advertising

There are various methods of advertising to find employees. Historically, and occasionally still today, employers have used newspaper advertisements. However, more commonly jobs are posted to online job sites such as Indeed.com, iHire, Monster, SimplyHired, and Glassdoor.

Special healthcare employment publications exist to serve national, regional, and local markets. Professional journals with national circulations often carry employment advertising. With all of these publications, longer lead times are involved because of publication schedules. This is especially true of professional journals. Organizations planning to use such focused advertising must often extend the length of their recruiting schedules.

An advertising executive once said that half of every dollar spent on advertising was wasted. Unfortunately, he was unable to identify which half was wasted. Some HR employment recruiters have said that they obtain no more than one-third of new employees as a result of print advertising. Others have commented that no more than 30% of all jobs ever get advertised in print.

Networking

A considerable proportion of the better-paying jobs, such as technical, professional, and managerial positions, are filled through networking. Networking ordinarily works in the following manner: someone seeking a position makes personal contacts among friends, relatives, acquaintances, and former colleagues. Individuals who are serious about networking contact people working within or in organizational proximity to their field of interest. These activities spread the word that one is seeking a particular kind of position. By forwarding networking contacts and referrals to other individuals, the original person often encounters a series of individuals who would otherwise have been unknown, unidentified, or unavailable, and who are then able to be directly accessed. This series of contacts, referrals, and subsequent contacts constitutes the network.

In attempting to establish networks, people should begin with the relevant personal contacts with whom they are best acquainted. They should follow leads or referrals to others through a series of networking or courtesy interviews. At each encounter or meeting, the job seeker should leave a current résumé. Serious job seekers are advised to carry a supply of business cards and several copies of their résumé at all times. The timing or existence of networking or potential employment opportunities cannot be predicted.

Employers engage in networking to find people to fill specific positions. Recruiters attend professional society meetings, conferences and conventions, and other gatherings of people who work in the occupation of interest to actively build networks of potential candidates. Many department managers have made initial contact with people they later hired at such gatherings. Considerable networking also takes place at job fairs.

Job Fairs

Job fairs are gatherings of employers who are interested in gaining exposure for their organizations and promoting them as good places to work. A typical job fair is organized in a fashion that resembles a vendors' room at a convention. All individual employers have tables and displays of information about their organizations. An employer's table will commonly be staffed by one to three people, usually an employment recruiter from HR and a department manager or employee of a particular specialty.

Job fairs are sponsored by municipalities, business organizations, trade associations, chambers of commerce, colleges and universities, and other organizations. They are usually well publicized. Candidates who attend job fairs are reminded to bring a supply of current résumés. Universities or other organizations that educate healthcare workers—for example, a school of nursing or a college of health and human services—hold job fairs that are attended by its graduating seniors. Local and regional healthcare employers are invited to attend.

Recruiting Trips

A department manager may become involved in recruiting trips. Human resources should be notified and involved with the planning of such excursions. These trips may involve going to conferences, conventions, colleges and universities, and other gatherings of persons that have the skills desired by an organization.

A department manager's participation in such trips may be essential when recruiting professional employees such as registered pharmacists, nurses, and physical therapists. Before leaving for such a trip, an HR recruiter provides information about the organization. During the recruiting trip, the department manager addresses questions asked on a professional-to-professional level. Experience has shown that recruiting trips involving a department manager or other professional from within the specific department that is seeking an employee tend to be more successful than trips made by an employment recruiter alone. After the trip has identified candidates, HR should provide the same services as when recruiting for any other position.

Search Firms

Search firms, frequently referred to as "headhunters," are often utilized to locate and secure employees for some hard-to-fill jobs. These are usually middle or upper management positions or professional positions for which applicants are in short supply on the labor market. The services of search firms are also used when an organization does not want to publicize a vacancy or wishes to conduct a confidential search.

The department manager may have occasion to suggest the use of a search firm. However, it is usually HR that engages the services of a search firm, and it usually does so only with administrative or executive concurrence. Search firm charges can amount to as much as 40% of the annual salary of the position being filled.

The Internet

By way of résumé-posting websites such as Monster.com or CareerBuilder.com, the Internet offers HR and department managers a sometimes fast and efficient means of assessing the state of the supply of job seekers in any given occupation. Few pertinent postings can indicate a seller's market in which the available few can expect to command generous offers; many pertinent postings can indicate a buyer's market, with more people seeking positions than there are available.

The Internet can also be used to some extent to assess supply and demand regionally, recognizing that available individuals in any occupation will not necessarily be evenly distributed throughout the country. We say "to some extent" because not all job seekers will be registered with these services.

The department manager is cautioned to coordinate the contacting of potential candidates located via the Internet with HR. It is HR that must do the actual contacting. Here is another caution to observe in looking up potential job candidates on the Internet: It is likely that not everyone who posts a résumé is seriously seeking new employment. Many, of course, are doing just that, but there are also those who are not actively looking to change jobs but have simply posted in case the "ideal" position should seek them out.

▶ Promotion from Within

Senior managers of most organizations endorse a philosophy of developing and promoting employees from within the organization. Many healthcare organizations have sent written copies of policies to this effect to all employees. Such policies recognize that one of the job-related conditions important to many employees is the opportunity for personal promotion and growth.

Despite having written policies, however, some department managers tend to initially look outside for their new employees. This practice frequently creates conflict because employees hear one message but see something different occur in practice.

It is necessary to strike a balance between internal transfer and promotion and external recruiting. To a considerable extent, an organization benefits by filling vacancies from within and promoting employees as vacancies occur. External recruitment is used to fill the entry-level positions vacated by those being promoted. However, filling all responsible positions by promotion from within can create organizational stagnation because people who think and act in the manner of their organizational role models simply perpetuate that behavior. From time to time, new personnel are necessary. Coming from outside of the organization, new people bring new or different ideas with them.

Filling all of the better jobs from outside can demoralize existing staff, many of whom desire to be promoted. After being passed over or denied promotion when management hires someone from outside, they become keenly aware of the contradiction between the espoused organizational policy of internal development and the actuality of external recruiting. In reaction to such a situation, the more promising employees tend to leave and seek employment elsewhere. The less promising employees stay, to the long-term detriment of an organization. Over time, employees from both groups find ways to seek personal equity.

As already mentioned, an important condition of employment for many people is the opportunity for growth and promotion within the organization. The important word in this statement is *opportunity*. Employees will know whether such opportunity is or is not present. Individuals who may never take advantage of it are nevertheless demoralized by its absence. The perceived absence of opportunity for growth and promotion imposes a figurative ceiling on potential advancement for all employees.

Most HR departments in healthcare operate a job posting system that provides information to employees about opportunities for promotion and transfer. These systems usually give existing employees a few days to bid on transfer or promotional possibilities before the jobs are made available to external applicants.

It is healthy for an organization to promote from within for nontechnical, nonprofessional positions, especially those for which most of an applicant's expertise is developed through on-the-job training and experience in departments that provide service and support for a larger organization. This leaves entry-level openings that can then be filled by outside applicants. This practice makes a great deal of sense because it permits managers to fill positions of increasing responsibility with people who are familiar with the organization and have proven themselves in entry-level positions.

Some department managers frequently tend to look externally because they are unsure that internal candidates, obviously untested at a higher level, can perform the required duties. However, this is a risk common to all placements whether from inside or outside. If a supervisor knew for certain that a particular person could handle a more responsible job, then the move might not represent a growth opportunity for the individual. Whether any particular employee comes from within or from the outside, there is always a risk associated with the placement. Some highly experienced managers have hired external candidates possessing marvelous qualifications who turned out to be disastrous. Growth and development require learning. Sometimes learning is not successful and results in mistakes. People learn from making errors. It should be a goal of every supervisor to limit the magnitude of possible mistakes.

There is an additional reason why department managers are encouraged to look closely at potential internal candidates before looking to the outside. When a qualified internal candidate who is a member of a protected class under the Equal Employment Opportunity Act does not get a desired position that subsequently is given to an external candidate, there is always the likelihood of a charge of discrimination. Many HR practitioners have received formal complaints that can be summarized by, "I didn't get the promotion because I was discriminated against because I am a member of a protected class." Protected classes include people identified on the basis of their race, creed, color, national origin, religion, gender, age, or sexual orientation. For this reason, and in support of development from within, department managers are always encouraged to look closely at qualified internal candidates before resorting to recruiting external candidates.

▶ Salary Bumping

Salary bumping ordinarily involves skilled occupations that are in short supply in a given community or for which the supply in an area is marginal. As a result, openings in these occupations usually take longer than average to fill. Salary bumping begins when a group of employees at one organization applies pressure for more money. They may exert this pressure themselves or use an advocate. An advocate may often be a physician whose income depends, in part, on the occupation in question. For example, an anesthesiologist may be an advocate on behalf of nurse anesthetists, or a surgeon may be an advocate for surgical physician assistants.

The group or the advocate requests higher pay for practitioners of the occupation, citing supposedly higher pay at other organizations in the area and expressing the fear that these better-paying employers are going to lure away some members of this group. Some present employees may even moonlight (use their professional skills and work for a second employer in the off-duty hours from their primary employers) for other employers in the area and can produce proof of higher pay at these other places. People who moonlight usually do receive higher hourly rates than regular employees to compensate for the absence of benefits. The group or the advocate attempts to trade on the fear that other local employers will lure away the best employees unless the group's salaries are increased across the board.

Some organizations do try to lure people with scarce skills away from other employers in their area, and sometimes they succeed. Pay rates for the occupation in question get bumped upward as organizations recruit each other's employees. However, this process does nothing to alleviate the short supply of individuals with the needed skill in the local area. It does nothing to recruit more help into the area. Salary bumping simply raises personnel costs for all local employers while the shortage continues to exist.

Some professional employees project an attitude of free agency. They behave as though considering themselves readily available to change organizations for what might appear to be a better deal. These employees feel greater loyalty to an occupation or profession than to an organization. They are prepared to move freely, usually for more money, among comparable employers as long as they feel that the professional experience remains about the same from one employer to another. Their profession, rather than any particular organization, holds their allegiance.

Free-agent employees are becoming more common among persons trained in occupations that remain in chronic short supply. As free agents move among organizations, they have the effect of raising the price for their skills in the community without altering the supply.

A department manager who hears stories to the effect that other local healthcare employers are threatening to recruit away the best people should consider the possibility that this may be true. However, an alternative explanation is salary bumping. When a manager hears such stories, he or she must resist the temptation to join the voices calling for increased salaries. Intelligent investigation is a more suitable alternative activity. Take the information to HR, which will have the means to verify or refute such claims.

▶ Recruiting During Periods of Shortage

Recruiting becomes more difficult during periods of low unemployment and at times when particular important skills are in short supply. When workers with particular skills become difficult to find or recruit, the specialists in demand have their choice of employers. Economists describe this as a seller's market. Under such conditions of shortage, a number of special approaches may be taken to attract new employees.

Internship programs have proven themselves to be effective for recruiting scarce professionals. For example, a hospital that provides an internship experience for one or two pharmacy students may find the students willing to return as employees after graduation. An individual who has had a pleasant internship experience as a student is more likely to become an employee than is a candidate for whom the organization is unknown.

Moving expenses may be paid or partial moving allowances offered to professional and managerial employees recruited from out of town. This is essentially a standard practice when recruiting top management personnel. As particular professionals become more scarce and in greater demand, organizations are more likely to offer such inducements when recruiting needed personnel.

Some organizations assist spouses in locating suitable employment as part of the recruiting process for scarce professionals. Dual-career couples are common. Supplying employment assistance to a spouse may determine the difference between success and failure when recruiting a sorely needed professional.

Signing bonuses have been used as incentives during periods of employee shortage. As of this writing, numerous advertisements for nursing personnel offer signing bonuses to new employees. A common industry practice is to pay one-half of the bonus when the person is hired and pay the second half when the individual has been successfully employed for a stated period of time, usually between 3 months and 1 year. Personnel shortages that continue often contribute to salary bumping.

During shortage periods, a finder's fee or bounty may be offered to employees who refer candidates for specific positions. The finder's fee or bounty is paid to the person making the referral when a new candidate is then hired to fill a vacancy in a shortage occupation. This procedure is often called an employee referral program. The finder's fee is ordinarily paid out in the same manner as a signing bonus, one-half of the bonus when the new person is hired and the second half when the new individual has been successfully employed for a stated period of time, usually between 3 months and 1 year. Occasionally, a signing bonus and a finder's fee are both paid to secure the services of a single new employee. A sound employee referral program increases in usefulness as the job market tightens and fewer good people are readily available.

In spite of the visible costs involved, an employee referral program can save money when compared with the costs of advertising. In many instances, a signing bonus and finder's fee together add up to less than the cost of a modestly sized display ad placed in an area newspaper. The savings generated by an employee referral program can be significant when compared with the cost of using a search firm. An employee referral program can often be shown to generate new employees at the lowest cost per hire of all recruiting practices.

Generally, hiring managers, executive managers, and HR personnel are not eligible for finder's fees. Other rules may apply in an employee referral program. For example, an employee will usually be barred from referring a family member or other relative into a job in the referring person's own department. Most organizations have policies governing nepotism or the employment of family members.

Finally, extremely specialized arrangements may be made with individuals who are needed to fill critical positions. It is common to employ physicians, for example, using individual or personal-service contracts. Another occasionally used practice involves an arrangement to pay off an individual's outstanding student loans in exchange for a contractual agreement to remain with an organization for a specific amount of time.

▶ Every Employee a Recruiter

All department managers can have a considerable impact on the extent to which their organizations appeal to prospective employees as reasonable places to work. A manager's leadership style and treatment of employees set the tone for the department and help to create a particular image for that work group. The attitudes of workers are clearly visible if they are comfortable with their working environment. Such an attitude is usually visible well beyond departmental boundaries. If enough departments project this kind of a positive image, then an organization earns a reputation as a good place to work.

Whether referral and reward programs do or do not exist, a fundamental truth of recruiting remains. Whether they are satisfied directly or indirectly, satisfied employees are often an organization's most effective recruiters.

▶ Conclusion

Legal constraints affect recruitment. The HR department provides services in partnership with other departments in the organization. An accurate position description and job requisition are usually required before HR can begin to recruit. The HR department provides a procedural template for organizational recruitment. This must be followed to avoid legal difficulties.

References are critical elements in any recruitment activity. They must always be checked by HR personnel. Responses to reference requests must be factual and objective, reflecting only information that is contained in written personnel records. Department managers are strongly advised to refer all reference inquiries to HR.

Several strategies are available for locating and recruiting suitable employees. These include print and media advertising, networking, job fairs, recruiting trips, and search firms. Promotion from within is a sound organizational practice that is not universally observed. Salary bumping occurs when organizations succumb to pressure to increase the salaries of scarce personnel beyond their market value. Other recruiting plans include internships, paying for moving expenses, assisting spouses of candidates to secure appropriate employment, paying a signing bonus or finder's fee, or making other, specialized arrangements to successfully recruit specific needed personnel. Happy, satisfied employees are often an organization's most effective recruiters.

CASE STUDY: Resolution

Returning to the case study, on the surface it appears as though newcomer Kathy knew more about some important aspects of management than did her boss. Believing that he was helping her because of her newness to the organization, Sam actually undercut what little authority Kathy may have had as a new supervisor. As long as Sam had put Kathy in place, he had an obligation to let her do her job as she saw fit, while he made himself available in the event that she asked for help. As long as Kathy knew the correct steps to take, Sam should have allowed her to take care of the hiring without his help or interference.

It is fundamental to the hiring process that the person who will directly supervise the new employee serve as the primary interviewer and make the hiring choice. Because Sam did the actual hiring, a case can be made that he should be the person to terminate the person's employment.

The relationship between Kathy Gray and Sam Weston may be influenced by this experience for some time into the future. At the very least, Kathy will have to be sensitive to the possibility of micromanagement on Sam's part. This will continue until she is able to prove to him that she knows the job and does not require his close supervision on an ongoing basis.

SPOTLIGHT ON CUSTOMER SERVICE

Customer Service, Department Managers, and the Recruiting Process

In most organizations, the initial opportunity to manage others accompanies a promotion to a first-line supervisor position. The newly promoted supervisor is often unsure of the responsibilities and expectations of the job. As experience accumulates, clarity concerning the job also arrives. A subsequent promotion to manage a department is easier to assimilate than the first. In such organizations, the position descriptions for each new job rarely mention customer service.

This scenario also describes wasted opportunities. Even in organizations that recognize the value of customer service, most position descriptions reflect a traditional approach and describe expected activities and responsibilities. When these documents are used in recruiting, the importance of customer service is not apparent to candidates. This omission continues as newly hired employees begin their new jobs.

The remedy for this wasted opportunity is relatively easy: include "Provides and supports customer service" as a duty in position descriptions. The relative ordering of such a duty reflects an organization's commitment to customer service. The presence of customer service in the recruitment process should remove any ambiguity as to its importance.

Questions for Review and Discussion

1. It has been said that an appropriately operated HR department actually hires no one in the sense of selecting a person who will be offered a position. Why is this so?
2. When an employee provides notice of termination or a manager otherwise learns of an employee's impending departure, a manager's very first action should be to submit a requisition for a replacement. Do you agree or disagree with this statement? Why?
3. Describe in detail at least three important uses of complete and up-to-date job descriptions.
4. Why is it important to begin the search to fill a position by considering persons already employed by the organization?
5. A colleague of yours who supervises a similar department in another local institution telephones you and asks for your assessment of a former employee of yours who is applying at his institution. Should you continue the call? Why? How much and what kinds of information should you provide? Why?
6. Explain the concept of negligent hiring and provide a hypothetical example of it.
7. Explain the rationale for insisting that all checking of employment references and providing of information in response to reference requests should be concentrated at a single point in an organization.
8. Describe the principal hazards in espousing a policy of development from within an organization while aggressively recruiting from the outside.
9. Provide three examples of the free-agent type of employee and describe the circumstances that create free-agent status for them.
10. How is it possible that employee referral programs, which often include the payment of signing bonuses and finder's fees, can often generate the lowest cost-per-hire of all recruiting practices?

Resources

Books

Dubin, S. (2015). *How to hire the right people.* Amazon Digital Services, LLC.
Evers, A., Voskuijl, O., & Anderson, N. (2005). *Blackwell handbook of personnel selection.* Malden, MA: Blackwell.
Herrenkohl, E. (2010). *How to hire A-players.* New York, NY: Wiley.
Sidney, E. (2005). *Managing recruitment* (4th ed.). London, UK: Ashgate.
Singer, M. (2005). *Fairness in personnel selection: An organizational justice perspective.* London, UK: Ashgate.
Widdop, D., & Jones, D. (2005). *34 activities for recruitment and selection.* London, UK: Ashgate.

Periodicals

Casey, B. R., Owens, J., Gross, D. A., & Dixon, L. M. (2005). Rural Kentucky's physician shortage: Strategies for producing, recruiting, and retaining primary care providers within a medically underserved region. *Journal of the Kentucky Medical Association, 103*(10), 505–513.

Ferris, G. R., Berkson, H. M., & Harris, M. M. (2002). The recruitment interview process: Persuasion and organization reputation promotion in competitive labor markets. *Resource Management Review, 12*(3), 359–375.

Gullatte, M. M., & Jirasakhiram, E. Q. (2005). Retention and recruitment: Reversing the order. *Clinical Journal of Oncology Nursing, 9*(5), 597–604.

HSJ awards 2005. (2005). Reducing health inequalities. Winner: Recruiting workers provides a valuable link with hard to reach groups. *Health Service Journal, 115*(5982[suppl.]), 48–49.

Lee, R. J., & Mills, M. E. (2005). International nursing recruitment experience. *Journal of Nursing Administration, 35*(11), 478–481.

Mathias, J. M. (2005). Hospital focuses on recruiting new grads. *OR Manager, 21*(10), 35–36.

Patel, D. (2017, March). 5 Tips for recruiting the best employees. *Forbes.*

Schmidt, L. (2018, January). A glimpse into the future of recruiting. *Forbes.*

CHAPTER 13

Conducting a Successful and Legal Selection Interview

CHAPTER OBJECTIVES

After studying this chapter, readers will be able to:

- Be familiar with the specific laws having implications for the interviewing process.
- Fully prepare for an interview prior to an applicant's arrival.
- Understand the interviewing process from the perspective of an interviewing manager.
- Differentiate the kinds of questions that can and cannot legally be asked in an employment interview.
- Recognize and apply methods useful when probing for additional information that could be helpful in arriving at an employment decision.
- Describe how an interviewer should react when receiving legally forbidden information provided voluntarily.
- Explain the present-day concept of "behavioral interviewing," and describe how it may or may not differ from "ordinary" interviewing.
- Recognize that some applicants have a tendency to interview the interviewer, and know how to address this behavior.
- Appreciate the potential for fraud and distortion on résumés and applications, and know how to address suspicions concerning such.

▶ Chapter Summary

Many laws, foremost among them Title VII of the Civil Rights Act of 1964, affect the interviewing process and provide a number of potential legal traps for an unwary interviewer. Interviewing is not to be entered into lightly; interviewers must be fully prepared. An interviewer must know about the job that an applicant is seeking and must learn as much about each applicant's

🔍 CASE STUDY: "It Wouldn't Be Fair to Her"

Nurse recruiter Carrie Taylor was experiencing some of the same problems as others in the region who did the same kind of work. Because of a widespread nursing shortage, she had positions that often required weeks or months to fill. Candidates of all skill levels and degrees of desirability were chronically in short supply. Carrie's needs were particularly acute in critical care areas and in her medical center's transitional care unit, where people were sent for rehabilitation services or to await placement in long-term care facilities. In view of these acute needs, Carrie was especially cheered when she received an application from an experienced nurse who desired a position in the transitional care unit.

The applicant was a registered nurse named Lynn Taylor. She was not related to Carrie, but their common name provided a perfect conversational icebreaker. Lynn interviewed well, but Carrie was dismayed by some of what she saw and much of what she heard. Lynn's small stature, frail build, and apparent age disappointed Carrie. Lynn Taylor appeared to be in her mid-fifties. Carrie was put off because she knew how demanding, both physically and mentally, the transitional care unit could be. When Carrie asked Lynn about a significant gap in her work history, without going into great detail Lynn said enough so that Carrie could readily conclude that Lynn had undergone breast cancer surgery.

Based on the interview, Lynn Taylor was not offered the position for which she applied. Carrie felt badly about not having anything to offer Lynn but was convinced that Lynn would be unable to keep up with the demands of the transitional care unit.

Some weeks after the Lynn Taylor interview, the transitional care position remained unfilled. At the same time, the medical center received a complaint Lynn had filed with the State Division of Human Rights. The document claimed that Lynn Taylor had been illegally denied employment based on age and disability. Because the complaint entered the organization via the human resources (HR) department, the HR director met with Carrie in an attempt to determine whether the charge of discrimination might be valid. Carrie explained the basis for her decision, adding, "She seems like a nice lady, and she's a knowledgeable nurse, but she's older and physically limited. It just wouldn't be fair to put her in a position where she's bound to fail."

Consider Carrie Taylor's reasoning. Was it sound? Should she have offered the position to Lynn? How would you respond to the allegations in the complaint?

background and qualifications as practical. Customary interviewing guidelines must always be followed. Interviewers must constantly be vigilant to observe legal boundaries when asking questions. An interviewer must always be conscious of the possibility that an applicant may interpret a statement or question as being discriminatory. Therefore, interviewers must always remember to keep the interview focused on the job and on the applicant's ability to perform it rather than on personal attributes. An experienced interviewer's strongest tool is often silence paired with effective listening. Selection interviewing is an acquired skill in which people can improve with time and experience.

▶ Legal and Other Prerequisites

There are many legal statutes affecting employment practices. The laws having the most effects on interviewing include Title VII of the Civil Rights Act (1964), the Age Discrimination in Employment Act (ADEA) (1967, amended in 1986), and the Americans with Disabilities Act (ADA) (1992). Most states and many municipalities have enacted laws and ordinances that address local issues; all requirements of this legislation must be met as well.

As employment legislation was enacted, many of the questions asked for years on application forms and regularly in employment interviews became illegal. Since the mid-1960s, approximately two-thirds of the information formerly requested on a typical employment application has become inaccessible because of legal constraints. As well as addressing information requested on paper, these prohibitions apply to interview questioning and designate what can or cannot legally be asked of job applicants.

This chapter encompasses the process of employee recruitment from preparation for an interview to appropriate follow-up after the interview. The concerns presented here extend beyond the legalities of an interview. The perspective is that of a department manager interviewing a prospective employee. Pertinent legal precautions are presented as appropriate to the process.

▶ Before the Candidate Arrives

Review the Job Description

All position descriptions in every department should be reviewed at regular intervals and updated as necessary. These reviews should be conducted each year. A job description should be reviewed for completeness and accuracy whenever a manager is preparing to interview a candidate to fill an open position.

Before interviewing any candidates for a position, the position description should be thoroughly reviewed and updated as necessary. Ideally, this should be undertaken as soon as authorization is received to fill a new or vacant position. Both the manager and the HR recruiter need the job description early in the process, so a revised or new position description should accompany the personnel requisition to HR to launch the recruiting process.

The individual who supervises an unfilled position is most familiar with its characteristics and requirements. An outside manager or HR recruiter may be only generally familiar with a particular job's structure and requirements if there are a number of different positions within a single area of responsibility.

An interviewer should review the appropriate job description shortly before an interview is scheduled so that pertinent information about the position is fresh in the interviewer's mind. Reviewing a job description for reference during an interview is sometimes acceptable. However, interviewers are cautioned not to rely on the position description during an interview. Recruiters are assumed to know about the position and what will be expected from employees hired for that position.

Review the Application or Résumé

An individual's application or résumé should be thoroughly reviewed before an interview begins. Reviewing an application or résumé for the first time during an interview is unprofessional and rude; such behavior is unsettling for the applicant.

Sometimes an applicant will be sent to an interviewing manager with a résumé or an application in hand. When this occurs, the interviewer should take a few minutes in private to go over the material before starting the interview. Human resources should not ordinarily send an application or résumé along with the applicant unless recruitment is urgent, and the organization has agreed to accept and interview applicants on a walk-in basis. Under normal recruiting conditions, an interviewer should have the résumé or application in advance of the interview. If this is not routine in the organization, then HR should review its standard operating procedures for recruiting.

In reviewing an applicant's information, the interviewer should be especially sensitive to any gaps in the individual's employment record and background. Periods of months or years for which no information is supplied should serve as a red flag. Such omissions often obscure information an applicant would prefer not to reveal. If you notice gaps, make a note to ask about them during the interview. Both the HR recruiter and the department interviewer should similarly look for gaps in the screening process.

Be alert for the possibility of exaggeration or out-and-out fraud in an applicant's background, especially in the areas of education and work experience. Résumé fraud is discussed in detail later in this chapter.

Arrange an Appropriate Time and Place

Arrange for a place to conduct the interview where the interviewer and applicant will be reasonably comfortable and can talk without interruption. Borrow a private office or use a conference room, if possible. A private office with a door is preferred. An open-topped or cubicle without a door is not private. If open space must be used, then a semi-enclosure or a corner table that is at some distance from the nearest person should provide a modicum of privacy. The area used should allow for interviewer and applicant to converse without being overheard. Trying to conduct an interview within the hearing of others can be distracting for an interviewer. To an applicant, it is not only unsettling but also unfair.

Physical comfort is a consideration. Surroundings do not have to be plush or elegant, but the seating should be comfortable, and the temperature should be reasonably controlled. If using a desk or table, the interviewer and applicant should face each other across a corner of the surface or out in an open area rather than across the full expanse of the desk or table. An expanse of surface between the parties can be intimidating to an applicant.

Make sure to allow adequate time for the interview. How long an interview should take depends on the kind of position being filled and the depth to which the interviewer wishes to probe. For entry-level positions, 30 minutes should be adequate. For technical and professional positions, an hour is most likely a minimum requirement. Promising candidates may be given more time, especially if other activities, such as providing a facility tour, are components of the interview.

Interruptions hamper the exchange of information. Experienced managers do not take or make telephone calls when conducting interviews. Drop-in visitors should be tolerated only in an absolute emergency because they disrupt the rhythm of an interview. In addition to being extremely disruptive to applicants, interruptions disturb an interviewer's train of thought and increase the difficulty of establishing a conversational rapport with the applicant.

Prepare Some Opening Questions

Have three or four relatively easy, nonthreatening questions prepared to initiate the conversation. A careful review of an applicant's résumé usually presents some useful elements for starting a conversation.

▶ Conducting an Interview

Remembering a few basic guidelines can assist interviewers in conducting professional, effective interviews.

Be on Time

Short of encountering a dire emergency, there is no reason for an interviewer to be late for an interview. If an interviewer is late, then the reason should be plausible and preferably visible. An employee selection interview is as important an event for the organization as it is for the applicant. By extension, it should be important to the interviewer. Casual tardiness by an interviewer displays disregard for the value of an applicant's time and can leave an applicant with a less-than-desirable impression of the organization.

If Possible, Help the Applicant to Relax

Most experts suggest beginning an interview with a bit of small talk or some inconsequential social chatter to help get the conversation started. With most applicants, this is sufficient to initiate a conversation. Although some applicants remain nervous, it is still best to make an attempt at helping them to relax.

Never forget that applicants may be intimidated by interviewers and the authority of their positions. An interviewer's position in an organization may not be particularly important, but to applicants, interviewers are authority figures who are perceived as having influence in determining whether they are hired.

An interviewer has a psychological upper hand in an interview situation. The interview is taking place in the interviewer's territory. The interviewer is a representative of the organization who may have the power to extend or withhold employment. Applicants react to perceived differences between themselves and their interviewers by becoming nervous, so any step an interviewer can take to relax the applicant and put the conversation on an equal footing will contribute to a more productive interview.

Adjust Language to Accommodate an Applicant

Successful interviewers put themselves on an applicant's level of education and sophistication when choosing their words by using terms an applicant is most likely to understand. Avoid the use of acronyms or abbreviations without explanation, and do not use jargon. Doing so helps to diminish the applicant's feelings of being an outsider. This suggestion can be ignored when an applicant is known to be an equal in terms of job experience. Overall, use language appropriate for the position under discussion. The use of appropriate language is important in health care, since a single manager may have direct responsibility for persons with a variety of educational levels. For example, interviewers use different language when conversing with nurse practitioners than with applicants for nursing assistant positions.

Avoid Both Short-Answer and Open-Ended Questions

An important interview objective is getting an individual to speak about knowledge, experience, reasons for seeking a particular position, personal likes and dislikes, and career goals. Interviewers will not learn much of substance if their questions can be answered by single words such as yes or no or by brief phrases. Effective questions require individuals to speak at least a sentence or two in response. In only a few instances are short-answer questions fully appropriate, as in, for example, "Do you have a current nursing license?"

In contrast, interviewers should not ask completely open-ended questions that provide no clear guidelines as to how much to say or when to stop speaking. A classic example is the opening line often used by interviewers who believe they are being clever and insightful: "Tell me all about yourself." A request of this nature has no recognizable boundaries, and any answer can ramble on for a considerable time without producing much of value. Because the question provides no guidelines as to how much a person is expected to say, it is inherently unfair to the applicant.

The most effective questions are those that require some thought and can be reasonably answered in three or four sentences. Interviewers should try to get applicants to talk about themselves relative to potential employment. However, they should do so in such a way that they can maintain control over the conversation and avoid causing an applicant to either talk without closure or freeze from confusion when asked an unfair, open-ended question. Examples of appropriate questions include the following: "How did you become interested in this occupation?" "What part of your most recent position did you like best, and why?" "Of what accomplishment of the last year or two are you most proud?" and "Tell me about something that went wrong on the job, and what you learned from it."

Interviewers should be sure to allow a pause between an applicant's response and the next question. This gives the applicant a chance to embellish the response; most applicants tend to fill in periods of silence.

Avoid Leading Questions

Be careful to avoid leading applicants toward a desired response. This is a particular hazard when interviewing someone who is making a positive impression. Interviewers in such a situation often begin to ask their questions in a manner that encourages an applicant to provide answers that they want to hear. A sharp applicant will recognize leading questions and cooperate by providing "correct" responses. For example, if the interviewer asks, "You left County Hospital because you weren't being sufficiently challenged, right?" the applicant knows the answer the interviewer wants to hear.

Avoid Writing During an Interview

Interviewers who find it necessary to make written reminders during an interview should limit them to one- or two-word notations. If more detailed notes are

---

EXHIBIT 13-1   The Manager and the Interview Process

Be on time
Help the applicant to relax
Adjust language to accommodate an applicant
Avoid both short-answer and open-ended questions
Avoid leading questions
Avoid writing during an interview
Promise and ensure follow-up

---

required, then the brief reminders can be expanded into sentences or paragraphs after the interview is concluded.

There are two sound reasons for not writing while an applicant is speaking. First, it is unnerving. In addition to causing the applicant to wonder what is being written down, it is impolite, it restricts eye contact, and it conveys the impression that an interviewer is giving the applicant less than complete attention. Second, it is not possible to listen carefully while writing. This is an attempt at simultaneously performing two important communication tasks. Few people can do this without either or both processes suffering. It is far better to give an applicant undivided attention and save writing until an interview has been concluded.

Promise and Ensure Follow-Up

At the conclusion of every interview, indicate to all applicants that they will be advised of the outcome after all interviews for the position have been completed. Pledge follow-up but provide nothing else. Do not promise that an offer will be forthcoming, even if the person who has just been interviewed is the leading candidate. A manager or supervisor should not make an offer or quote a salary without confirmation from HR. An applicant's specific questions about pay and benefits should be answered by HR and not by an interviewing department manager.

Having promised follow-up on behalf of the organization, interviewers have an obligation to ensure that the steps or activities are undertaken and delivered. It is extremely important that all applicants who have given their time for an interview receive closure within a reasonable period following the interview. Allowing unsuccessful applicants simply to fade away without acknowledgment creates ill will toward the employer.

The foregoing interview steps are summarized in **EXHIBIT 13-1**.

▶ Interview Questioning: To Ask or Not to Ask?

Inquiring about an applicant's personal life, beliefs, values, and attitudes is illegal. In an employment interview, the focus must remain on the position and whether an applicant has the skills needed to accomplish a given task for the organization. Experienced interviewers speak of evaluating interpersonal chemistry. To the extent that this is assessed, the evaluation cannot be made using words. In short, an employment interview provides an opportunity to develop some knowledge of what a prospective employee can contribute to an organization.

As a general rule, keep all interview questions related to an applicant's capacity to perform the job in question. The following sections discuss subjects and provide commentary about the legal status of topics that may arise in an employment interview.

Race, Color, Religion, Creed, National Origin, Sex, Marital Status, Birth Control Practices

These subject areas are addressed together because there are no questions concerning them that can legally be asked. This means that an interviewer may not ask questions about the origins of a person's name or where the individual's family came from. Asking about the existence of a family is not permitted. This prohibition extends to questions that can be interpreted as fishing for forbidden information. Information of this nature cannot be requested or collected on an employment application.

The reasoning behind these prohibitions is the need to eliminate the possibility of discrimination based on such information. For example, at one time it was common to ask young female applicants if they were engaged, and if so, when they planned to marry. Married women of childbearing age were asked if they planned to have children. Divorced or separated women were asked if they were single parents and how many children they had. Information obtained in responses to such questions was used to make hiring decisions. Many managers believed that avoiding people who might not remain with an organization for very long or who might experience more absences than others who lacked particular responsibilities simply reflected prudent business practices.

Antidiscrimination legislation has imposed changes. It is now illegal to make employment decisions based on personal information. Contemporary interviewers must do their best to determine whether an individual is capable of performing a given job, not to determine the likelihood of a person being absent from work or leaving employment.

Age

The only legal question that an applicant can be asked about age is: "Are you at least 18 years old?" It is permissible and sometimes necessary to ask this because the employment of workers younger than 18 years is governed by state child labor laws. Many employment situations are prohibited for persons younger than 18 years. With the exception of this question, prohibitions on questions about age relate to discrimination laws. The Age Discrimination in Employment Act, passed in 1967 and amended in 1986, prohibits discrimination on the basis of age. Under the law, only a small number of *bona fide occupational qualifications* (BFOQs) exist under which age can be considered a legitimate employment criterion. For the vast majority of employment situations, the single criterion that prevails is an individual's ability to perform the job.

Disability

The Americans with Disabilities Act prohibits employers from asking whether an applicant has a disability or has ever been treated for any number of specific medical conditions. Employers are forbidden to ask about an applicant's Workers'

Compensation history at any time prior to making an offer of employment. The only questions that can be asked before an offer of employment has been made are questions concerning a person's ability to perform the duties of the job under consideration. Questions asked prior to employment cannot be phrased in such a way as to solicit information about medical conditions or physical limitations. For example, if a job requires driving, then an interviewer may ask if an applicant has a driver's license but may not ask if the person has any visual limitations.

When inquiring into an applicant's ability to perform the major duties of a job, an interviewer can ask whether the person has any medical, physical, or mental impairment that might interfere with the individual's ability to perform the specified job duties, or whether there are positions for which one should not be considered because of an impairment. It is illegal, however, for an interviewer to inquire about the nature of any impairment. The key to questioning in this area is to focus on ability, not disability.

Name

It is permissible for an interviewer to ask whether an applicant has ever worked for the organization under a different name. Employers have this right because they are entitled to have access to an applicant's prior work record. Interviewers may ask whether additional information is available concerning a name change or the use of different names to adequately complete reference checks. An interviewer is forbidden to ask a female applicant's maiden name or the original name of any applicant whose name has been changed by court order.

Address and Duration of Residence

It is permissible to ask an applicant's place of residence and how long the person has been a resident of that municipality.

Birthplace and Date of Birth

No questions can legally be asked concerning an applicant's place of birth or the birthplace of an applicant's parents or any other family members. In most instances, because age cannot legally be considered when making hiring decisions, it is illegal to ask an applicant's age. For similar reasons, employers are prohibited from requiring applicants to submit birth certificates, baptismal records, naturalization records, or any other proof of age.

Photograph

The practice of requiring applicants to supply photographs with their applications is illegal. Even suggesting that a photograph may be submitted at an individual's option is blatantly illegal.

Citizenship

It is lawful to ask whether an applicant is a citizen of the United States, but it is unlawful to ask of what country an individual is a citizen. This question is construed as asking about national origin. Applicants who are not citizens can legally be asked whether they intend to become citizens or if they have the legal right to remain and work in the United States. It is not permissible to ask whether an applicant or an applicant's parents or spouse are naturalized or native-born U.S. citizens. An applicant cannot be required to produce naturalization papers.

Language

It is legal to ask what foreign languages applicants are able to speak and write with fluency. However, it is not legal to ask them about their native language or to ask individuals how they acquired the ability to read, speak, or write a foreign language.

Education

It is legal to ask applicants about their academic, vocational, or professional education and the public or private schools that they attended. This discussion can and should include the relevance of particular programs or courses taken.

Experience

Interviewers should concentrate most of their questions in this area. The primary objective during this phase of the interview conversation should be to gather sufficient information about an applicant's work history to make an informed decision as to whether an individual's experience is applicable to the position being discussed. When talking about employment experience, it is usually most helpful to begin with an applicant's present or most recent position and work backward in time.

Salary History

Salary history is steadily becoming forbidden information; it is one of the most prominent present-day issues concerning recruitment and employment activity. It has long been a practice of employers to ask job applicants how much they earn at their present jobs or what they earned in prior employment. This practice, it is now regularly charged, serves to continue the disparity in salary that exists between women and men in the workforce. For essentially most job applicants, whether male or female, it has long been a practice to base salary offers on what the applicant was most recently earning rather than on some scale indicating the monetary worth of the position. Thus, this approach is seen as perpetuating the gender gap in salaries.

Although there has long been federal legislation in place requiring equal pay for persons doing essentially equal work—specifically the Equal Pay Act of 1963 and the Civil Rights Act of 1964—there have been no truly effective enforcement mechanisms in place to address wage discrimination. Existing legislation essentially calls for equal pay for all persons doing the same work, although legitimate disparities could exist based on valid merit-increase systems or seniority-based pay scales. However, past efforts to require equal pay for equal work have proven ineffective.

Managers should now consider that requesting salary information from job applicants is generally forbidden; though not yet an illegal practice nationally, it most likely will eventually be just that. Massachusetts became the first state to pass legislation addressing the salary disparity issue. The new law, effective in July 2018, requires hiring managers to state a compensation figure based on the job—what a person in that position is worth to the organization—rather than what the individual earned in previous employment. Some municipalities, Philadelphia and New York City foremost among them, have banned questions about salary history in recruitment activity.

There are, however, a couple of sets of circumstances that make the salary history issue somewhat easier for some managers who do interviewing and hiring. First, in an organization of any appreciable size, there is a compensation function in human resources that provides guidance as to how much can be offered (and official offers usually come from human resources). Second, most such organizations have published pay scales that essentially predetermine how much an individual of certain qualifications and a particular amount of experience should be offered.

For the present, it should be sufficient to remember that asking for salary history in an interview or on an application is to be considered forbidden. As to how much to offer, follow the organization's published pay scales or, better still, let human resources address the salary issues.

Relatives

It is permissible to ask the names of an applicant's relatives who are already employed within the interviewer's organization without specifying their relationship. This includes a spouse. This is relevant when an organization has rules about nepotism. However, prospective employers may not ask about relatives and specify the relationship, as this is interpreted to be discriminatory on the basis of family status. It is illegal to solicit any information concerning an applicant's spouse, children, or other relatives who are not employed by the interviewer's organization.

Notify in Case of Emergency

In the pre-employment stage of recruiting, it is illegal to ask an applicant for the name and address of a person to be notified in the event of an emergency. This is one of the elements of information (along with date of birth, marital and family status, and other personal information) that organizations are not permitted to solicit until an offer of employment has been extended and accepted.

Military Experience

It is permissible to ask about the nature of an applicant's military experience in a branch of the armed forces of the United States. However, interviewers may not ask about general military experience without specifying armed forces of the United States or a branch thereof. Furthermore, interviewers are not permitted to ask applicants about the character or terms of discharge or separation from military service.

Arrest

Although the question of arrest was standard on employment applications and during interviews for many years, it is no longer legal to ask whether one has been arrested. For some time, it was generally permissible to ask whether the applicant had ever been convicted of a crime, but this practice is presently under fire from several directions. These days, one may hear references to the "box," that is, the check-off item on an application asking whether the applicant has ever been convicted of a crime, amid mounting pressure to eliminate this question altogether. Much prevailing opinion suggests that if one has been convicted and paid the penalty, then one should not be penalized by being refused employment for this reason.

However, an individual may be rejected for employment because of a criminal conviction if there is a reasonable relationship between the nature of one's crime and the position for which the person is applying. For example, an organization may be acting reasonably and properly by rejecting a convicted embezzler for a finance position or by rejecting someone with a drug-related conviction for a pharmacy position. The same organization would be likely to encounter a claim of discrimination for rejecting someone with a felony driving while intoxicated (DWI) conviction for a position as a cook or housekeeper but may successfully reject an applicant with a felony DWI conviction or a record of traffic infractions for a position requiring driving.

Organizations

Past employment applications routinely asked applicants to list all clubs, societies, and other organizations to which they belonged. This is now illegal, because the names of many organizations allow prospective employers to infer personal information such as national origin or religion.

One absolute prohibition concerning external memberships involves inquiries into whether an applicant is or ever has been a member of a labor union. Employers, especially those who may be union-free, ordinarily do not want to knowingly hire people they fear might attempt to spread interest in union organizing. Legal history has provided many instances of applicants claiming that they were rejected for employment because of union affiliations. Asking about prior membership in a labor union is considered discriminatory and an unfair labor practice under labor law.

To remain legal, any inquiry about organizations must be limited to asking about membership in groups that applicants consider relevant to their ability to perform the duties required by the position under consideration. For all practical purposes, this limits questions about organizations to technical and professional societies related to an applicant's occupational field.

Job applicants may reveal personal information during the course of an interview. Such admissions are legal and within the realm of their personal rights, but interviewers may not respond with questions on the same topics. Potential employers may not use such information when making hiring decisions. As an example, a female applicant may talk about her recent divorce, her three dependent children, and the fact that her church is assisting her to pay for cancer treatment that is thought to be due to benzene exposure on her last job. An interviewer may not ask for any details and must not use any of the offered information when making a hiring decision. The only relevant consideration is whether the applicant has the ability to perform the duties and responsibilities of the position for which she is applying.

EXHIBIT 13-2 provides a number of specific questions as examples of prohibited inquiries. These questions, or variations of them, may not be asked of a job applicant whether in an interview or on a job application. **EXHIBIT 13-3** provides a number of examples of legal pre-employment interview questions.

EXHIBIT 13-2 Examples of Forbidden Pre-Employment Questions

General

Concerning an applicant's general history, in a pre-employment interview, a potential employer may not ask the following:

1. Do you attend church regularly? What church do you go to, and who is the pastor?
2. What religious holidays do you observe?
3. What is your nationality, ancestry, descent, parentage, or lineage?
4. Of what nationality are your parents? Your spouse?
5. What is your native language?
6. Are you married? Divorced? Separated?
7. Where does your spouse work? What does he (or she) do for a living?
8. Do you have children? What are their names and ages? Do you have a reliable arrangement for child care?
9. Was your name ever changed by marriage or court order? If so, what was your original name?
10. When were you born? How old are you?
11. Where were you born?
12. Where were your parents born? Where was your spouse born?
13. Of what country are you a citizen?
14. Are you a native-born or naturalized citizen of the United States?
15. Do you own your own home or do you rent?
16. How did you acquire the ability to read, write, or speak English?
17. What are the name, address, and relationship to you of the individual to be notified in case of accident or emergency?
18. What kind of discharge did you receive from the U.S. military?
19. To what clubs, societies, lodges, or fraternal organizations do you belong?
20. How many children do you plan to have?
21. Have you ever had your wages garnished or attached?
22. Have you ever filed for bankruptcy, either personally or as a business owner?
23. Has your spouse ever worked here?
24. What is your height? Your weight?
25. Would your spouse approve of your employment here should you be hired?

Medical

Concerning an applicant's medical history, in a pre-employment interview a potential employer may not ask:

1. How is your health in general?
2. Do you have any relevant medical problems or conditions?
3. Have you or any member of your family ever been treated for any of the following diseases or conditions? (This is followed by a checklist that may include cancer, heart disease, high blood pressure, diabetes, epilepsy, AIDS, back problems, carpal tunnel syndrome, hearing loss, contact dermatitis, drug or alcohol abuse, tendonitis, arthritis, tuberculosis, sexually transmitted diseases, and mental illnesses.)
4. Are you taking prescription medication? What drugs, prescribed for what conditions?
5. Have you ever been hospitalized? For what conditions?
6. Are you in any way disabled, or do you have a disability? If so, how did you become disabled?
7. What is the prognosis of your disability?

(continues)

EXHIBIT 13-2 Examples of Forbidden Pre-Employment Questions *(continued)*

8. Will you require time off for treatment or medical leave due to anticipated incapacitation because of your disability?
9. Have you ever been injured on the job or had any other work-related accidents?
10. Check off on a list of potentially disabling impairments any physical limitations that you may have.
11. Is any member of your family disabled?
12. Have you ever filed a Workers' Compensation claim?
13. Have you received any payment for a Workers' Compensation claim?

EXHIBIT 13-3 Examples of Legally Permissible Pre-Employment Questions

Concerning an applicant's personal information, in a pre-employment interview, a potential employer may legally ask the following questions or request the following information:

1. What is your full name?
2. What are your address and the telephone number at which you can be reached?
3. What is your prior work experience? For each prior employer, this may include:
   - Employer's name and address
   - Jobs or positions held
   - Duties performed
   - Skills needed to perform job duties
   - Tools, machinery, equipment, and vehicles used in job performance
   - Name of immediate supervisor
   - Rate of pay received
   - Length of time on the job
   - Reason for leaving
4. What do you know about the requirements of the job for which you are applying?
5. What skills, education, training, or experience have you had that are relevant to performing the duties of this job?
6. Do you hold the licenses or certifications that may be required for employment in the position in question (e.g., a driver's license, an electrician's license, a registered nursing license)?
7. What were the primary duties and most important responsibilities on your most recent job?
8. What do you believe was the most difficult part of the job you have been most recently doing? Why?
9. What safety procedures were you required to follow at your most recent employment?
10. Are you applying for full-time, part-time, or temporary work?
11. Are you able to work the particular shift or shifts on which this job is ordinarily used?
12. Are you able to work overtime or weekends when it is necessary?
13. Are you able to meet this organization's attendance standard?
14. If hired, when are you able to begin work?

Probing for Intangibles

After discussing more concrete subjects such as qualifications and experience, interviewers often spend some time discussing less tangible issues. They are attempting to develop an overall impression of an applicant's personality and attitude toward work and career. Because too much cannot be asked in an interview, it is important to develop a gut feeling or personal sense about each candidate. Gut feeling is highly subjective, but it is a legitimate part of the interview process, as it refers to the feeling an interviewer develops about an individual during an interview. Such feelings can provide clues as to how other employees will regard the new person if an offer of employment is extended.

EXHIBIT 13-4 offers a number of possible questions that can be used when assessing an applicant in areas other than specific qualifications and experience for the position under consideration. In addition to assessing intangibles, an interviewer should keep another question in mind throughout the conversation: "How well do I believe this person would fit into the present work group?" Whoever is hired will have to work, often closely, with current employees on a daily basis. Concern for how a new person may relate to existing employees is highly appropriate.

EXHIBIT 13-4 Examples of Questions to Use in Probing for Intangibles

Concerning the information supplied by an applicant in a pre-employment interview, a potential employer may legally ask the following questions or request the following less tangible information:

1. What aspects of a job are most important to you?
2. What are your own personal criteria for your success?
3. What are your short-term career goals? What are your long-term career goals?
4. What are you seeking in the position under discussion that you are not getting from your present position?
5. What past goals have you set for yourself, and what have you done to accomplish them?
6. In what way would a position with our organization help you meet your career goals?
7. What factors do you believe have contributed the most to your growth?
8. What has prevented you from moving ahead as rapidly as you would have liked?
9. What job would you choose if you were completely free to do so?
10. Which of your jobs did you enjoy the most? Why?
11. How did you get each of the positions you have held?

What Is an Applicant Really Seeking?

While assessing intangibles and throughout an interview, an interviewer should be attempting to judge whether the applicant is trying to obtain a more desirable position or escape from something that is dissatisfying. In other words, the interviewer is trying to determine whether the applicant's driving force is positive or negative. Is the applicant seeking advancement, more interesting work, better compensation, a preferred occupation, growth, or personal satisfaction? Conversely, is the applicant trying to get away from an unpleasant environment, undesirable hours, an unpleasant supervisor, a quarrelsome mix of personalities, or some other unknown factor?

It is not always easy to determine whether a person's motivations for seeking a new position are positive, negative, or mixed. However, the time allocated to making a decision is still worth the investment. A person who is seeking a more desirable position is more likely to remain as a positive performer over time. An individual whose primary motive is to escape something is more likely to simply become a turnover statistic.

▶ Very Few Exceptions

There are some legitimate exceptions to the prohibitions against making hiring decisions based on some of the categories of forbidden information discussed in this chapter. For example, physical condition and age can legitimately be considered as BFOQs for police officers, fire fighters, airline pilots, and surgeons. Gender may be relevant for applicants applying for a position as an attendant for a men's or women's fitting room or to model gender-specific clothing. Having a driver's license is a legitimate requirement for operating a taxicab.

▶ When Forbidden Information Is Volunteered

As already noted, forbidden information must never be used as the basis for an employment decision, even when it is voluntarily provided.

Most interviewers receive forbidden information at one time or another. This puts the interviewing manager in an uncomfortable position of having heard unsolicited information and then having to ignore it. This is easier said than done. The situation is similar to a comment made in court followed by a judge's admonition to "Disregard that last remark." It is easy to disregard something that has not been heard, but it is not so easy to ignore something that has been heard. The information is known. The best advice is conscientiously to avoid using it when making a decision.

An occasional applicant may often volunteer personal information in a plea for sympathy, hoping it will lead to a job offer. Examples of such pleas include, "I really need this job because I'm a single parent," "I've been out of work for months and my husband is ill," or "We get our health insurance through my wife's employer, so I could save you some money on benefits."

On occasion, applicants deliberately drop items of personal information and later claim they were the victims of discrimination when the job is given to someone else. An example of such an assertion is, "I happened to mention I was pregnant. I know that's why I didn't get the job." Interviewers who hear comments including personal information are encouraged to report them in writing to their supervisors as soon as is practical after the interview is concluded. They should later file documentation summarizing the strengths and weaknesses of each candidate and rank all persons in the applicant pool. Finally, interviewers should note the reasons for recommending an offer of employment to the successful hire and the reasons for not recommending other applicants.

To reiterate, no matter how it is obtained, forbidden information must never be used as a factor in an employment decision. Because interviewers may be required to defend a particular employment decision, an HR recruiter and hiring manager should always be able to state succinctly and honestly why one person was hired in preference to others.

▶ After the Interview

Ordinarily, an employment recruiter in HR has the responsibility to make a formal offer of employment. This includes the starting pay, which will have been settled upon in conjunction with the department manager. It is fairly common practice for the offer to be conveyed by telephone and then followed with a formal written offer by letter.

Human resources usually has the duty to notify unsuccessful applicants and thank them for applying and making themselves available for interview. When conveying regrets, HR personnel will not tell unsuccessful candidates why they did not get the position. Each is simply told that someone who appeared to be more suitable or more appropriately qualified was given the position.

Occasionally, unsuccessful applicants will call the interviewing manager directly and ask specifically why they were not hired. Managers who receive such calls can handle them in one of two ways. The caller can be politely referred to HR for the official response, or the manager can simply say that the position went to the applicant who seemed best suited for the position. Organizations must always be able to defend their reasons for rejecting any particular candidate should that become necessary. However, an organization is under no obligation whatsoever to explain to unsuccessful applicants why they were not chosen.

It is often helpful to maintain a brief written record of the reasons for rejecting candidates in a recruiting process, especially if many applicants are involved and the final hiring decision might be seen as close or arbitrary. However, interviewers should exercise care about what is written and how it is expressed. Such notes can be made public in the event of a legal action that follows a hiring decision. A good rule of thumb is never to write anything about an applicant or employee that would be embarrassing if it appeared in the daily news.

▶ Behavioral Interviewing

The concept of behavioral interviewing is growing in popularity and is seen in many quarters as generating a greater degree of reliability than so-called ordinary interviewing. And it is receiving increasing visibility in management literature. One needs to ask, however, if behavioral interviewing is truly something new or if this is but a new label describing a practice that should have been followed all along and has in fact been followed by better (meaning more successful) interviewers. In other words, how much of behavioral interviewing is genuine improvement over older ways, and how much simply represents a new name attached to a process that has acquired a measure of tarnish for having been carelessly practiced by many? Just as "delegation" became so abused through improper application that thorough and proper delegation became redefined as "empowerment," so much interviewing was so poorly accomplished that some apparently felt the need for a unique label for proper, effective interviewing.

The fundamental underlying premise of behavioral interviewing is the belief that the most accurate predictor of an individual's future performance is past performance in a similar situation. It has been described as a relatively new style of interviewing developed by industrial psychologists during the 1970s. It was perhaps given that name during the 1970s, but long before it was so labeled, numerous insightful interviewers practiced the process without the benefit of a special name. Many of the numerous sources of information about behavioral interviewing describe traditional interviews as including questions such as "Tell me all about yourself" (which is not a question, but rather an open-ended instruction and grossly unfair to the applicant). Recall that an earlier section described questions like "Tell me all about yourself" as highly inappropriate. The same section included a pair of examples that might have come directly from a list of behavioral interviewing questions, specifically: "What accomplishment of the past year or two are you most proud of?" and "Tell me about something that went wrong on the job, and what you learned from it." Other examples include questions like: "Describe an instance in which you had to go above and beyond the call of duty to get a job done," and "Have you ever had to sell an unpopular idea to others? How did you proceed, and what were the results?" Also note that many of the questions listed in Exhibit 13-4, "Examples of Questions to Use in Probing for Intangibles," are applicable to behavioral interviewing.

A behavioral approach to interviewing is preferred in the majority of instances of dealing with candidates for technical, professional, and managerial positions, especially when the candidates are experienced. The approach may have to be narrowed somewhat in interviewing, for example, new graduates who have had no work experience in their fields. And one's interviewing approach may have to be further narrowed in assessing personnel for entry-level positions, especially those who are new to the workforce.

Regardless of what the approach may be called, the premise is undoubtedly sound: past performance in a similar situation is probably the best predictor of future performance. However, behaviorally oriented or not, selection interviewing is far from being a perfect process. No one has yet devised a reliable way to separate the applicants who simply *talk* a good job from those who will later *do* a good job.

▶ The Interviewer's Behavior: A Second Possible Direction

Occasionally, the process of an employee selection interview becomes reversed and the applicant takes the lead and interviews the interviewer, effectively interviewing a department or organization. Some applicants seem to do so naturally, whereas a smaller number of sharp applicants deliberately turn the focus of an interview around. This process requires the interviewer to be able to recognize such a situation and then reclaim control of the interview to end the reversal.

More Silence than Talk

Some interviewers tend to dominate the conversation and speak at length about the organization, their departments, and themselves. The object of an employment interview is to get applicants to talk about themselves and to discuss appropriate job-related topics. An interviewer must control the interview with proper questions and must concentrate on what the applicant is saying.

Nonstop talking by the interviewer limits the information that can be gained from the applicant. It sends an inappropriate message about the organization. The proper role of an interviewer involves more silence than speech. From the perspective of an interviewer, the most productive parts of an interview occur with one's mouth shut and ears open.

More Points to Keep in Mind

Effective interview technique includes being in complete control of an interview situation without obviously appearing to do so.

Successful and experienced interviewers resist the temptation to make a hasty judgment concerning a job candidate. Research has demonstrated that a majority of interviewers make up their minds about candidates during the first few minutes of contact. The remainder of the interview does little to change that mind-set. Always keep in mind that even though first impressions are sometimes proven correct, they are just as often proven incorrect.

Never encourage an applicant to criticize a present or past employer and be wary of an applicant who voluntarily does so. Conversely, one indicator of a promising applicant is how diplomatically an individual describes an apparently unpleasant employment experience.

Remain aware of the nonverbal clues that may be exhibited during the course of an interview. Remember, too, to recognize the need of applicants to compensate for normal nervousness. This is especially true for applicants who have little or no interviewing experience.

Be conscious of the halo effect when interviewing. This occurs when interviewers allow one or two obviously positive traits to bias their judgment favorably when assessing unrelated characteristics.

In every interview, try to convey an overall positive picture of the organization offering the employment opportunity. By espousing the belief that the organization is a good place to work, some of the positive viewpoints will be communicated to the applicant.

Be honest about the negatives of the job, if any. Most jobs include duties that are boring or repetitive. Some jobs include decidedly unappealing tasks or situations that may be physically or emotionally discomforting. Remain upbeat overall, but do not overlook the negatives during an employment interview. Applicants who accept a position only to discover the unpleasant parts after starting work are likely to feel they have not been treated honestly.

References

To reiterate, a department manager should never become directly involved in checking references. This is stressed because many department managers have been told, even in some of the management literature, to check references themselves. They are advised to go directly to applicants' former supervisors and bypass the HR departments of an applicant's former employer and of their own organization. Some of the same sources will pointedly advise them to avoid their organization's HR department. A common rationale for these recommendations is that HR is usually too frightened of legal repercussions to request any usable information. Following this advice can easily place them at the center of a legal action. As long as an organization has an HR department, HR should be making the reference checks.

▶ Résumé Fraud: Lies and Embellishments

At times it seems that writing an employment résumé involves putting nearly as much fiction as fact on paper. Experts have estimated that up to 40% of résumés include exaggerations or outright untruths. As many as 75% include some degree of fluff designed to make certain selected facts appear more significant than they actually are. This is accomplished by putting a favorable spin on information.

Deception on employment résumés can take a number of different forms. These involve positive spin, embellishment, exaggeration, lying, or a combination of these devices. Many variations exist.

A résumé may be deliberately ambiguous. One of the most frequently encountered examples of ambiguity has to do with education. An individual will claim to have "attended Prestige University in the BS Program in Chemistry." The hope is that readers of this résumé will assume that the applicant received a BS degree in Chemistry. In truth, the length of attendance is not known, no major was completed, and the person was not awarded a degree.

Another deception is to shift dates of education or experience deliberately to conceal periods of unemployment or, occasionally, a period of imprisonment. An honest résumé may well include one or more gaps. Applicants know that they are likely to be questioned about these gaps.

A variation on date shifting is using years to create the impression of having worked longer in a place than was actually the case. For example, a résumé may report working for "Ajax Hospital, 2010–2011." The hope is that readers of this résumé will assume that employment essentially covered the better part of 2 years. In truth, the length of employment may have been from November 2010 through January 2011. The same approach is used to conceal gaps in employment.

Another common strategy is to exaggerate job responsibilities, claim inflated job titles, and provide inflated salaries. In truth, this is a dangerous practice because basic employment information such as titles and position responsibilities is easily verifiable through reference checks. Salary data are also relatively easy to verify. These actions are intended to make applicants seem more appealing than might otherwise be the case.

Interviewers occasionally encounter claims of a more prestigious institution awarding an individual's degree. For example, an applicant may list "Stanford MBA" on a résumé. In truth, the person has been awarded a master of business administration (MBA) degree from Obscure University. This practice is openly fraudulent. Official copies of educational transcripts are often required as a condition of employment. Presenting fraudulent documentation is usually a reason for immediate discharge from a position when the misrepresentation is revealed.

Candidates may claim to have degrees and other credentials they do not possess. Honors and awards may be invented. Numbers of publications and conference presentations may be inflated or openly invented. However, such claims are easily verified.

Résumé fraud increases during periods of job scarcity. However, it is present to some extent on a continuing basis, so employment recruiters and other interviewers should be alert to the possibility of fraud in every résumé they review.

Spotting Embellishments and Inconsistencies

There is no reliable way to uncover every instance of fraud, exaggeration, or untruth that may appear in the résumés an organization receives. The task of verifying every fact on every line would be extremely time consuming and costly. However, interviewers who remain alert to subtle signs and signals are likely to know when closer examination is warranted.

Look for gaps in a person's record. It is common for someone who wants to cover something up simply to omit it. Be alert for overlapping dates and inconsistent details. An occasional untruth can upset the chronology of one's experience, and the person manipulating the facts often fails to adjust other information to match the untruth. Ask questions about the prestigious school an applicant claims to have attended or the city in which the applicant claims to have worked. Many people who have put themselves in the position of making things up as they go along will fumble, stumble, or hesitate in coming up with responses.

Always consider an applicant's reason for leaving a particular position and ask for clarification, especially if the job being sought represents a downward or lateral career move. The majority of people who have been terminated from a job for cause, not laid off, will use wording that characterizes their departures as voluntary.

During an interview, question the applicant about specific details that appear in the résumé. People who have lied or exaggerated will often find it more difficult to remember everything they have written. Try to decide whether a job candidate's answers seem memorized or rehearsed. Someone with nothing to conceal does not need to have pat answers prepared in advance.

Always be conscious of nonverbal clues. Excessive nervousness, failure to look an interviewer in the eyes, or physical fidgeting in a chair can be an indicator of fraud. However, be careful not to confuse simple nervousness with fraud. Ask an applicant for permission to have specific information verified. This will usually be done by HR. An applicant who has faked something significant will often withdraw from the process right after the interview.

Upon request, HR will frequently become involved in verifying résumé information. This is done when work references are checked. However, verification must sometimes go beyond ordinary reference checks. When confirming information by telephone, an HR representative will go through a company's operator or HR department rather than using a telephone number that the applicant may have provided. Some people who fake their experience have friends or relatives pose as former employers. If there is any doubt as to whether a reference's address is genuine, HR may test the address by mailing something there.

▶ An Acquired Skill

Many who are new to recruiting responsibilities are initially uneasy about interviewing prospective employees. Because of this uneasiness, and because of being too careful and worrying excessively about the process, interviewing becomes more difficult for them than it has to be. Individuals who take interviewing seriously and conscientiously try to do it effectively and endeavor to learn from each interview experience will find that their skills improve with practice. Being too casual or disorganized when interviewing can result in the loss of a potentially good employee and can leave that person with a poor impression of the organization. In contrast, being overly careful, dragging out the recruitment process by interviewing too many candidates, and delaying a decision also can lead to the loss of a potentially good employee.

It is useful to remember that when selecting employees, there is no guaranteed perfect choice. Some risk of error is always present. Experts remark that while a personal interview is a problematic and marginally reliable means of filling a job vacancy, no better means are available.

▶ Conclusion

The parameters of a recruitment interview are proscribed by legal statutes. Preparation for an interview begins before an applicant arrives. Interviewers should review the relevant position description, review the applications and résumés of all candidates, arrange for a room or area suitable for interviewing, and prepare opening questions.

🔍 CASE STUDY: Resolution

Returning to the initial case study involving interviewer Carrie Taylor and applicant Lynn Taylor, Carrie has placed the organization at risk by the manner in which she allowed herself to be influenced by Lynn's "frail build, small stature, and apparent age." Lynn revealed enough personal information for Carrie to conclude that Lynn had received surgery for breast cancer. Carrie allowed this personal information to influence her thinking about Lynn's capabilities. Carrie's motives may have been honest and her concern for Lynn genuine, but her actions were illegal. Carrie did not have the right to conclude that Lynn was "bound to fail." She was not legally entitled to base an employment decision on that subjective conclusion. As long as the specifications of the nursing position in the transitional care unit did not delineate specific physical requirements that Lynn could not meet, Carrie had no basis for rejecting Lynn as a viable candidate.

Lynn could be legitimately rejected for the position on physical grounds, but doing so is not within Carrie's scope of authority. Such rejection must come from the organization's employee health physician and would ordinarily occur when an applicant who has a tentative offer of employment fails a pre-employment physical examination.

In response to the human rights complaint, the organization should attempt to negotiate a settlement that includes an examination of Lynn by employee health to determine whether she is physically capable of handling the transitional care position. Using an occupational physician from an outside agency would minimize bias. When an individual is turned down for employment on the basis of a personal observation or forbidden information, the final determination appropriately involves an assessment of the individual's ability to perform the job.

SPOTLIGHT ON CUSTOMER SERVICE

How Customer Service Contributes to a Successful and Legal Selection Interview

Full disclosure: we are not aware of any statute that mandates customer service.

Although privately, we feel such a concept (requiring good customer service) has merit, we will defer any discussion of it for now.

Contributing to a successful selection interview is a different matter. An organization that has a reputation for providing good customer service is likely to have a good reputation in the minds of the public. That fact is likely to attract individuals who want to work in such an environment. This is likely not only to increase the number of applicants for a given position but also to improve the quality of the applicant pool.

This assertion can be supported. The Walt Disney Company (entertainment) and L.L.Bean (clothing and household products) have both had reputations for providing good customer service. Both companies routinely attract large numbers of applicants when they have positions to be filled. Because this has been the case for many years, applicant pool size cannot be attributed solely to recent problems with the economy and unemployment. A reputation for good customer service does provide unexpected consequences.

Modified from Segal, J. A. (1990). Did the Marquis de Sade design your discipline program? *HR Magazine, 35*(9), 90–95.

Interviews should begin on time, with initial questions designed to help candidates to relax. The language used should be appropriate for the candidate. Leading questions and inquiries that result in excessively long or very short responses should be avoided. Writing during an interview should be kept to an absolute minimum if not completely avoided. Closure and follow-up should be promised and promptly delivered.

Guidelines concerning legal and forbidden topics must be closely followed. Interviewers must be alert for irregularities in documents or the intent of applicants. Interviewers must remember that others have the responsibility to extend job offers and check references. Guidelines for appropriate behavior at all points in the interviewing process must be followed. Interviewing is an acquired skill that usually improves with practice.

Questions for Review and Discussion

1. In interviewing a prospective employee, why should you consider it important to inquire about the presence of information gaps or time periods that are not accounted for in the applicant's work record?

2. Why should an interviewing manager review all available information about an applicant before beginning an interview? Managers are busy people. Is arriving for an interview with an application in hand and then beginning an interview on time not sufficient?

3. If an interviewer wants the applicant to do most of the talking, what is wrong with opening an employment interview with the question, "Tell me all about yourself"?

4. Provide three examples of interview questions that are legal but which provide an interviewing manager with little or no useful information.
5. Why do you believe it is no longer appropriate to ask whether a job applicant has ever been arrested? Is it not in an employer's best interests to avoid taking on workers who have criminal records?
6. Can you make use of personal information in rendering an employment decision if the information was voluntarily provided to you? Why or why not?
7. An interviewing manager should be prepared to respond in considerable detail to any unsuccessful job candidate who calls asking why he or she was not offered employment. Do you agree or disagree with this statement? Why?
8. Why do experts recommend that the proper role of an interviewer involves more silence than speech?
9. Develop a brief procedure or protocol (a simple list of points to be covered) for reviewing an employment application or résumé for possible inaccuracies or embellishments.
10. Write (or quote from the chapter) a concise statement that, if conscientiously applied in interviewing, will ensure that only legal questions will be asked.
11. Why should an interviewing manager attempt to assess an applicant's intangible factors that are not directly reflected in the record of education or experience?
12. Why is it advisable to keep writing to a minimum while interviewing an applicant? Is it not helpful to capture as much information as possible about the person?

Resources
Books

Bunting, S. (2005). *Interviewer's handbook: Successful techniques for every work situation*. London, UK: Kogan Page.
Cook, M. (2004). *Personnel selection: Adding value through people* (4th ed.). New York, NY: John Wiley.
McConnell, C. R. (2019). *The effective health care supervisor* (9th ed.). Burlington, MA: Jones & Bartlett Learning.
Schell, M. (2004). *Human resource approved job interviews and résumés*. Vancouver, BC: Approved Publications.
Taylor, P., & O'Driscoll, M. P. (2005). *Structured employment interviewing*. London, UK: Ashgate.

Periodicals

Blackman, M. C. (2002). Personality judgment and the utility of the unstructured employment interview. *Basic and Applied Social Psychology, 24*, 241–250.
Cook, K. W., Vance, C. A., & Spector, P. E. (2000). The relation of candidate personality with selection-interview outcomes. *Journal of Applied Social Psychology, 30*, 867–885.
Lunenberg, F. C. (2010). The interview as a selection device: Problems and possibilities. *International Journal of Scholarly Academic Intellectual Diversity, 12*(1), 1–7.
Ryan, A. M., & Ployhart, R. E. (2000). Applicants' perceptions of selection procedures and decisions: A critical review and agenda for the future. *Journal of Management, 26*, 565–606.
Smith, D. B., Hanges, P. J., & Dickson, M. W. (2001). Personnel selection and the five-factor model: Reexamining the effects of applicant's frame of reference. *Journal of Applied Psychology, 86*, 304–315.

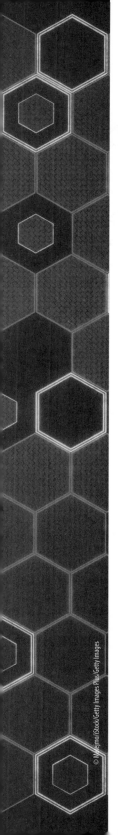

SECTION IV

Problems, Correction, and Discipline

It is an unfortunate reality of organizations that their employees can at times be troublesome and occasionally require some form of correction. The chapters included in Section IV address various aspects of the disciplinary process. Chapter 14 (Managers and Employee Problems) introduces problems that employees may have. All too often, these problems accompany them to work and are manifested as effects on productivity and relationships. Chapter 15 (Addressing Problems Before Taking Critical Action) provides guidance for all managers but is especially useful for first-line supervisors who are most likely to encounter troubled employees. Chapter 16 (Terminating Employees) covers the steps associated with separating employees from the organization.

CHAPTER 14

Managers and Employee Problems

CHAPTER OBJECTIVES

After studying this chapter, readers will be able to:

- Accept the inevitability of people problems in any work group and understand some common origins of such problems.
- Understand that the primary purpose of most means of addressing employee problems is correction of behavior.
- Differentiate problems of performance and problems of behavior and be familiar with processes for addressing each.
- Address excessive absenteeism.
- Understand the purpose and applicability of an employee assistance program (EAP).
- Address different common forms of termination for cause: discharge for behavior problems and dismissal for performance problems.
- Appreciate the necessity of emphasizing problem prevention whenever possible.

▶ Chapter Summary

People problems are an inevitable concern for anyone who manages others. Some first-line supervisors, especially those who are relatively inexperienced, are inclined to regard people problems as intrusions on their work. They eventually learn, however, that addressing the problems and the needs of employees is at the heart of a manager's role. Employees are individuals; although all are different from each other to some extent, some are sufficiently different as to pose behavioral problems and other difficulties their managers must address. In pursuing the ongoing goal of having people produce goods or deliver services, a manager must maintain employees as producers. Doing so requires managers to address people problems arising from both issues related to their work and difficulties arising outside of work.

The primary objective of a manager's actions in response to people problems should always be the correction of behavior. Depending on the nature of a specific problem, behavioral issues are addressed through individual coaching, counseling, activities aimed at improving performance, or disciplinary actions. Problems of performance and behavior can both be corrected. Behavior issues often constitute breaches of rules or policies.

Disciplinary action is customarily applied in a progressive manner. The extent or severity of the corrective action is proportional to the gravity of the problem or infraction. Correcting behavior is the main objective of disciplinary action except under extreme conditions or instances in which an employee must be removed from the organization.

🔍 CASE STUDY: Always Is a Dangerous Word

"I know what I heard, period," staff nurse Molly Stern said curtly. Her face was a mask of anger, and she spoke in the righteous tone that head nurse Penny Jerome had heard so many times.

"Dr. Benson says otherwise, Molly," said Penny. "She told me she was certain the instructions she left for you were just the opposite of what you actually did. And she really came on strong."

"She's wrong," snapped Molly.

"She seems just as certain that you were wrong." Penny paused before adding, "She explained the whole situation to me, and I have to admit that I understood her instructions. At least I was able to repeat them in my own words so she was satisfied that I understood."

Molly shrugged and said, "Then Dr. Benson changed her story between the time we talked and the time she spoke with you."

"Are you suggesting that she lied to me?"

"I didn't say that. I'm only saying that she told me one thing and then apparently told you something different. Maybe she didn't realize what she said. You know how she just rattles off something quickly and runs away."

Penny said, "Did you consider the possibility that you didn't understand? It isn't hard to misinterpret a message when things happen so fast and—"

"I know what I heard," interrupted Molly. "When I know I'm wrong, I say so. But in this case, I know I'm right. I could not have misinterpreted Dr. Benson."

Feeling that Molly had given her cause to bring up something that had been nagging her for quite some time, Penny said, "It seems to me that you're never wrong, Molly."

Molly glared at her supervisor. "What do you mean by that?"

"I've been head nurse of this unit for 3 years, and in all that time I've never known you to admit being wrong about anything. This problem with Dr. Benson is just one more example of how you always turn things around so that you look innocent. Is it so necessary that you be right all the time?"

In icy tones, Molly said, "As I said, when I'm wrong I'll admit it—but only when I'm really wrong. And I want to know the other times you're talking about, the times you said I 'turned things around.'"

"I don't have any specifics in front of me, but you ought to know what I'm talking about. Think about it, and you'll know what I'm saying. You seem to have an answer for everything, and it's always an answer that places you in the right."

"You can't think of any specific incidents because there haven't been any," said Molly. She rose from her chair and continued, "You may be my supervisor, but I don't have to listen to this. Is there anything else you wanted to say about *Dr. Benson's* problem?" She glared down at Penny.

Penny stood. "Just that the incident isn't to be considered closed. Dr. Benson insists that it be written up as a formal warning."

"I'll protest, of course," said Molly. "I won't accept a warning that I don't deserve, and I won't say I'm wrong when I know I'm right."

When Molly left the office, Penny began to regret having spoken as she did. She was convinced, however, that she had to try to get through to Molly about her apparent need to be right whenever a disagreement or a misunderstanding arose.

What critical error did head nurse Penny Jerome make in her one-on-one exchange with Molly Stern? Why was that particular action of Penny's wrong? How would you recommend that Molly and Dr. Benson resolve their misunderstanding? How would you respond to employees who are always right?

▶ People Problems Are Inevitable

Consider the following typical vignette. A chronic personnel problem involving differences between some staff members of two adjoining departments had surfaced once again. This time it affected two department managers, several rank-and-file employees, and an employee relations manager. A discussion meeting had been scheduled to explore the situation. After more than an hour of animated discussion during which charges and counter-charges flew back and forth, the employees were excused and the others continued for another half hour. When the meeting finally broke up, an hour and a half had elapsed, and only the most tentative of conclusions had been reached. As the participants rose to leave the room, one department manager's pager sounded. The manager checked the message and muttered, "I was expecting this. It looks like another of my pet troublemakers is acting up again." As he left the room, the manager also remarked, in a voice strained with frustration, "You know, I could probably get some real work done around here if it weren't for all these people problems that keep popping up."

Most managers have more than enough to do without spending time tending to the problems of the adults they supervise. However, any manager who feels frustration because of people problems must appreciate the fact that people-related problems are part of the job of anyone who supervises the work of others. A first-line manager supervises people who perform hands-on work and provides an interface between rank-and-file employees and the organization's management. If maintaining rank-and-file employees as effective producers did not include addressing the frustrations and issues that employees bring to their jobs, far fewer managers would be needed in work organizations. As long as there are people in the workplace, those who are responsible for getting work done through these people can expect people problems. Although it is a less than appealing aspect of being a manager, coping with people problems is an inevitable and unavoidable part of the department manager's role.

Problem Sources

Problems presented by employees can come about because of job-related difficulties, personal problems experienced largely outside of work, or a combination of the two. Some people are more successful than others at keeping the working side and the personal side of their lives separate from each other. However, it is not possible to completely and unfailingly separate the person on the job from the person off the job. Personal problems accompany people to their jobs and often affect job performance and employment relationships. Work-related problems go home and often affect personal lives and relationships.

One might be tempted to say that an employee's personal problems are no business of the manager. Such a position is correct but only up to a point. If an individual's personal problems are affecting work through deteriorating performance, reduced productivity, or disruption of a department's ability to operate normally, then a supervisor must become interested because of the negative effects on operations.

When an employee who has performed satisfactorily for a prolonged period and has always gotten along with others reasonably well begins to show signs of performance and relationship problems, the manager has every reason to suspect an underlying problem behind the changed behavior. It may not initially be evident whether the problem has its basis in the workplace or on the outside, but the results of the changed behavior are a manager's legitimate and immediate concern. Performance or relationship problems that affect the work environment are always of vital interest to managers.

Supervisors who suspect that personal problems are behind declines in performance must approach their employees in a manner respectful of their right to privacy. Although the performance resulting from an individual's behavior must be addressed for the sake of the department and the people being served, events in an individual's private life are not the business of the manager.

Managers must always address the *results* of behavior and never attempt to infer the *causes* of that behavior. As necessary, tell an individual, through whatever channel is used, about current behaviors or actions that appear to be causing problems. Point out errors of judgment or improper actions and offer suggestions as to how these can be corrected. Using the resources that are available, provide whatever help is needed to take appropriate corrective action. Do not, under any circumstances, probe for personal information. Managers must forever make it clear that they are there to listen if or when a person wants to talk, but managers must not ask individuals about problems that seem to lie outside of the working situation.

If employees volunteer information concerning personal problems, listen and be prepared to refer them elsewhere as necessary. Even if employees reveal their problems and ask for advice, wise supervisors will not respond to such requests. Even supervisors who are trained professionals working in a human service function are advised to keep their advice to themselves. Some of the most troublesome statements a manager can make begin with, "If I were you . . ."

Refer troubled employees to an appropriate person or agency from which they can be directed toward an appropriate source of knowledgeable help. This will most often mean referral to the employee health service or the organization's employee assistance program (EAP).

▶ Primary Purpose: Correction

Throughout this chapter reference is made to corrective processes. Although there are instances in which the action taken in response to an employee problem is punitive, the primary purpose of the action is to correct employee performance or behavior. Although discipline involves punishment or the perception of punishment, its underlying purpose is to teach or to correct problem behaviors. The root of discipline is the word *disciple,* which is a learner, pupil, or follower.

Correction is always the primary intent of what is referred to as the *corrective process.* Nevertheless, there is an unavoidable punitive dimension in most corrective processes. Policies that are violated or rules that are broken result in warnings. Even though we may acknowledge the punitive aspect of true disciplinary action in some instances, we must recognize that it is not applicable to all employee problems. It is essential to separate problems of performance from true behavior problems.

Separate Issues of Performance and Behavior

Department managers will find it necessary to address different kinds of problems presented by employees on the job. Some will involve behavior issues, while others will involve issues of performance. These two kinds of problems must be addressed using different approaches.

Performance problems are manifested in an employee's failure to consistently meet the expectations or requirements of a job and generally show up as difficulty doing the work and producing the minimum level of quality or output required. *Behavior problems* involve violations of policies or work rules; these are conduct issues. Usually issues of conduct are unrelated to performance; they may have no bearing on how an employee is performing on the job.

It is sometimes necessary to determine whether a particular employee *cannot* perform as expected or *will not* perform as expected. The former requires the employee's immediate supervisor to address a performance problem; the latter may require disciplinary action. These areas occasionally overlap when an individual's deliberate acts of recklessness, negligence, or carelessness cause performance to fall below accepted standards. In other words, when an employee *cannot* perform, the issue consists of a performance problem. When an individual *will not* perform, then the issue consists of a problem of conduct or behavior.

A thorough orientation to the organization is—or most certainly should be—a requirement for all employees. Workers are entitled to know what is expected of them, whether related to performance or behavior. Concerning behavior, it is essential that employees are informed of all applicable policies and work rules. Concerning performance, it is equally essential that all employees be thoroughly trained and given every opportunity to learn their jobs. Such opportunities must be consistent among all employees. Whether behavior or performance is involved, the first area of concern for a department manager to examine should be the expectations of an employee: was this person fully knowledgeable of the expected behavior or performance? This is a critical question; all employees at every level from the chief executive officer to the newest entry-level laborer are entitled to know what is expected of them.

Addressing Performance Problems

Employees who do not meet their expected performance levels commonly fall behind in output, produce poor-quality work, or simply do not follow established procedures. The first step a department manager should take is to look for the source (not the *cause*) of the problem. The initial critical issue to address is whether the immediate supervisor (and perhaps predecessor) did everything reasonably possible to help this employee succeed. That is, the first place that supervisors must review is their own actions or behavior.

Performance problems, especially those occurring early in a person's employment, are often the result of a weak or sketchy orientation to the job. To address a performance problem, a department manager must positively identify the problem and proceed to work out, preferably with the participation of the employee, what must be done to correct the difficulty and a time frame for action.

The performance improvement process should proceed in the following manner. A manager observes a problem situation involving substandard performance in some form. Common issues include unacceptable quality of work, poor service quality, insufficient productivity, complaints by customers or others receiving services, complaints by visitors, or other less-than-acceptable results. The manager next conducts an investigation to verify the existence and nature of the problem. Prudent managers ensure that their facts are correct before addressing the situation with an employee. A supervisor next meets privately with the problem employee. The purpose of the meeting is to define and discuss the perceived difficulty with the employee and to elicit the employee's views and perspectives.

The manager should next make every reasonable effort to secure the employee's agreement concerning the nature of the problem and what should be done to correct the unacceptable performance. Ideally, the two should agree on a brief written description of what is wrong and what is needed for correction. The agreement should include a timetable for correction, with both parties agreeing on a date by which corrective action must be accomplished. Part of this agreement should specify whether interim checkpoints will be needed at which to review progress. Some corrective processes may require a brief period, while others may require more time. When the evaluation points are reached, the supervisor must follow up in good faith, completely, and on time. One of the greatest shortcomings encountered with corrective processes in general is a manager's failure to provide timely follow-up.

At the end of the evaluation period, the manager must decide whether the employee's performance improved as required, improved partly, did not improve, or deteriorated further. The desired result of an evaluation period is returning an employee to an acceptable level of performance. Depending on the actual outcome, however, other steps can be taken. These include extending the improvement period in the case of partial improvement or dismissal for failure to meet expected evaluation standards.

How should managers treat employees who modify their performance well enough to get by the correction period and then go back to substandard performance some weeks or months later? Some department managers may elect to repeat the performance improvement process with such employees, but most will not look forward to going through it for a third time. The documentation created the second time through the process should include wording to the effect that subsequent performance must remain at or above standard or the person will be at risk for dismissal.

EXHIBIT 14-1 presents a model procedure for addressing the need for improvement in performance.

EXHIBIT 14-1 Model Policy and Procedure: Performance Improvement Process

The following procedure is provided to establish clear direction for the resolution of problems concerning an employee's substandard job performance.

Substandard performance is defined as a demonstrated lack of acceptable work performance, or chronically unsatisfactory results that prevent an employee from attaining or maintaining the job standard.

Job standard is defined as the average or acceptable level of output provided by employees in the same or similar position or classification, or the standard level of results defined in advance by the department manager clearly identifying the quality or quantity of output expected.

In the event that nonprobationary employees exhibit substandard performance of job duties or fail to fulfill all the responsibilities of their positions, a department manager should make a sincere and adequate effort to guide them in returning to an acceptable level of performance. The first steps in this process include the following:

- Verify the job standard for accuracy and applicability and make any necessary adjustments
- Advise and guide employees to create a plan for their return to standard performance and a time frame for doing so, documenting this effort using a Counseling Form (Attachment A)
- Guide and monitor employee efforts to attain standard performance
- Remove obstacles to employee progress where possible

In the event an employee does not attain the job standard within the agreed-upon time, department managers should next:

- Complete a Work Improvement Evaluation (Attachment B)
- Repeat the creation of a mutually agreed upon plan of action, this time including referral to Employee Relations or Employee Health, if applicable (should there be some documentation of an underlying difficulty or problem to warrant such a referral)

If the second effort is unsuccessful in returning the employee to standard performance within the agreed-upon time:

- Complete a Performance Expectations form (Attachment C), placing the employee on notice of probationary status and calling for dismissal on the grounds of substandard performance no later than 30 days following this final notice unless standard performance is attained during that period

Note: Once an employee has been through the Performance Expectations stage and has again achieved standard performance, that person's performance is expected to remain at standard or better. Without extenuating circumstances (e.g., undergoing a corrective or rehabilitative process under the Employee Assistance Program or the auspices of Employee Health), reversion to substandard performance will result in dismissal.

(continues)

EXHIBIT 14-1 Model Policy and Procedure: Performance Improvement Process *(continued)*

Attachment A: Counseling Form

___ Performance Counseling

___ Probationary Counseling

___ Other _____

Employee Name: _____ ID No.: _____

Department: _____ Hire Date: _____

Job Title/Grade: _____ Job Date: _____

Summary of Discussion:

Action to Be Taken by Manager:

Action to Be Taken by Employee:

Date of Follow-Up Meeting:

Employee Signature: _____ Date: _____

Manager Signature: _____ Date: _____

Attachment B: Work Improvement Evaluation

This document summarizes a work improvement discussion between manager and employee. An initial effort to correct a documented performance problem was unsuccessful, indicating the need for additional corrective action represented by the numbered objectives that must be met to return the employee to an acceptable level of performance.

Description of Objective and the Agreed-Upon Criteria for Achievement

1.

2.

3.

Referral to Employee Relations or Employee Health as appropriate: _____

Date of Next Review: _____

Employee Signature: _____ Date: _____

Manager Signature: _____ Date: _____

Attachment C: Performance Expectations

Employee Name: _____ ID No.: _____

Department: _____ Hire Date: _____

Job Title/Grade: _____ Job Date: _____

Summary of Performance-Problem Discussion:

Follow-up was performed on the following dates: _____

Continued substandard performance makes it necessary to place this employee in probationary status subject to dismissal during or after 30 days from the date of signing unless fully satisfactory and lasting improvement is demonstrated by the employee.

Employee Signature: _____ Date: _____

Manager Signature: _____ Date: _____

▶ Addressing Behavior Problems

Disciplinary Action

A chief reason why many supervisors do not confront problem employee behavior is their discomfort with the traditional punitive discipline systems many are required to use (Segal, 1990). This comment says a great deal about why supervisors frequently shy away from disciplinary action even when it may be deserved. Regardless of how a system is designed, most employees, supervisors, and managers perceive their disciplinary systems as punitive. To repeat, the goal of disciplinary action is to correct behavior. Few managers ever look forward to delivering disciplinary action.

The mere thought of having to take disciplinary action is unsettling to many managers. Impending disciplinary action can make managers apprehensive. Some managers simply ignore situations, postponing action until events resolve themselves (least likely) or the problems can be entirely forgotten (rarely occurs). Others approach disciplinary action with hesitation, watering it down so much that it becomes ineffective.

Disciplinary action is similar to any other difficult task. Conscientious attention to the process and practice eventually leads to a degree of familiarity. At that stage, a manager can apply disciplinary action honestly and confidently when needed. Most managers never become entirely comfortable with the process. Given that disciplinary action has the potential to affect one's employment or damage a career, a certain level of discomfort or uneasiness with the process is healthy in that it heightens the supervisor's awareness of the importance of the action to the employee. Phrased differently, a manager who can freely dispense serious disciplinary action without experiencing qualms or doubts is ill suited for the responsibilities inherent in managing people.

The Process of Progressive Discipline

The complete progressive disciplinary process consists of counseling, one or more oral warnings, one or more written warnings, suspension with or without pay, and termination. A considerable range of possible violations is subject to progressive discipline. Not all infractions are subject to the entire range of progressive discipline. Lesser violations—for example, absenteeism or chronic tardiness—may include some but not all of the steps. With minor infractions, it may be advisable to repeat a step if a significant time lapse has occurred between infractions. Some infractions may involve only two steps. For example, sleeping on the job might call for a written warning for the initial offense and termination for a second offense.

The initial step in many instances is informal counseling. Counseling is best undertaken when a manager observes an employee headed for difficulty but is not yet at the point of requiring disciplinary action. An oral warning is the first formal step in the progressive disciplinary process. Although it is delivered orally to an employee, a supervisor should create a written record and ask the affected employee to review and sign it so that evidence that this step was followed is available if needed. Many organizations have forms specifically designated for documenting oral warnings.

The requirements for documentation and associated procedures can be confusing. Although a record is created, in many instances this record never goes into an employee's personnel file unless the problem is repeated and a written record is required. Documentation is essential to prove that an organization's processes were followed. If a disciplinary policy states that an oral warning is the first level of response for a given infraction, it may later be necessary to prove that the oral warning was actually given.

At all steps of the disciplinary process, the affected employee is asked to review and sign the documentation created. The manager should stress that signing does not necessarily indicate agreement with the action. Rather, signing simply acknowledges that the employee has seen the document, has discussed the problem with the manager, and has been provided with a copy. It is not unusual for an employee to refuse to sign a warning or even to acknowledge its receipt. When an employee refuses to sign a warning, the supervisor simply notes that fact in the signature area, "Employee refused to sign," and ensures that the document is dated. In difficult circumstances when a manager has reason to believe that disagreement may escalate and involve others, another manager should witness an employee's refusal to sign and so note on the document. The second supervisor should also sign the document.

When Discipline Is Not Progressive

Disciplinary action cannot always be progressive. Some infractions, usually clearly defined in policy manuals and employee handbooks, call for immediate termination. These may move to immediate suspension pending investigation as necessary. Such transgressions ordinarily include fighting or physical assault, using illegal drugs or alcohol on the job, carrying a weapon on the premises, theft, or threatening other employees or managers. Immediate termination with no chance to change an individual's behavior is hardly corrective. Experts note, however, that when an employee is released for a serious infraction, the problem has been corrected by removing its cause.

EXHIBIT 14-2 presents a sample progressive discipline policy and procedure for a healthcare organization, including the recommended treatment for different infractions.

EXHIBIT 14-2 Model Policy and Procedure: Progressive Discipline

This organization is committed to providing the best possible working conditions for all employees. Rules of conduct have been established to assist the organization and its employees in achieving organizational goals as well as providing a safe and productive work environment. All employees are expected to observe all rules of conduct and to follow the instructions provided by their immediate supervisor. Supervisors and managers are responsible for applying the rules to all employees in a fair and consistent manner.

When an employee appears to have violated a rule, the immediate supervisor should address the specific problem through the progressive discipline process.

A. Steps in Progressive Discipline
    1. Counseling
        Before informal or formal disciplinary action is taken, the employee's supervisor has the responsibility to counsel the employee to correct the undesirable behavior. Use the Counseling Form (Exhibit 14-1, Attachment A), which is retained in departmental files until the employee terminates employment, at which time the form is forwarded to human resources (HR).
    2. Oral Warning
        a. An informal disciplinary conference may be scheduled when an employee repeatedly displays undesirable behavior and does not respond to counseling. The conference should be summarized on

the Record of Oral Warning (Attachment A), which is retained in the department manager's files.
   b. If further disciplinary action is necessary for the same offense, then the Record of Oral Warning should be forwarded to human resources for inclusion in the employee's personnel file.
3. Written Warning
   a. If counseling and oral warnings fail to correct employee behavior, a written warning should be generated. The employees will be informed that the Record of Oral Warning and the Written Warning will be included in their personnel file and they will perhaps be ineligible for transfer for some period of time. Repetition of the offense will lead to more serious disciplinary action such as suspension without pay or termination of employment.
   b. An employee whose inappropriate behavior has not been corrected by counseling, oral warning, or written warning will be referred to Employee Relations for further counseling or to Employee Health or Employee Assistance for evaluation and referrals if appropriate.
4. Suspension Without Pay
   a. A temporary termination of work at the will of the employer may be initiated if an employee fails to respond to the foregoing steps. Time off may be waived at the discretion of the manager if staffing needs require the employee's presence. However, waiver of time off does not lessen the severity of the disciplinary action.
   b. At the discretion of the manager, indefinite suspension pending investigation may be utilized to provide time and a thorough opportunity to investigate an alleged violation that has the potential to result in termination.
5. Discharge
   Termination of employment for violation of organizational rules may apply after repeated counseling, warnings, referrals, and suspensions or after initial commission of specific severe violations.
6. General
   The organization reserves the right to amend these rules as necessary. Each manager has the right to initiate the progressive disciplinary process at any step, depending on the severity of the offense. All violations leading to potential suspension without pay or discharge must be reviewed with human resources.
B. Violations and Severity
1. Carelessness: Careless acts that could result in personal injury to patients, employees, or visitors, or damage to property.
   a. First violation: Written warning
   b. Second violation: Up to 5-day suspension without pay
   c. Third violation: Discharge
2. Insubordination: An employee's refusal to comply with a reasonable and safe work instruction as required by an immediate supervisor.
   a. First violation: Up to 5-day suspension without pay, and referral to Employee Relations
   b. Second violation: Discharge
3. Absenteeism: Excessive absenteeism is the frequent use of sick time that in the judgment of the department manager adversely affects the operation of the department, regularly occurs before or after scheduled days off, weekends, holidays, or scheduled vacations, or that results in sick time

(continues)

EXHIBIT 14-2   Model Policy and Procedure: Progressive Discipline   *(continued)*

being used as it accrues. Unexcused absenteeism is absence without timely notice to a manager or designee prior to the start of a scheduled shift, per departmental policy.

   a.   First violation: Oral warning
   b.   Second violation: Written warning and referral to Employee Health for counseling
   c.   Third violation: Up to 3-day suspension without pay
   d.   Fourth violation: Discharge

   Note: Failure to appear at work or call in per policy for 3 consecutive work days will result in discharge for job abandonment.

4.   Tardiness: Consistent tardiness is the patterned failure to report for work at the designated starting time.

   a.   First violation: Oral warning
   b.   Second violation: Written warning and referral to Employee Relations for counseling
   c.   Third violation: Up to 3-day suspension without pay
   d.   Fourth violation: Discharge

5.   Misconduct: Actions detrimental to the interests of the organization or that cause harm or disruption to any person or organizational activity. Some examples include threatening or discourteous behavior toward patients or visitors; sexual harassment; misuse of confidential information; leaving the work area without permission; gambling; possession of explosives, firearms, or other weapons on organization property; and violation of safe practices in the performance of work.

   a.   First violation: Written warning and up to 5-day suspension without pay, plus referral to Employee Relations for counseling
   b.   Second violation: Discharge

6.   Sleeping: Sleeping on the job is prohibited unless it is recognized as a legitimate part of an employee's extended shift.

   a.   First violation: Written warning and up to 5-day suspension without pay, plus referral to Employee Relations or Employee Health for counseling
   b.   Second violation: Discharge

7.   Solicitation: Employees may not engage in unauthorized solicitation, distribution, or posting of materials on organization premises.

   a.   First violation: Written warning
   b.   Second violation: Written warning and up to 3-day suspension without pay
   c.   Third violation: Discharge

8.   Falsification of Information: Falsification of information on employment applications or in other work situations is prohibited. This prohibition includes the making of false entries on time records or punching another employee's time card.

   a.   First violation: Indefinite suspension pending investigation prior to possible discharge

9.   Alcohol and Illegal Drugs: Possession, use, or being under the influence of alcohol or illegal drugs on organization premises is prohibited. Employees using prescription medications while at work are requested to report such use to the appropriate manager. Because of the considerable responsibility that all employees have for the organization's patients, a manager who has

probable cause to believe an employee to be under the influence of alcohol or drugs may ask the employee to submit voluntarily to an appropriate test arranged by either Employee Health or the Emergency Department. Refusal to submit to such reasonable request may result in disciplinary action.
   a.   First violation: Indefinite suspension pending test results and, if necessary, the employee's willingness to enter an approved rehabilitation program as determined by the employee's personal physician and Employee Health
   b.   Second violation: Discharge
10.   Unauthorized Possession of Property: The unauthorized use, possession, or removal of organization property or the property of patients, visitors, employees, or others.
   a.   First violation: Indefinite suspension pending investigation prior to possible discharge

Attachment A: Record of Oral Warning

Employee Name: _____ ID No.: _____

Department: _____ Hire Date: _____

Job Title/Grade: _____ Job Date: _____

Specific problem or incident, and rule or policy reviewed and discussed:

Dates of previous discussions or counseling relating to the foregoing:

Action Required of Employee:

Employee Signature: _____ Date: _____

Manager Signature: _____ Date: _____

This record will be maintained in departmental files. If further action is required for the same offense, it will be forwarded to the human resources department for inclusion in the personnel file.

Attachment B: Written Warning

Employee Name: _____ ID No.: _____

Department: _____ Hire Date: _____

Job Title/Grade: _____ Job Date: _____

Specific problem or incident, and rule or policy reviewed and discussed:

Dates of previous discussions, counseling, or warnings relating to the foregoing:

Action Required of Employee:

Employee Signature: _____ Date: _____

Manager Signature: _____ Date: _____

This record puts the employee on notice that additional violations will result in more serious disciplinary actions, such as suspension without pay or discharge.

Attachment C: Suspension Without Pay

Employee Name: _____ ID No.: _____

Department: _____ Hire Date: _____

Job Title/Grade: _____ Job Date: _____

Specific problem or incident, and rule or policy reviewed and discussed:

(continues)

EXHIBIT 14-2 Model Policy and Procedure: Progressive Discipline   *(continued)*

Previous Actions Taken:

Date Action Taken: _____

Suspended for _____ days from above date. Report back on _____.

Time off waived by manager for the following reason (waiver does not lessen the severity of the action):

Employee Signature: _____ Date: _____

Manager Signature: _____ Date: _____

This is a final warning. Failure to respond appropriately may result in discharge.

Attachment D: Notice of Discharge or Dismissal

Employee Name: _____ ID No.: _____

Department: _____ Hire Date: _____

Job Title/Grade: _____ Job Date: _____

You are being terminated from employment for the following reasons:

Previous Actions Taken:

Date Action Taken: _____

____ Check here to indicate that the employee desires an exit interview to discuss benefits. If the employee declines this opportunity, then continuation of benefits information will be mailed to the employee's home address.

Employee Signature: _____ Date: _____

Manager Signature: _____ Date: _____

▶ Employee Absenteeism

Some degree of absenteeism is accepted as a fact of organizational life. People become legitimately ill or experience family emergencies and other urgent matters that sometimes keep them away from work. As many department managers have discovered, however, the line between acceptable and unacceptable levels of absenteeism is extremely fine and difficult to recognize.

Some department managers appear to pay little or no attention to employee absenteeism. Such attitudes set the standard for a department. Managers who seem to ignore absenteeism usually wonder why their absenteeism rates are higher than normal for their organization.

Absenteeism costs money. While someone may be receiving paid time off for being away from work, a job that must be covered incurs the direct cost of a temporary replacement or staff overtime. For nonessential positions, a replacement may not be needed for an absence of 1 or 2 days. However, a department will experience lost productivity as a result of the absence.

Experience with traditional sick-time benefit programs has suggested that an organization's sick-time benefit often generates its own usage. Consider the experience of two healthcare organizations in the same community. One provided a benefit of 12 sick days per year, and the other provided 5 days per year. In the facility where employees received 12 sick days per year, the average usage per employee was approximately 7 days per year. In the facility where employees received 5 sick days per year, the average usage per employee was slightly more than 3 days per year. The organization with the higher rate of sick-time consumption did not necessarily have fewer healthy employees than did the other facility.

Such experiences with sick time have encouraged an increasing number of organizations to reduce their absolute sick-time benefit and combine it with vacation and other personal time in a paid-time-off (PTO) bank. Under these plans, a person who uses little or no time off for illness has the time left for other uses. Critics point out that such a policy encourages ill people to come to work and potentially infect other workers. Both sides in this argument have merit.

A department manager's conscientious attention to absenteeism is a significant component of controlling employee absences. Some employees will be inclined to abuse sick time if they see that their manager pays no attention to their absences. They interpret the lack of attention as approving their conduct. In truth, this interpretation has merit; such behavior by the manager is in fact approval by default.

For controlling absenteeism in a department, a supervisor cannot clearly remember everyone's attendance, so accurate attendance records are required. Effective managers do not rely on other departments to maintain their attendance records. By personally monitoring attendance, they stay in closer touch with their employees. They check in with employees after they return from any absence, even a single day. A simple question or statement, such as "Feel better today?" or "Good to have you back," tells employees that their supervisors are aware of their attendance.

Attentive supervisors watch for patterns of absences. Patterns are among the more reliable signs of sick-time abuse. Common examples of sick-time abuse include holiday stretching: being absent the day before or the day after a scheduled holiday. Weekend stretching involves being absent on a Friday or Monday. Employees tend to be "sick" on Monday more than on any other day of the week.

Counsel any employee who appears to be getting close to a level of absences that can trigger disciplinary action. For example, if the policy says that five instances of unexcused absence in a 12-month period call for the start of disciplinary action, meet with an individual who has been absent four times in 8 months, explain the policy, and point out the consequences of the next unexcused absence. Effective supervisors do not wait until disciplinary action is required before speaking up. They do not avoid taking disciplinary action for absenteeism when it is deserved. Finally, they are not punitive. A progressive system allows more than ample room for improvement. A supervisor's intent should be to help employees improve and succeed.

Employee Assistance Programs

An EAP sends a message to employees that their employer cares about them beyond the usual demands of the organization. An EAP provides information, assessments, advice, and referrals for employees who are experiencing personal problems that can affect them as individuals and as producers of goods or services. Employees who take advantage of an EAP will receive a confidential assessment that is ordinarily followed by a referral to an appropriate source for professional help.

It is common practice to use an external assessment and referral agency rather than have organizational employees—for example, someone in HR—perform this task. This helps to preserve employee confidentiality and allows employees to build a level of confidence in the EAP. For obvious reasons, many employees are more likely to share personal issues with someone outside of their organization than with another employee.

Improvements realized through intervention by an EAP ordinarily require some time. There is often a temptation to look for short-term improvement, rather than long-term benefits for both an employee and the organization. Quick fixes for the kinds of problems addressed through an EAP are unlikely. The EAP frequently addresses difficult issues such as substance abuse (drugs or alcohol), marital or family problems, financial troubles, compulsive gambling, and other addictions. Most EAPs ordinarily provide two or three counseling sessions to determine an appropriate referral path. After these initial visits, an individual's health insurance or other applicable program takes over.

Employees can enter an EAP through self-referral, meaning that they voluntarily approach the EAP themselves. Alternatively, employees can be referred by a supervisor, a manager, or by an employee health office. If an individual's problem has the potential to negatively affect performance or presents a danger or risk to people or property, then the organization can mandate referral to the EAP and require completion of a subsequent program as a condition of continued employment. An example of a potentially dangerous problem is alcohol abuse that requires rehabilitation. Managers and supervisors do not need to know details of a problem. However, when a problem affects the performance or safety of other patients, visitors, or employees, it becomes a manager's business.

An EAP usually costs an organization a set, nominal amount of money per employee or full-time equivalent (FTE) per year. Often the cost of an EAP for an entire year is less than the costs associated with replacing one or two employees. Most HR experts agree that an EAP is cost effective. To serve its intended purpose completely, an EAP requires support from senior and executive managers, adequate funding, an efficient and confidential assessment and referral process, record keeping that ensures confidentiality, and educating employees and managers about the EAP program and how to access it.

An EAP can relieve department managers of difficult problems involving ordinarily good employees who encounter personal difficulties. An EAP can effectively assist a person for whom termination would be the alternative. Department managers usually agree that there is far more satisfaction in helping to salvage one or more employees who might otherwise fail than there is in firing any of them.

▶ When Termination Is Necessary

Discharge Versus Dismissal

It is helpful to distinguish between the two most common kinds of involuntary separation. These are dismissal and discharge. Dismissal is related to performance, while discharge is related to conduct or behavior.

Dismissal is the appropriate path for an employee who must be released because of performance problems. This will apply to newer employees who are unable to gain sufficient control of their jobs to pass the probationary period. Dismissal may also be appropriate for employees who experience performance problems and do not respond to corrective processes. Dismissal should be the final resort following all reasonable efforts to improve performance.

A dismissal is the equivalent of a layoff; it is a separation that does not involve fault. Human resource experts often refer to this as no-fault separation. A no-fault separation concedes only that a person did not fit a particular kind of work and makes no judgments about the person's ability to succeed elsewhere. Similar to the situation of a layoff, a dismissed employee is eligible for unemployment compensation.

Discharge is related to conduct or behavior. Discharge is termination for cause, more commonly referred to as being fired. Discharge should occur only after all elements of an organization's progressive disciplinary process have been applied and failed to correct the offending behavior. Employees who are discharged for cause are usually ineligible for unemployment compensation. However, an outside agency ultimately determines eligibility for unemployment compensation.

An Important Caveat

No employee should ever be summarily discharged, fired on the spot, or fired in anger. The nature of any given infraction does not negate this rule. An appropriate reaction to the most blatant of offenses that are punishable by immediate discharge is to place the offender on indefinite suspension or administrative leave pending investigation and discharge. This provides a cooling-off period for all concerned, and it provides time for a fair and thorough investigation if needed.

▶ Partnership with Human Resources

Disciplinary action is one area in which department managers and human resources (HR) personnel frequently collide. Such controversy, however, can be minimized by having clearly stated policies governing who is responsible for each part of the process. A significant number of organizations require managers to coordinate all disciplinary actions with HR. This is a reasonable requirement. Human resources can help to ensure that the elements of a progressive discipline program are consistently applied and to confirm that all legal requirements are observed.

Human resources should be allowed to serve as a central monitor for disciplinary actions, initially rendering an opinion as to whether a proposed action is appropriate to the situation. Another important aspect of the HR role in discharge is to ensure that all of the proper steps called for in the policy have been fairly applied.

▶ Prevention When Possible

Active prevention is important in reducing the need for disciplinary actions and keeping them to a minimum. Two important keys to prevention are information and education.

Be certain that all new employees are familiar with the work rules and applicable policies, all of which should be identified in the employee handbook. These may have been covered during the organization's general new-employee orientation, but do not assume so. It certainly will not hurt to go over them a second time.

Make sure each new employee goes through the employee handbook and signs and turns in the handbook receipt as required. Employees will rarely read an employee handbook if they are determined not to do so. However, a signed receipt shifts the responsibility for knowing the contents to employees.

Managers should periodically review rules and policies with the entire staff. This can be conveniently accomplished by covering one or two items at every regular staff meeting. Personnel policies should be periodically revised and updated. Publication of a revision presents a good opportunity for a review. If the rules and policies are kept fresh in employees' minds, they will be less likely to ignore them.

Preventive employee relations has the potential to avoid disciplinary actions. Successful supervisors remain alert to signs or signals that indicate the possibility of employee problems. They talk to their employees when they sense problems. Actual problems are far more difficult to manage than are avoided issues.

Managers who remain visible and available to employees can help to prevent the need for disciplinary actions. When a department manager is present, many issues that might otherwise escalate into behavioral problems can be identified and addressed. The presence of a manager tends to have a stabilizing effect on a work group. A supervisor who stays in touch with employees and maintains solid one-to-one relationships with them helps to prevent disciplinary problems.

Elements of Effective Corrective Action

Knowledge

Supervisors must be thoroughly familiar with their organization's policies and work rules. Thorough familiarity means that they do not have to look in a book whenever questions or problems arise.

Likewise, they must be completely familiar with the progressive disciplinary process and know the contacts in HR with whom to coordinate disciplinary actions. To keep their knowledge current, they take advantage of training in these processes whenever it is offered within the organization.

Timing

Effective supervisors do not delay deserved criticism or disciplinary action any longer than is necessary. Delay only weakens the impact of actions taken and lessens their importance. Immediate actions are more likely to be effective.

Consistency

Managers must strive for consistent treatment of employees. Work rules and policies must be applied consistently regardless of who is involved in a particular problem or infraction. This can be difficult to accomplish in situations involving people with other personal issues or involving friends. Consider the situation of two employees: one has long-standing health problems, and the other routinely abuses sick time, but they must be treated equally if they are chronically absent.

Intimidation

Effective supervisors do not allow themselves to be influenced by employees who try to outsmart or intimidate them. The job market and the attendant scarcity of certain kinds of employees can cause intimidation. Supervisors must react to problems as they arise without being influenced by issues such as scarcity of employees with particular skills. No matter how specialized or valuable they may think they are, no employees are indispensable. What applies to one must apply to all. A department or organization cannot maintain a double standard of employee conduct. This again raises the issue of consistency, which is arguably the most important single factor in a department manager's handling of corrective processes.

▶ Document, Document

Most HR practitioners can relate to the following situation. A department manager came to HR prepared to discharge a particular employee. The HR representative heard a ringing indictment of the employee. The individual is never cooperative, is the department's worst performer, has the worst attendance record of anyone in the department, is frequently insubordinate, and is constantly making trouble for other employees. The employee has once again caused a problem. The angry manager demands, "I want this person discharged, now." The HR person begins to consider the manager's request by pulling the employee's personnel file and going through it item by item. The HR representative finds no warnings, no discussions about performance or behavior issues, and no record of disciplinary actions. The file contains middle-of-the-pack satisfactory performance appraisals covering several years. The discussion of discipline for behavioral issues is over at this point. Without supporting documentation of similar past difficulties, those past problems simply do not exist.

There are lessons in the foregoing story. Instances in which an employee deserves some form of reprimand or formal disciplinary action must not be ignored. Every instance of reprimand or disciplinary action must be properly documented and submitted for inclusion in an employee's personnel file. If an employee's file contains nothing about a particular problem, then for all practical purposes, it never happened. Finally, less-than-honest performance appraisals are never appropriate; when the record appears to support the employee, it can be used to challenge almost any disciplinary action. Documentation is critical for every disciplinary action.

Supervisors should never attempt or proceed with a personnel action without ensuring the existence of the appropriate documentation. Managers must always remain aware that any employee-related document generated can be made public should an employee become involved in a legal proceeding against the organization.

▶ Conclusion

Problems related to employees are inevitable in any organization. No employee is immune to experiencing personal difficulties. Supervisors must respond to behavior, and personal opinions or predispositions must be set aside. The rules, procedures, and penalties for noncompliance must be clearly explained to all employees.

The primary objective of disciplinary actions is correction. Performance problems relate to meeting the expectations or requirements of a job and difficulty doing the work and producing the minimum level of quality or output required. Behavior problems involve violations of policies or work rules. In other words, when an employee is *unable* to perform, the issue involves a performance problem. When an individual *will not* perform, the issue involves a behavior problem.

Performance and behavior problems should both be addressed in a progressive manner using a protocol that has been approved in advance. The steps for each type of issue differ. Discipline should be progressive. All actions taken by any supervisor or manager must be documented. EAPs provide confidentiality for workers.

Separating employees is occasionally required in most organizations. Dismissal is a no-fault separation. Dismissed employees are usually eligible for unemployment benefits. Discharge is separation for cause, and discharged employees are usually not eligible for unemployment compensation. Eligibility for unemployment compensation is ultimately determined by an external agency. All separations require documentation. Discharges must never occur immediately, and no one, regardless of circumstances, should ever be discharged in anger. Suspensions can be immediate for actions in unusual and well-defined situations. Discharges should occur only after allowing time for anger to dissipate and thorough investigations to be made.

Preventive measures can help to avoid some disciplinary actions. Thorough and ongoing education is important for prevention to occur. Supervisor availability has the potential to open lines of communication. Documentation is an absolute requirement for any employee action involving human resources. The importance of documentation cannot be overstated.

🔎 CASE STUDY: Resolution

Returning to the opening case study, Penny Jerome's damaging error relates to generalizing. When delivering criticism, do not generalize. "Always" is a dangerous assertion to make; in the sense of being absolute, two of the most dangerous words in the language are *always* and *never*, because rarely is either state provable. Penny was doing fine while talking about the specific problem Molly had with Dr. Benson. When she generalized, she greatly reduced the chances of engaging in meaningful communication.

When criticizing an employee or delivering disciplinary action, a supervisor must be specific. Valid criticism must include a constructive element. It must indicate or suggest a direction for correction.

If Penny pursues the matter, she must try to have a joint meeting with Molly and Dr. Benson. Having all concerned parties together is the only realistic way to resolve this kind of issue. If Penny shuttles between the parties, she is likely to accomplish little or nothing.

Penny should have already learned that when interacting with Molly, she must be clear, specific, and detailed at all times. Furthermore, Penny must always be prepared to explain the reasoning or logic of any criticism directed at Molly. Finally, Penny must be absolutely certain that her documentation concerning Molly is both correct and complete.

SPOTLIGHT ON CUSTOMER SERVICE

Customer Service Aspects Related to Managers and Employee Problems

Customer service includes both external (members of the general public) and internal (organizational employees) individuals. Troubled employees present an uncommon situation in terms of customer service because they can affect both external and internal constituencies.

Employees with personal problems are often distracted, and they frequently exhibit unfriendly behavior. This translates to rudeness toward customers, patients, clients, or other individuals seeking services from the organization. Such behavior reduces the probability that the individuals being served will return in the future. Over time, revenue, reputation, and goodwill are likely to be lost.

Distracted or troubled employees usually treat their coworkers to the same spectrum of unacceptable behavior. Over time, colleagues come to resent such treatment and learn how to avoid the irritating persons. At best, this can result in service delays for external customers. At worst, it can disrupt internal operations.

All managers have an obligation to promote good customer service. This means getting to know the people whom they supervise. Being vigilant in this situation includes providing adequate training and making referrals to EAPs as appropriate. Any successful restaurant owner will agree that the negative impact of a single dissatisfied customer more than offsets the positive impacts of 20 people who enjoyed their meals. These numbers also apply to organizations that provide services related to health.

Modified from Segal, J. A. (1990). Did the Marquis de Sade design your discipline program? *HR Magazine, 35*(9), 90–95.

Questions for Review and Discussion

1. Comment on the claim that "like it or not, people problems are the legitimate terrain of a first-line manager." Why is this often true?
2. Why do experts strongly recommend that regardless of the apparent severity of an infraction, no employee should be summarily discharged but rather be placed on indefinite suspension pending an investigation?
3. Why do we stress that an employee's personal problems are no business of the manager? Under what conditions and to what extent can a department manager be concerned with any facet of an employee's personal problems?
4. We repeatedly stress that the primary purpose of disciplinary action is *correction of behavior*. If this is so, why have we delineated specific behavioral problems that call for loss of employment upon a single occurrence?
5. Explain why corrective action should be taken as soon as possible and practical following an infraction.
6. Why do experts strongly recommend that performance problems be considered separately from conduct or behavior problems?
7. Why is it necessary to have a completely documented history leading up to an employee's involuntary termination? With what must this documented history agree?
8. Why is a department manager's timely follow-up so important in the performance improvement process?

9. Why do senior executives require that no significant disciplinary action be implemented without the involvement of the HR department?
10. Describe the approach you would take with employees who you feel are repeatedly coming close to termination because of tardiness or absences but correcting just enough to avoid discharge?
11. Why is it inadvisable to skip steps in the disciplinary process leading up to an employee's involuntary termination?
12. Why is it necessary to create and retain a written record of an oral warning?
13. How would you address the problem of a pleasant, likeable employee whose normally marginal performance repeatedly becomes substandard a few weeks after corrective action is applied?
14. Describe two hypothetical situations in which it is appropriate for a department manager to direct an employee into the EAP as a condition of continued employment.
15. Where should a department manager first look for clues to corrective action when an employee exhibits problems in meeting the job's minimum standards of performance?

Reference

Segal, J. A. (1990). Did the Marquis de Sade design your discipline program? *HR Magazine, 35*(9), 90–95.

Resources
Books

Delpo, A., & Guerin, L. (2005). *Dealing with problem employees: A legal guide.* Berkeley, CA: NOLO.
Maiden, R. P. (2005). *Accreditation of employee assistance programs.* Binghamton, NY: Haworth Press.
McConnell, C. R. (2019). *The effective health care supervisor* (9th ed.). Burlington, MA: Jones & Bartlett Learning.
Shepard, G. (2005). *How to manage problem employees: A step-by-step guide for turning difficult employees into high performers.* New York, NY: John Wiley.
Tate, R., & White, J. (2005). *People leave managers . . . not organizations: Action based leadership.* Lincoln, NE: iUniverse.

Periodicals

Anthony, A. E. (2017). Effects of discipline management on employee performance in an organization: The case of county education office human resource department, Turkana County. *International Academic Journal of Human Resources and Business Administration, 2*(3), 1–18.
Batt, R. (2002). Managing customer services: Human resource practices, quit rates, and sales growth. *Academy of Management Journal, 45,* 587–597.
Brooke, L. (2003). Human resource costs and benefits of maintaining a mature-age workforce. *International Journal of Manpower, 24*(3), 260–283.
Ellens, J. H. (2005). Emotional reason, deliberation, motivation, and the nature of value. *Journal of Psychology and Christianity, 24*(2), 179–180.
Thomas, D. (2005). Manpower problems. *British Dental Journal, 199*(9), 545–548.
Vest, M. J., Tarnoff, K. A., Carr, J. C., Vest, J. M., & O'Brien, F. P. (2003). Factors influencing a manager's decision to discipline employees for refusal to work with an HIV/AIDS infected coworker. *Employee Responsibilities and Rights Journal, 15*(1), 31–43.

CHAPTER 15

Addressing Problems Before Taking Critical Action

CHAPTER OBJECTIVES

After studying this chapter, readers will be able to:

- Recognize the importance of preventing employee problems whenever possible.
- Understand that visible attention to chronic absenteeism and tardiness can reduce both.
- Recognize and address potentially troublesome issues concerning employee privacy and confidentiality.
- Respond to legal orders such as subpoenas, summonses, and warrants.
- Understand the organization's policies and legal posture concerning searches of employees' desks and lockers.
- Know the rules governing access to employee personnel records and health records.
- Understand the actual and perceived hazards of personal relationships in the workplace.
- Know the causes and possible means of preventing violence in the workplace.
- Appreciate the power and value of employee participation and involvement in avoiding potential problems.
- Understand the use of counseling for preventing certain circumstances from becoming genuine problems and for resolving small problems before they become large problems.

▶ Chapter Summary

The best time to address a problem is before it occurs. In terms of time, cost, and aggravation, problem prevention—finding solutions for problems in their earliest stages or avoiding problems altogether—is most effective. Many contemporary workplace problems concern issues of privacy and confidentiality that have been

🔍 CASE STUDY: A Good Employee, Except for—

Supervisor Alice Ross faced a situation that left her feeling uneasy about the action she might have to take. In discussing the matter with fellow supervisor Ed Wilson, she began by saying, "I have no idea what to do about Jane Lawson. I just don't recall ever facing one like this before."

Ed asked, "What's the problem?"

"Excessive absenteeism. Jane has rapidly used up all of her sick time, and most of her sick days have been taken immediately before or after scheduled days off."

"What's unusual about that? Unfortunately, we have any number of people who use their sick time as fast as it accrues. And most get sick on very convenient days. I should say convenient for them, not us."

"What's unusual is the fact that it's Jane Lawson. She's been here for 7 years, but the apparent sick time abuse has all been within the recent few months. She's used up her whole sick time bank in 6 months, and most recently she was out for 3 days without even calling in."

Ed said, "You can terminate her for that."

"I know," said Alice.

"Especially when you take her other absences into account. Have you warned her about them?"

After a brief hesitation, Alice said, "No, not in writing. Just once, face to face."

"Is there any record of it? Any form she had to sign?"

"No," said Alice. "I really hated to make her sign a form. I know I should have taken some kind of action by now, but I can't seem to make myself do it."

"Why not?"

"Because she's always been such a good employee. She's always been pleasant, always done what she's told, and always done quality work. She's still that way, when she's here. She's also a friend. I guess what I'm hung up on is, um, how do I discipline someone who's usually a good employee and do it in a way that doesn't destroy any of what's good about her?"

Ed said, "Good performer or not, you should be going by the policy book. That's all I can suggest."

How has Alice's failure to take action as troubles emerge or do anything about the signs of impending problems hampered her ability to take effective action now? What has Alice actually done by allowing matters to proceed as far along as they have? What impact will their friendship have on the situation?

addressed in legislation. Sexual harassment, workplace violence, and personal relationships create problems for managers at all organizational levels. Many difficulties can be avoided through employee participation and involvement in programs that raise awareness of these issues. Astute managers offer some counseling to their employees or refer them for other assistance when indications of problems begin to emerge.

▶ Prevention when Possible

The best time to address a problem is before it becomes a problem. Managers cannot accurately anticipate difficulties in specific forms or at particular times, but by developing an awareness of behavioral patterns and learning how to spot signs of trouble, a manager can catch many actual or would-be problems in their early stages.

An example illustrates the value of prevention in a proactive approach to absenteeism: Consider a policy concerning absences that specifies a supervisor must start disciplinary action after an employee has five instances of unexcused absence within a 12-month period. A supervisor learns that a particular employee has just been absent for the fourth time in 8 months. The supervisor has two options: ignore the problem but prepare to begin disciplinary action as soon as absence number five occurs, or hold a conference to warn the employee about the possibility of disciplinary action.

Why simply ignore the issue now? Why let it go further if there is a course of action that can be taken to prevent more serious consequences in the future? The supervisor should take the employee aside and address the recent absences before formal action is indicated. Prevention should be practiced whenever possible. In addition to being less stressful for both supervisor and employee, prevention improves morale by showing that the manager cares enough to pay attention to employees and their circumstances and behavior.

Employee tardiness and absenteeism deserve a department manager's visible attention. If employees see their manager paying attention to these problem areas, some will be deterred from abusing the rules. Conscientious and common-sense management can help minimize or avoid many problems.

▶ Employee Privacy and Confidentiality

Issues of employee privacy and confidentiality are pervasive in contemporary organizations. This is especially true in health care. Human resource professionals are familiar with the debate between employee privacy on one hand and the right to know on the other hand. In other terms, the conflict frequently amounts to individual rights versus business needs. The rights of individuals to privacy and confidentiality have been a growing concern in contemporary American society.

▶ Privacy and the Changing Times

There is an increasingly strong belief in society concerning the right of an individual to privacy. There is also increasing apprehension about how the government might use information it gathers about individuals. This stems from a number of concerns. Many observers feel that agencies are intruding more deeply into peoples' lives as the government enacts new legislation and increases demands for information. Businesses are widely perceived as exercising their legal right to review computers and electronic documents and to monitor telephone conversations as they strive to learn more about the people they employ. Advancing and expanding computer technology is simplifying the collection, storage, and retrieval of personal information. Since September 11, 2001, the government has been responding to a perceived need to monitor many individuals and their movements.

Because employees are becoming increasingly aware of their rights, they are coming to expect their privacy to be protected. At the same time, organizations are requesting an increasing amount of information from people when making decisions about hiring, promotions, benefits, and security. When individuals seek employment, work organizations want information about past and present employers and often additional information. Depending on the requirements of a particular job, the application process may involve detailed security screening. Employees continue to grow more sensitive to the issue of privacy rights, and they perceive that organizations are delving continually deeper into their personal lives.

Many individuals believe that organizations collecting data about them ask for more personal information than is legitimately needed. Petrocelli (1981) offers a classic definition of the right to privacy: "It is the right to be free from the unwarranted appropriation of one's personality, the publicizing of one's private affairs with which the public has no legitimate concern, or the wrongful intrusion into one's private activities, in such a manner as to outrage or cause suffering, shame or humiliation to a person of ordinary sensibilities" (112).

Consider the rights of privacy and drug testing. Individual rights are continually giving way to perceived needs for drug testing, especially for people in occupations having responsibility for public health and safety. Consider AIDS and testing for the presence of HIV. This represents a constant collision of individual rights with the need to have information about people seeking treatment and employees' coworkers. Concern about HIV was largely responsible for the adoption of universal precautions under which all bodily fluids are regarded as potentially hazardous.

Many organizations once routinely used polygraph (lie detector) tests to screen potential employees and randomly test existing employees. Adverse reactions to that practice led to passage of the Employee Polygraph Protection Act of 1988.

Most controversies that arise concerning employee information and organizational management involve business needs versus employee expectations of privacy.

Privacy in the Computer Age

Many of today's privacy issues arise from the ever-expanding use of electronic means of creating, capturing, storing, and transmitting information. Means of protecting data in electronic form (statistics, records of all kinds, correspondence, and information of essentially every conceivable kind) and providing security and ensuring privacy have steadily improved. However, the techniques of hackers and data thieves have likewise continually advanced, so unwanted intrusions into our programs and files continue to present problems.

We hear much in the news about major data breaches that occur from time to time involving the exposure of massive amounts of personal information, much of it of a financial nature (credit card numbers, bank account numbers, and such). What we do not hear about are the multitude of smaller breaches affecting the records of individuals or specific organizations.

Data breaches, even major breaches, are readily accomplished in very little time; it has been claimed that more than 90% of data breaches are accomplished in minutes or even seconds by data thieves who know what they are doing. And one highly unsettling estimate suggests that as many as 7% of data breaches exist undiscovered for a year or longer.

It has been established that at the level of the working manager, looking at individual computer use and an organization's business systems, more than 60% of identified and confirmed breaches involve weak, stolen, or default passwords. The lesson here, of course, is for those who control access to electronic files or data systems to get serious about applying passwords that are not easily compromised.

Legislation Affecting Privacy

Since 1975, employees have developed stronger voices in the workplace, and government has responded to those voices. Large amounts of personal information were formerly requested on job applications and in employment interviews. Curtailment of such practices commenced when antidiscrimination laws began to limit the kinds of information employers could request.

Title VII of the Civil Rights Act of 1964 was the first major law to have a significant bearing on individual privacy. The next major attack on this issue resulted in passage of the Privacy Act of 1974. Officially applying only to agencies of the federal government (but often regarded as a model for other employers), this legislation stated that an agency may obtain and retain only information relevant and necessary to accomplish its official purposes. Furthermore, it requires that as much essential information as possible be obtained directly from individual rather than from secondary sources. The law ensures record confidentiality, guarantees employees the right to examine their personnel files, and requires that no information be disclosed without the consent of affected employees.

In addition to providing a useful guideline for most employers, the Privacy Act has served as a model for the privacy laws of many states. In the majority of states, privacy laws allow employees to know that a personnel file is maintained and to examine it when desired. Most state statutes permit employees to enter information in their files to clarify whatever they may consider to be inaccurate.

The Polygraph Protection Act of 1988 proclaimed the practice of routinely administering lie detector tests to be an invasion of privacy. The act prohibited the use of lie detectors in most screening situations, stated that employees cannot be randomly tested during their terms of employment, permitted polygraph use if there is a reasonable suspicion of involvement in workplace incidents resulting in economic loss or injury to an organization, and exempted government employers from the provisions of the law. The Polygraph Protection Act does allow testing of selected employees in positions of responsibility for significant dollar value, including armored car employees, employees of alarm and security-guard firms, and current or prospective employees of firms handling controlled substances.

The Fair Credit Reporting Act limited the extent to which an organization can delve into the personal finances of an individual. This legislation regulates the conduct of consumer reporting agencies and users of consumer credit reports, prevents unjust damage from inaccurate or arbitrary information in credit reports, and keeps employers from receiving reports about employees, with the exception of specifically defined purposes related to work.

Legal Orders

It is a relatively common practice for agencies to serve subpoenas, summonses, and warrants to employees in the workplace. While many such orders are served at employees' homes, officers frequently attempt to serve them at job sites because no one can be found at an employee's last known home address. If they enter via administration, they will probably be referred to human resources (HR). In either administration or HR, they will frequently ask for directions to the employee's department. Although the practice may vary, many organizations prefer to have HR arrange for such an order to be served in private and avoid unnecessary embarrassment to an employee.

Managers who become aware of an attempt to serve a legal order on an employee in the department should send the serving officer to HR. Human resources will arrange for the order to be served in private or, in some instances, be permitted to accept it on behalf of the individual. The latter possibility is usually restricted to an employee being summoned as a witness in a legal proceeding.

Any external request for information about an employee should be referred to HR. Occasionally, human resources will receive a legal order calling for employee information required in legal proceedings. With the exception of responding to legal orders, HR should not release any information to outside persons or parties without first securing a signed release from the affected employee.

Employee Searches

It is sometimes necessary to conduct searches of areas within a facility such as desks and lockers that legitimately contain the personal property of employees. Organizations should have a published policy governing such searches. The organization should publicize the policy so employees know searches can occur and the basis for the surveys, specifically whether they are to occur at random or for reasonable cause or both. Steps should be taken to ensure that the search policy is justified and that there are good reasons for random searches. All search policies must be applied evenly and consistently to eliminate any perception of discrimination. No employees should be exempt from a search. Employee consent should be requested before a search. While it may not be legally required, consent can often avoid charges that might arise after the fact. Every search should be conducted discreetly and with respect for individual persons and property.

Access to Employee Information

Employee confidentiality always involves questions of access to information. Once information is collected, who is entitled to see it? Although arguments can be made about the need to know, legitimate needs can usually be determined by answering the question: What will be the result if this information is not made available?

Employees have a legally protected right to examine their personnel files and add clarifications they believe are necessary. Organizations ordinarily have policies governing employee access to records, usually including a requirement that files may not leave the HR department. Most such policies require that files must be reviewed in the presence of an HR employee to ensure that no material is removed.

Employee personnel files may be made available to managers who are considering particular persons for transfers. The need to know in such an instance is a legitimate requirement to review the employment history of persons being considered for a position in a manager's own department.

All organizations should have a written policy governing the release of information concerning both employees and others, such as patients for whom they provide services. Although department managers often maintain files concerning their own employees, it should be generally known that this practice is followed. Similar information should be kept for all employees, with no exceptions. Supervisors should not maintain secret files on selected individuals.

Employee Health Records

Many organizations formerly kept records related to Workers' Compensation, disability, and the like in employees' personnel files. Because they relate to employee health or physical condition, these documents and records are now considered to be medical records and are subject to stricter rules of accessibility. Employee health records are now customarily filed separately from personnel information, often in a separate office such as the employee health service. They are commonly retained by the employee health office and are subject to the same rules of access that govern patient records in a physician's office.

▶ Personal Relationships

Some organizations have rules governing personal relationships, particularly those of a romantic nature. The likelihood of such rules increases as the size of an organization increases. It is not uncommon to have a prohibition against employees being involved with each other or being involved with employees of direct competitors. Generally, however, employers can do nothing regarding the conduct of employees off of the job. They typically do nothing as long as there is no adverse effect on job performance or on the organization's reputation. Employees should be encouraged to disclose the existence of romantic relationships involving coworkers voluntarily to their supervisors. Organizations often require employees to disclose the existence of personal or romantic relationships with individuals employed by direct competitors.

There are legitimate concerns about the appearance of favoritism and an increased likelihood of sexual harassment claims and employee unrest when romantic relationships exist between management and nonmanagement employees. Such relationships may create conflicts between an employee's right to privacy and the organization's legal responsibility to prevent sexual harassment. An organization is particularly vulnerable when a member of management is involved. Courts have held organizations liable for sexual harassment by a manager even if senior managers did not know about the specific relationship. As many organizations have discovered, relationships that begin as consensual can go sour and lead to charges of sexual harassment.

Many organizations have policies that prohibit having one spouse under the supervision of the other, or even placing both spouses in the same department or group. Experience has shown that harmful perceptions often arise in the group when these prohibitions are ignored. Little or no inappropriate behavior may occur; however, because the possibility of discriminatory behavior is present, perceptions arise. To the perceiver, perception is reality.

A rule against having spouses in a superior–subordinate relationship will ordinarily hold up under scrutiny, but prohibiting spouses in the same department may be challenged. Generally, a no-spouse rule will prevail if it can be shown that the rule is designed to avoid aggregation of family members, is applied evenly and consistently, and results in no adverse impact on either gender. However, inconsistent or uneven enforcement of this and similar rules can result in discrimination charges. Overall, all rules concerned with personal relationships are especially vulnerable to challenge under privacy and antidiscrimination laws.

▶ Sexual Harassment

The risk of sexual harassment charges was mentioned in association with personal relationships on the job. In reality, this risk extends far beyond the boundaries of failed consensual personal relationships.

Under Title VII of the Civil Rights Act of 1964, sexual harassment is a form of sex discrimination. Many kinds of actions can result in charges of discrimination against employers; sexual harassment relates to just one particular area of troublesome behavior. However, sexual harassment has for some time been one of the two most frequently charged forms of discrimination for employers in the United States. (The other is discrimination based on age.)

The increasing number of cases and increasingly large monetary settlements involved make sexual harassment a concern of every employer. Thus, it becomes important for every department manager. Without exception, all employees of any organization must understand sexual harassment and know about organizational policies relative to it.

We hardly need to point out that in recent times, sexual harassment and sexually related interpersonal conduct have been showcased prominently in the news, especially as more and more individuals have felt encouraged to claim past transgressions they had previously been hesitant to reveal. This surge in complaints some time ago reached a stage at which careers have been damaged or destroyed by allegations of past sexual conduct. The lesson in this for managers in healthcare organizations is to take all such complaints seriously but do not automatically accept them as truth. Investigate every such allegation following the organization's policy for doing so. Surely there is some truth in most allegations of such conduct, but investigation is always essential. In the eyes of the law, we still remain innocent until proven guilty.

Sexual Harassment Defined

Sexual harassment consists of unwelcome sexual advances, demands or requests for sexual favors, or other conduct of a sexual nature. It is harassment if acceptance of or submission to such conduct is either explicitly or implicitly a term or condition of employment, if acceptance or rejection of such conduct is used as a basis for making employment-related decisions, or if the conduct can be viewed as unreasonably interfering with work performance or creating an offensive or intimidating work environment. The latter condition is often referred to as a hostile environment.

Sexual harassment can be as direct and blatant as offensive touching or making direct sexual propositions. Alternatively, it can be as indirect as exhibiting sexually suggestive posters or calendars, or allowing sexually related humor to be overheard by parties who find it offensive. Both extremes and any behaviors in between constitute sexual harassment. A list of concrete examples, specific instances of behavior that could be interpreted as sexual harassment, could easily fill several pages without covering all of the possibilities. A particular mode of behavior might constitute sexual harassment at one time but not at another time. For example, it is ordinarily not considered sexual harassment for an individual to ask a coworker for a date. If the person who is asked declines and the other party repeatedly makes the same request, this may then be construed as sexual harassment. Often, determining whether some mode of conduct is or is not considered sexual harassment rests with how the conduct is perceived. Much behavior that is judged to be sexual harassment is generally unwelcome, unwanted, and repeated.

All organizations should have policies that prohibit sexual harassment and also specifically prohibit retaliation against anyone complaining of such harassment. Department managers and all supervisors have the responsibility to know the sexual harassment and antiretaliation policies in sufficient detail. They must be able to train employees in the contents of the policy and the procedures for reporting sexual harassment. Human resources should include a briefing on sexual harassment in the new-employee orientation. Organizations should also have printed guidelines in their employee handbooks and their personnel policy manuals. These documents are often available on an organizational website. All employees should be offered copies of the sexual harassment policy or otherwise have direct access to this information. It is essential that all employees know the process for reporting sexual harassment and be aware of the processes by which any charges of such behavior are investigated. Most organizations require a complaining employee to report any issues relating to sexual harassment to the immediate supervisor. Alternative procedures usually allow employees to make harassment complaints directly to HR or to another point in the organization should an employee's immediate supervisor be the subject of the complaint.

It is difficult to say whether sexual harassment is declining overall or continuing at its previous levels. It is clear, however, that since the passage of antidiscrimination legislation, sexual harassment has become more visible because people who once had no recourse to such behavior now have legal channels through which they may lodge complaints. Sexual harassment has long been prevalent in business and industry, but before 1964 there was little its victims could do about it. In other words, before the emergence of legal channels through which to complain, sexual harassment was entirely "underground," and for the most part it was shrugged off or deliberately ignored. Surely anyone who has been in any portion of the American mixed-gender workforce for a few years can attest to the continuing presence of significant sexual harassment.

Sexual harassment remains a major concern throughout business and industry. It must remain a key concern of every manager in every organization. Sexual harassment cannot be condoned or tolerated. Every manager should maintain a zero-tolerance policy toward sexual harassment; to do otherwise is to leave employers open to the possibility of huge financial penalties and some of the most negative publicity an organization can experience.

▶ Violence

Violence in the workplace is often the result of stress. It frequently occurs when individuals become stressed to an unbearable level. When stress becomes unbearable, some people become ill, some break down, and some walk away from the situation. However, some become violent. Violence is similar to other forms of human behavior in that it is action in response to a condition, need, or demand.

Every organizational change that alters expectations held by employees becomes fertile territory for anger. Over time, chronic anger can lead to diminished productivity, reduced quality, increased fatigue, burnout, depression, and violence. In 2002, the Federal Bureau of Investigation reported that on average 12.5 of every 1000 employees are the victims of violence in the workplace.

A department manager's best approach to workplace violence involves awareness and prevention, but this advice introduces the manager to another potential source of trouble: there is no consistent profile to describe persons who commit violent acts in the workplace. Individuals who perpetrate workplace violence may be experiencing family problems; have a history of abuse; have problems stemming from substance abuse involving alcohol or drugs; have a history of violence; have an aggressive personality; experience mental conditions such as depression, paranoia, or schizophrenia; or have a poor self-image or low self-esteem.

According to the Occupational Safety and Health Administration (OSHA), workplace violence consists of any act or threat of physical violence, harassment, intimidation, or other threatening disruptive behavior that occurs at the work site. It ranges from threats and verbal abuse to physical assaults and even homicide (Lebron, 2018). And the most dangerous setting in which to work is health care. Although employees in health care account for about 12.2% of the working population, nearly 75% of all workplace assaults occur in a healthcare setting (Lebron, 2018). Experience has shown certain healthcare personnel, specifically nurses and nurse aides, to be at greatest risk when employed in emergency departments, psychiatric settings, and dementia units.

There are no all-inclusive reasons why people commit violent acts. Reasons driving workplace violence include the inability to cope with unbearable levels of stress; drug reactions; problems involving job, money, or family; reaction to the loss of employment; reaction to the loss of a relationship; frustration with long waits or with what may be perceived as rude or indifferent treatment; confusion or fear; and perceived violations of privacy.

Managers, psychologists, and criminal justice professionals cannot with unfailing accuracy identify persons who may resort to violence. However, there are steps that can be taken to prevent violence. Treat everyone, including employees, patients, visitors, and customers, with respect and consideration. Keep all objects that could be used as weapons stored out of easy access. Employees should remain beyond the reach of patients and visitors in tense situations and take all threats seriously, immediately reporting them through proper channels. All managers must know the organization's security procedures, alarms, and warning codes and unhesitatingly initiate these when an apparent threat arises.

Employees and managers should be extra alert to the possibility of violence if a person appears under the influence of alcohol or drugs, appears to have been in a fight, is brought into a facility by law enforcement, or is already being restrained.

Visible indicators of potential violence include obvious possession of a weapon; nervousness; abrupt movements; extreme restlessness, pacing, or obvious agitation; hitting walls or objects; or breaking things.

When observing an individual who appears to be on the edge of losing control, notify other staff and call the security department. Remain alert but remain calm. Always maintain a safe distance, giving an agitated person plenty of space. Under no circumstances should an untrained employee touch an agitated or upset person. Obstacles between an upset person and others provide some protection. Untrained employees in the vicinity of an agitated person should always be certain of a clear way out; dead-end corridors or corners are especially dangerous. Listen to the agitated individual, never display anger or defensiveness, and do not argue. Speak calmly, slowly, and quietly.

Some departments, a case in point being emergency rooms, are relatively more likely than other departments to experience violence. However, violence is possible anywhere in any facility or organization. Therefore, all employees should receive training in how to react to violent behavior. If violence does occur, employees should protect themselves to the extent necessary; sound an alarm, call the appropriate code, or call security. Employees should help remove others from the vicinity, if necessary. Employees who lack specific training must not try to disarm or restrain an agitated person. If possible, meet the violent person's demands if these are within reason.

▶ Employee Participation and Involvement

True employee participation has the potential to influence behavior positively and avoid potential problems. Participative management is not a program with a beginning and an end; rather, it is a continuing relationship between a manager and the employee group. It requires management commitment. Individual managers must be willing to allow employees to participate in decisions. Employees must know that managers genuinely want their input and that it is valued. Involving employees requires that management listen to them. Managers should be both visible and available. Walking around and visiting with employees at their workstations is valuable. The more employees feel that managers are interested in what they do and in their thoughts, the more they will feel respected, challenged, and constructively utilized.

A few employees prefer to simply do just as they are told, put in their hours, and go home. The majority of employees, however, usually prefer to be challenged. They have the potential to become engaged in their jobs. Many people are capable of managing their own work if they are provided with a supportive environment and given the opportunity to perform. Effective managers remember that nobody knows the inner detailed workings of a job better than the person who does it every day. This is the source of knowledge that a manager should try to access through honest participation.

The primary factor in employee involvement is supportive managerial behavior. Managers must be able to empower their employees. They will not necessarily always get to make the decisions or develop the solutions, but employees must understand how they can influence processes and whom they will help decide. Decisions that relate to individual jobs are usually best made by the people who perform the jobs. The more levels of management separating a decision maker from the person affected by the decision, the greater the chances the outcome will be unfavorable.

Effective employee involvement requires a gradual transition as mutual trust develops between managers and employees and each becomes more willing to help the other succeed. An organization or department that can achieve effective employee participation will usually experience a significant increase in productivity and a noticeable decrease in employee problems. Interested, stimulated, and challenged employees constitute the best possible means of preventing problems.

▶ Counseling

Counseling is appropriate for addressing problems and potential problems at their early stages to keep them from becoming larger problems. Sometimes counseling is informal guidance and work-related advice provided by a supervisor. Overall, counseling may be employed to identify problems in their early stages and attempt to resolve them before they become overwhelming. Counseling can be used to strengthen weaknesses in employee performance and provide ongoing guidance. Counseling may enable a manager to recommend developmental activities for an employee or improve communication between supervisor and employee.

Supervisors should try to counsel employees when problems appear to be developing rather than letting them continue to grow until some form of corrective action is required. A need for counseling may be signaled by a noticeable decline in an individual's performance or a person's failure to continue meeting job standards. A decline in performance, especially in an employee who has performed well for an extended period, often indicates the presence of a personal problem. A counseling session can afford employees the opportunity to talk. This provides a manager the opportunity to make an appropriate referral. Employees should not be allowed to continue on a path toward disciplinary action when a friendly one-to-one counseling session may be able to head off further trouble. Changes in individuals relative to their jobs are often indicators that counseling may be appropriate. Changes in interpersonal relationships are another indicator of potential trouble. Complaints about an employee from other people, especially those involving alleged rude or inappropriate behavior, are often indicative of personal problems.

Discussing a need for counseling with a subordinate is not easy for every manager. Managers should remember that they are primarily conduits to trained professionals. Effective counseling requires training. However, managers can provide basic advice and guidance to their employees. A first rule is to understand the boundaries. Supervisory counseling encompasses coaching on job-related topics or on behavior relative to policies or work rules. Counseling must never become personal—that is, it should never involve intrusions into private lives.

Many common obstacles to counseling success may be overcome. Practice and experience should overcome uneasiness and a lack of experience. Lack of time can be addressed by making appointments and clearing a calendar for 30–60 minutes at a time. Friendships are more difficult. Counseling friends is not much easier than disciplining friends, so many managers tend to avoid both activities. Counseling a person with more seniority than the counselor is often awkward. If awkwardness at counseling is not overcome with practice, it will likely not disappear with the passage of time. A reasonable fear of making mistakes is healthy and helps managers respect appropriate boundaries and guidelines. Fear of a lawsuit should reinforce the directive to refer people with problems to qualified professionals.

To provide effective advice in appropriate settings, managers must be knowledgeable and credible. Managers must know what they are talking about and avoid trying to bluff their way through unfamiliar situations. Effective counselors stick to known facts and avoid generalizations. Timeliness is appreciated by all concerned. As with delaying disciplinary action, delaying counseling until a later time dilutes the message and diminishes its impact.

Effective managers are alert for employee defensiveness and do not argue with them. Some employees will interpret any effort at counseling as direct criticism and will immediately become defensive. Should this occur, hear an employee out and avoid contradicting the person. Successful counselors are as positive as possible. Counseling may indeed contain elements of criticism, but a positive direction to a discussion is always helpful. Effective counselors listen, really listen. When an employee is speaking, they provide their undivided attention and focus on what is really being said.

At all times, department managers must remember that their primary goal should be focusing on the results of behavior, not on the supposed causes. In talking with subordinates, managers should never attempt to infer the cause of behavior and should not attempt to look for it. Focusing on the results of behavior and correcting inappropriate behavior help managers to avoid entering an employee's personal life.

Wise managers document each counseling session briefly and informally, making note of employee name, date, and nature of the discussion. The aim of such informal and personal notes is to capture the essence of the discussion objectively and using anecdotes. These notes are not considered permanent records but should be retained for 1–2 years in the event the problem recurs. These personal notes should be destroyed if the problem has not recurred within 2 years.

▶ Conclusion

Many employee-related problems can be prevented by timely and appropriate interventions. Employee confidentiality and privacy must be respected and protected; federal legislation has reinforced this need.

Personal relationships involving colleagues or supervisors present significant problems. Most organizations have established policies to address such situations in an effort to protect all concerned. Sexual harassment is one of the most serious problems facing workers in contemporary organizations. All employees must understand and follow organizational policies and procedures that address sexual harassment. Zero tolerance for such activities is the only defensible position an organization can adopt.

Violence has become more common in the workplace. All employees must be instructed in how to respond to threats of violence because violence is possible anywhere in any type of facility or organization. Employee involvement can facilitate and improve organizational operations. Supervisors should be able to provide advice or limited counseling to their employees.

🔍 *CASE STUDY: Resolution*

Returning to the initial case study, Alice Ross has made additional work for herself by allowing the situation with Jane to continue without intervention. Alice faces a sticky problem because she did not use early opportunities to head off the worst before it could develop. She has made a classic error by avoiding confrontation. Alice does not wish to antagonize an employee who is otherwise doing a decent job. Maintaining a personal friendship with a subordinate complicates the situation.

It is likely that there is a reason behind Jane's behavior. She may be experiencing a personal problem. If so, privacy issues must be considered. An element in Jane's personal life could be causing her frequent absences, but as a supervisor Alice cannot ask about personal issues. While she could ask about personal issues as a friend, her supervisory responsibilities should take precedence. Alternatively, the pattern of Jane's absences might suggest that she is simply playing the system for time off, possibly having lost interest in her job. Alice should offer to listen to anything Jane wishes to talk about and then refer Jane to sources of help such as an employee assistance program.

Because she has not taken any formal action on the apparent problem, Alice has little choice but to start over with Jane and apply the organization's disciplinary policy. However, Alice should first tell Jane exactly where she stands and explain the consequences of continued absenteeism.

Alice's colleague Ed pointed out that the prescribed response to 3 days of unexplained absences is discharge. This circumstance, commonly referred to as "three days no-call no-show," is identified as job abandonment in many organizations' personnel policies and calls for immediate termination. Alice must watch the breaks she gives to any individual. Policies must be applied consistently, and Alice cannot be allowing Jane to slide by without consequences for doing something for which others would be disciplined. The fact that their friendship interferes with operations is the basis for organizational policies restricting personal involvement with coworkers.

Alice should have recognized signs of a developing problem before Jane hit the threshold for an initial warning under the progressive discipline policy. An ideal course of action would have been counseling at an earlier stage in an effort to avoid a more serious problem.

Some managers will allow an employee to wander deeply enough into trouble before starting to deliver warnings. Thoughtful managers, however, will take reasonable steps at the earliest signs of trouble to prevent small concerns from becoming full-scale problems.

SPOTLIGHT ON CUSTOMER SERVICE

Customer Service and Addressing Problems

Prevention is synonymous with taking steps to avoid an unwanted or undesirable consequence or outcome. The concept is well known in health care. Clinical providers offer advice and counseling to their patients. The goal of their activities is to maintain or improve their patients' health. Immunizations are used to prevent disease. Public health personnel work in communities and schools to present information about healthy personal habits, food sanitation, and avoiding diseases. Sanitarians inspect restaurants and similar establishments to ensure that appropriate methods and procedures are used by individuals preparing and handling food.

This chapter has focused on a different form of prevention: trying to address employee behavior problems before legal or other actions become necessary. Managers should gather data and review facts before contemplating disciplinary or other corrective actions. Because they should not act in anger, supervisors are advised to simply wait (assuming that other people or organizational assets are not in danger) and reflect before initiating any form of punishment.

Customer service is also a form of prevention. People appreciate being treated well and with respect. However, unintended consequences have been documented. Physicians and other healthcare providers who treat their patients with respect and take time to provide explanations about diseases and treatments have a lower than average incidence of malpractice suits. In states that allow voter-approved tax levies for supporting public health, agencies that provide good customer service are more likely have their levy requests approved than are agencies that do not back their stated commitment to the public with good customer service.

Modified from Lebron, L. (2018). *The latest on workplace violence statistics.* Rave Mobile Safety (American Software Company). Retrieved from https://www.ravemobilesafety.com

Questions for Review and Discussion

1. Why should supervisors and managers be most interested in the results of employee behavior? Why should they not try to eliminate the causes of such behavior?
2. How do the needs of an organization and the privacy rights of an individual differ? When do these needs conflict?
3. How could a department manager prevent excessive absenteeism among employees?
4. Under what circumstances is polygraph testing of employees legal?
5. Why is it advisable to maintain documentation having a bearing on employee health issues separately from regular personnel files?
6. When may a department manager be granted access to the personnel files of employees of other departments?
7. Why is employee involvement frequently recommended as a strategy for preventing problems?
8. Why should supervisors take time to counsel employees when a disciplinary problem appears to be developing? Why should they not wait until definitive disciplinary action is permissible under an organization's policies?
9. How should managers prepare their employees to react to violence in the workplace? Why is the preparation necessary?
10. Why must an organization obtain an employee's written permission before releasing any information concerning that employee? When may such information be released without employee permission?

References

Lebron, L. (2018). *The latest on workplace violence statistics.* Rave Mobile Safety (American Software Company). Retrieved from https://www.ravemobilesafety.com

Modified from Petrocelli, W. (1981). *How to avoid the privacy invaders.* New York, NY: McGraw-Hill.

Resources
Books
Elliott, C., & Turnbull, S. (2005). *Critical thinking in human resource development*. New York, NY: Routledge.

Ghodse, H. (2005). *Addiction at work: Tackling drug use and misuse in the work place*. London, UK: Ashgate.

Goldsmith, J. (2005). *Resolving conflicts at work: Eight strategies for everyone on the job*. New York, NY: John Wiley.

Joy-Matthews, J., & Surtees, M. (2004). *Human resource development*. London, UK: Kogan Page.

Kaye, B., & Jordan-Evans, S. (2005). *Love 'em or lose 'em: Getting good people to stay* (3rd ed.). San Francisco, CA: Berrett-Koehler.

MacLennon, W. (2005). *Counselling for managers*. London, UK: Ashgate.

Periodicals
Hogan, R., Hogan, J., & Roberts, B. W. (1996). Personality measurement and employment decisions. *American Psychologist, 51*, 469–477.

Huffcutt, A. I., Conway, J. M., Roth, P. L., & Stone, N. J. (2001). Identification and meta-analytic assessment of psychological constructs measured in employment interviews. *Journal of Applied Psychology, 86*, 897–913.

Munn-Giddings, C., Hart, C., & Ramon, S. (2005). A participatory approach to the promotion of well-being in the workplace: Lessons from empirical research. *International Review of Psychiatry, 17*(5), 409–417.

Riolli, L. (2003). Optimism and coping as moderators of the relation between work resources and burnout in information service workers. *International Journal of Stress Management, 10*, 235–252.

Schaeffer, C., Booton, L., Halleck, J., Studeny, J., & Coustasse, A. (2017). Big data management in U.S. hospitals: Benefits and barriers. *The Health Care Manager, 36*(1), 7–95.

Talbot, T. (2005). "Working interviews": The human resources perspective. *Journal of the Michigan Dental Association, 87*(5), 17–20.

CHAPTER 16

Terminating Employees

CHAPTER OBJECTIVES

After studying this chapter, readers will be able to:

- Understand the roles of human resources and department managers in terminating employees.
- Explain the concept of constructive discharge.
- Know the sequence of steps to consider before deciding to lay off personnel.
- Understand how to determine who is released and who remains in a legal and equitable layoff.
- Understand the actions and processes related to termination.
- Discuss the potential effects of a reduction on the survivors, and suggest how management can address these issues.

▶ Chapter Summary

Terminations of employment are inevitable. There are positive terminations, specifically retirements and resignations, as well as negative experiences such as discharges (firings) and layoffs. Involuntary termination is the end of employment upon the decision of management. There are two types of such terminations. Dismissals occur when individuals fail to meet the standards of the job or as part of a layoff. Discharges occur when employees are released for reasons of conduct or behavior that usually involves violations of policies or work rules. Discharges are an ongoing concern because they may be necessary at any time. Most dismissals, other than a relative few related to job performance, are layoffs for reasons such as reengineering, downsizing, merger or other organizational affiliations, or cutbacks driven by economic forces. Layoffs are traumatic occurrences that sever personnel from their employment and adversely affect the morale and motivation of survivors. Properly conducted layoffs require the guidance of human resources (HR) and the active participation of all levels of management.

🔍 CASE STUDY: The Case of Joan von Willebrand

Joan von Willebrand was a phlebotomist at City Hospital. Her supervisor, George Parker, worked as a member of the phlebotomy team. George reported to Gloria Garcia, a unit manager of the laboratory.

Joan had been employed at City Hospital for 5 months when she was discharged for chronic tardiness. Gloria initiated the discharge with the concurrence of George. When the matter was turned over to HR, Gloria told HR that Joan had been given written warnings for clocking in more than 30 minutes late on three prior occasions. Gloria also said, "There were numerous other occurrences that had been overlooked or that had resulted in undocumented oral warnings."

Joan complained that the 6:30 A.M. starting time for the morning blood-collecting rounds was too early for her. She stated that as a single mother, she had the responsibility of looking after one child. Even though she lived with relatives, she had difficulty getting to the hospital on time. She also stated that when she was hired, George had led her to believe that the blood-collecting job was temporary and that a regular opening in the lab, starting at 8:00 A.M., would be available in 2 or 3 months.

Gloria had criticized George for being too lenient and for not following organizational policies. He had delivered an initial oral warning as required. However, on subsequent occasions, he repeated the oral warning and never issued written warnings. She said that George was inconsistent in his behavior, often not reprimanding Joan for behavior that did not comply with the organization's policy. George started delivering written warnings after Gloria prompted him to do so. According to hospital policy, four written warnings for tardiness constituted grounds for discharge. George gave this information to Joan each time she received a written warning. After receiving the fourth written warning, Joan was fired.

Although George and Gloria both admitted to the possibility of mentioning a regular technician job in the future, they were both convinced that there had been no promises. The HR recruiter supported these facts and said that he had also mentioned to Joan the possibility of moving into a different job should one become available but had made no promises.

Joan took her complaint to the State, claiming that her firing was unwarranted and unfair. Although she had been late a few times, she said, she never failed to stay and make up the time and she had always performed her assigned duties. However, George cast some doubt on this claim. He said that on days when Joan was late, he and another technician had to cover extra territory to make up for the missing employee.

Joan charged that the written policy meant very little because early in her employment she had been late several times, but on these occasions she had not received warnings. She charged management in general, and Gloria in particular, with using the tardiness policy as an excuse to get rid of her.

What procedural errors were made in the handling of Joan von Willebrand's case? How would you rule on Joan's claim? What would be the basis for your decision?

▶ Involuntary Termination

This chapter addresses involuntary terminations. These include discharges for cause, such as violations of policies or work rules, and dismissal for reasons of substandard performance or because of reduction of the work force (layoff). Questions occasionally arise concerning some supposedly voluntary terminations such as resignations and retirements.

▶ Individual Terminations

Discharge: Termination for Cause

Discharge and dismissal are different, although both result in separation from the organization. *Discharge* is commonly referred to as being fired. Discharge usually occurs after employees break the organization's work rules or violate organizational policies. *Dismissal* typically occurs for reasons of job performance, such as failure to pass the probationary period or failure to meet the minimum standards of a job.

Most managers dread having to fire someone, even if the employee clearly deserves the termination. Dismissal is likewise not easy for most managers, and it rarely becomes easier with time. Before a termination is undertaken, the manager must work with HR, must be in agreement with HR concerning the details of the termination, and must agree that all required information is complete and available.

From an employer's perspective, terminations involving the least risk to the organization are those for which good cause is evident. Managers must ensure that the organization closely followed its own policies, and that the organization can demonstrate that a discharged employee was given every reasonable opportunity to correct the offending behavior. The manager or HR must ensure that the organization's policies have been followed. Adherence to the progressive disciplinary policy is critical; it is essential to ensure that all required documentation is complete and in place. The most critical dimension of termination for cause is ensuring that management and HR observe all essential steps of the process. Despite the best efforts of department managers and HR, unexpected circumstances can cause problems for the organization. For example, a written passage in an employee handbook stating that an employee who passes probation becomes a "permanent" employee has at times been interpreted as constituting an employment contract—that is, a guarantee of employment. Such an interpretation has at times been used to protest discharge. Most organizations that have encountered this problem addressed it by dropping the "permanent employee" in favor of "regular employee" or "regular employment status." A department manager must always be mindful of the possibility that a member of a protected class may claim discrimination when being discharged. A wrongful termination lawsuit can be frustrating, costly, and time consuming. An organization's best protection against wrongful termination charges is fair personnel policies consistently applied. Performance appraisal systems also must be fair. All documentation must be complete and available. Above all, the organization must always have clear evidence of employee wrongdoing to support a discharge.

Dismissal: Inability to Meet Job Standards

Dismissal is used to describe a termination when an individual is not considered to be at fault. This is an essential difference between dismissal and discharge; dismissal relates to performance, not conduct or behavior. Because no rule is broken or policy violated, dismissal for inability to meet the standards of the job or failure to pass the probationary period is treated as a layoff. The distinction becomes important when dismissed employees apply for unemployment compensation. A discharged employee is technically ineligible for unemployment compensation, but a dismissed employee is eligible for unemployment compensation.

The majority of employees who are involuntarily separated apply for unemployment benefits regardless of the circumstances leading to their termination. They do so because they feel they have nothing to lose. Discharged employees are frequently granted unemployment compensation contrary to the fact that they were discharged for cause. This usually occurs when an individual who is discharged nevertheless files a claim for unemployment compensation but the organization (usually HR) fails to protest the claim. When a claim for unemployment compensation is not protested, such compensation is usually granted. A protested claim often leads to a hearing at which an administrative law judge listens to both sides and decides whether the claim is or is not valid.

Constructive Discharge

An occasional manager will behave as though believing that the most effective way to get rid of an underproducing or uncooperative employee is to keep piling on work, or generally to make life miserable until the person finally quits. A manager may reason that since an employee who voluntarily resigns is not eligible for unemployment compensation, this potential expense is avoided and a problem is solved without cost to the employer. However, there is a significant risk in using this approach to getting rid of an employee.

Constructive discharge becomes an issue when a former employee registers a legal complaint alleging that the organization, as represented by one of its managers, made life so difficult and unbearable that the individual had to resign for the sake of his or her physical and mental health and well-being. A resignation forced by extreme or intolerable conditions or treatment specifically imposed to get rid of the person is considered a constructive discharge. Thus, a resignation tendered under such conditions is not considered strictly voluntary.

Another similar-but-not-quite-the-same situation occurs when an individual who is approaching termination for cause is allowed to resign "for the record" in lieu of discharge. A well-intended manager may suggest that an individual be allowed to resign for the record, believing it is better for one to avoid having a discharge in the personnel record. Thus, one's record will be seen as relatively "clean" when references are checked. However, doing so can expose the organization to a claim of constructive discharge by the employee ("I was forced to resign") and possibly a claim of negligent hiring against the organization taking on the released employee. It is far more prudent for the organization to stick to the truth and utilize a well-documented discharge in accordance with organizational policy.

▶ Reductions in Force

There are several reasons that compel organizations to reduce the numbers of their employees. Growth supports increases in employee counts; other forces cause organizations to reduce the numbers of their employees. These latter forces include downsizing, reengineering, mergers, acquisitions, and combinations and variations of these. Organizations use several methods to reduce the number of employees, including layoffs and terminations.

Reengineering

Reengineering is the systematic redesign of a business's core activities, starting with desired outcomes and establishing the most efficient possible processes to achieve those outcomes. Healthcare organizations entered into reengineering a few years after it peaked in manufacturing. Reengineering is often referred to—usually incorrectly—by other names including *downsizing, rightsizing, reorganizing, repositioning, revitalizing,* and *modernizing,* although reengineering is in fact a considerably more complex undertaking than these other named processes. Nevertheless, to most employees, reengineering has a single significant result: job loss. Mention of the term alerts employees to the likelihood of layoffs. Organizations in the healthcare sector have long been making changes that affect their employees. To provide some examples, by 1998, 81% had reduced their staffs through layoffs or attrition, and nearly half had laid off managers (Serb, 1998). Data provided by the Bureau of Labor Statistics reveal that changes affecting employees continue. A 2011 report issued by the Advisory Board Company noted that "the sluggish economy and looming provider payment cuts have driven more hospitals to consider reducing staff as a way to stabilize their bottom lines" (Advisory Board, 2013). Increasing demand for healthcare services associated with decreasing reimbursement payments for such services has led hospitals to turn to less costly staff to deliver certain needed services. Steady rates of new unemployment claims by displaced hospital staff coupled with slow but steady increases in total numbers of employees illustrate these changes (Bureau of Labor Statistics, 2013).

Employee morale is likely the most severe HR problem in the healthcare sector, with layoffs and the mere possibility of layoffs the main cause of morale problems.

Mergers, Acquisitions, and Other Affiliations

Mergers, acquisitions, and other forms of affiliation have become common in contemporary health care. Because these recombinations most often occur in response to financial pressures, they usually mean the loss of jobs.

Systems often promote diversification and breadth of services. Not-for-profit systems are usually more diversified than for-profit systems. For-profit systems are more likely to be specialized; they are far less likely to maintain services that are not profitable. Not-for-profit systems are more likely to carry unprofitable services for the sake of remaining full service to the communities they serve. Little evidence exists to suggest that hospitals belonging to multiorganizational systems are any more efficient than freestanding hospitals. In some parts of the country, systems and alliances have been the salvation of certain endangered rural hospitals, but usually at the cost of job loss in the affected communities.

Mergers usually lead to the reduction of management jobs as well as staff positions. Consider the merger of two small-town hospitals located not far from each other. The merger involved combining parallel departments at both institutions under a single management structure. For example, two clinical laboratories with two managers were combined into a two-location laboratory department with a single manager. Because of this merger, 12 managers were eliminated, and each of the managers who remained was left with a greatly enlarged span of control.

The process of consummating a merger is usually considerably more difficult and more expensive than what was originally anticipated. Employees of one organization usually fear absorption by the other organization and the loss of their identity. This happens even in a merger of so-called equals; one organization absorbs the other or is at least perceived as having done so.

Consolidation expenses can be high. Organizations can require an extremely long time to recover their merger expenses through lower operating costs and improved efficiency. Organizational recombinations can be highly disruptive to staff in a number of ways as conflicting organizational cultures are forced to mix. The human side of merger or acquisition is rarely given sufficient attention. Emotional issues that can make or break a merger usually take a distant second place to the financial issues.

When organizations explore the possibility of merger or affiliation, little information is likely to be available. Once the possibility of a merger becomes known, however, employees become uneasy. Thoughtful managers maintain a dialogue with their employees. They listen to their concerns and keep them informed. They keep lines of communication open and provide the best information available. Honesty is an absolute requirement for maintaining personal credibility.

Layoffs
Other Considerations First

Department managers and HR staff experience considerable stress when ordered to implement significant layoffs. When a layoff is impending, the organization should examine other possible steps to take before releasing employees. All realistic steps that do not involve layoffs should be taken before employees are actually released. One early step should be eliminating the use of all temporary employees. Another early step is the imposition of a hiring freeze. By stopping the influx of all but essential staff, such an action provides time to consider possible internal reallocation of personnel.

Following a hiring freeze, closing open positions can reduce the total number of employees "on the books" without releasing people. If the reduction in staff is to be extensive and likely to be permanent, executive management should consider offering a voluntary termination incentive. The organization might also consider offering an early retirement incentive. Early retirement incentive plans are helpful but can be risky. Specific individuals or groups cannot be targeted, as to do so is discriminatory. An additional risk is that key employees may actually leave.

Who Goes and Who Stays?

A department manager is usually involved in determining which employees leave and which ones stay. Personal preferences must be subordinate to established organizational guidelines. All organizational guidelines should be established with the guidance of legal counsel. Selection for layoff is most often accomplished according to seniority, although this is not an absolute requirement unless a contract governs selection for layoff. Seniority may not be the sole factor. For example, assessment mechanisms might consider a combination of factors that could include performance as reflected by appraisals, attendance, conduct as reflected by disciplinary actions, and seniority.

Many organizations have determined that seniority is the fairest and safest means of determining who leaves and who remains. Using seniority alone, questions remain as to how it is determined. Seniority can be determined by time in an organization, time in a specific department, or time within a particular task or job class.

Related to the degree of seniority is the process of bumping or displacement. Bumping occurs when the job of an individual is eliminated. Persons of greater seniority are allowed to displace or bump persons having lesser seniority from their positions. This process continues until the person having the least seniority is laid off. Bumping can be simple or extremely complex, depending on the rules that are in place.

In addition to utilizing temporary employees, healthcare organizations actively use many part-time employees and carry on the rolls some who work only when called upon (per-diem employees). An official approach taken to selecting employees for layoff may include guidelines governing the order of reduction based on work status. For example, temporary employees are released first, followed by regular part-time employees, while per-diem employees are simply not called upon.

Whatever combination of factors is used, consistency in how the guidelines are applied is critically important. Ideally, the organization should have a personnel policy governing staff reductions. Such a policy should be in place well before reductions become necessary. However, in many organizations, no policy is created until the need for reductions becomes apparent. **EXHIBIT 16-1** contains a sample reduction-in-force policy illustrating how one organization has addressed most of the foregoing concerns. If employees are represented by a union, a collectively bargained agreement between employer and union usually determines how employees are chosen for layoff.

Once a layoff plan has been created, personnel from administration and HR and the organization's legal counsel must assess the proposal to ensure the absence of bias. Charges of discrimination are likely to arise if patterns based on age, gender, or race emerge among those slated for layoff. For example, some organizations wanting to reduce personnel costs have laid off higher-paid employees. As higher-paid employees tend to be older, the resulting process can be considered discriminatory on the basis of age. All scenarios must be examined before a layoff plan can be considered workable and nondiscriminatory.

The goal of an ideal layoff will be a resulting organization that has reduced its personnel costs but retained its best employees. However, rarely is such an ideal outcome fully realized. Compromises must be accepted as a consequence in fairness to all employees. Older employees tend to earn higher salaries, and they are often protected by seniority. Younger employees may earn lower salaries but possess critical skills. While these traits are desirable in an organization, younger employees lack seniority. Layoffs should not be undertaken without considerable deliberation.

EXHIBIT 16-1 Model Policy and Procedure: Reduction in Force Policy and Practice

Policy

The relative security of the organization's employees is best served by continuous employment. However, occasions may arise when reducing staffing levels is necessary because of changing financial or operational circumstances. The objective of this policy is to provide a rational basis for reducing staffing levels in the event such adjustments are necessary.

Definitions

Department: A cost center or a set of cost centers having common positions, tasks, functions, or duties that report to the same manager.

Department seniority: An individual's uninterrupted service time as a full-time or part-time employee of the present department or unit, adjusted for approved leaves of absence.

Incumbent employee: An employee currently occupying an approved full-time or part-time position.

Organizational seniority: An individual's uninterrupted service time as a full-time or part-time employee, adjusted for approved leaves of absence.

Qualified employee: An individual who possesses the stated qualifications for a specific position by virtue of education, experience, or both, and can either presently perform in that position or achieve standard performance within the normal introductory period.

Determining Staff Reductions

1. Workforce Composition
   a. Establishing the size, composition, and distribution of the workforce remains a prerogative of management.
   b. Before deciding that staff reductions are necessary, management will investigate alternative processes that can avoid a reduction or lessen its impact. Staff reductions will proceed only after all reasonable alternatives have been either implemented or eliminated from consideration.
   c. When circumstances necessitate staff reductions, management shall determine the numbers and kinds of positions to be eliminated.
2. Guidelines Affecting Incumbent Employees
   a. Nonexempt employees, excluding those in designated essential positions that may be designated by management, shall be subject to layoff generally by job assignment and by department according to staffing needs.
   b. Employees working within a specific job assignment and department will be ranked using the following criteria:
      - Appropriateness of individual qualifications and experience in meeting the hospital's needs
      - Past personal performance (average of the three most recent performance appraisals)
      - Disciplinary counseling or warnings within the past 12 months
3. Organizational Seniority
   a. Each of the foregoing criteria may account for up to 25% of the ranking decision for an employee. From time to time, depending on circumstances

and need, management may devise rating scales to facilitate employee ranking.

b. After all employees within a department or job assignment are placed in rank order, selection for layoff will proceed in reverse order of the list.

c. Employees remaining in a department following a staff reduction may be subject to changes in hours, shift schedules, and work assignments, as necessary.

d. Management may exercise the right to displace less senior nonexempt employees in one department with qualified nonexempt employees from another department who have greater organizational seniority, providing that this is accomplished within similar job assignments and without significant disruption of departmental operations.

e. Management, physicians, and other exempt positions, and particular technical and professional nonexempt positions that may be designated, are subject to position-specific reductions without regard to seniority or other factors. The principal criterion for determining the status of such positions will be their appropriateness in meeting the needs of the organization.

f. Any employee identified for layoff will be considered for other possibilities such as transfer or demotion to a position in an area of need. Whenever possible, employees will be allowed to choose from available alternatives. Employee requests for reassignment to alternative positions shall be honored solely at management's discretion. Displaced employees who decline an alternative position will be dismissed.

4. Administration of Reduction

a. Department managers will identify the positions to be eliminated and will furnish administration with a list of those positions and incumbent employees.

b. Administration and HR will review potentially affected employees proposed for possible transfer or reassignment to areas of need, if any, and will make recommendations as appropriate.

c. Human resources will submit departmental lists of employees recommended for layoff to the appropriate vice president and the president.

d. Following executive approval of layoff, HR will coordinate with department managers to arrange for providing employees with proper notification of termination date and information concerning terminal benefits.

e. Each affected employee will be offered an exit interview intended to cover:
   - Method and timing of payment for accrued vacation time
   - Status and conversion of insurance coverage
   - Pension plan vesting, if appropriate
   - Unemployment compensation procedures
   - Reinstatement rights, if any
   - Recommendations or referrals for external placement, if any

5. Other Considerations

a. Every effort should be made to eliminate the use of all temporary employees before regular employees are considered for layoff.

b. An employee who is still in the introductory period (the first 6 months of employment) does not need to be re-ranked with others according to 2.b. If such an employee's job is eliminated, the individual is to be considered dismissed due to lack of work.

(continues)

EXHIBIT 16-1 Model Policy and Procedure: Reduction in Force Policy
and Practice *(continued)*

    c.   In the displacement of an employee as described in 3.d, a full-time employee
        may displace another full-time employee or a part-time employee, but a
        part-time employee may displace only another part-time employee with
        equal or lesser hours.
    d.   For employees about whom a recommendation for layoff depends in part on
        performance or disciplinary issues, appropriate supporting documentation
        must be in the personnel files.
Attachment: Employee Ranking Scale

Employee Ranking Scale

a.	Qualifications/experience	
	Still learning the job	0
	Fully trained but limited experience	2
	Fully trained and experienced	4
	Fully trained in multiple areas, cross-functional capability	6
b.	Past performance	
	Average of three most recent evaluations <3.50 (standard)	0
c.	Average of three most recent evaluations 3.50–4.25	2
	Average of three most recent evaluations 4.26–4.70	4
	Average of three most recent evaluations >4.70–6.00	6
d.	Disciplinary counseling/warnings (recent 12 months)	
	Multiple problems; suspended one or more times	0
	More than two counseling, or no more than two warnings	2
	One or two counseling, or one warning	4
	No counseling, no warnings	6
e.	Seniority (organizational)	
	Less than 1 year	0
	1–2 years	2
	2–5 years	4
	More than 5 years	6

NOTE: This ranking scale is applied to groups of employees who work within the same job description and are engaged in the same general activities. Employees in the group should be arrayed from highest (possible 24) to lowest, with the lowest rankings receiving first consideration for reduction.

The Timing of Layoffs

The timing of reductions is an issue for which there are no easy or unambiguous solutions. From the perspective of employees, timing is irrelevant because layoffs contain no positive benefits. Consultants and HR professionals who develop reduction plans and policies disagree on whether it is best to phase in reductions over a period of time or accomplish all layoffs at once. Both approaches have shortcomings.

When layoffs are phased in over a period of time, morale and productivity decrease as everyone waits and wonders who will be next. Teamwork becomes a distant second to worries about individual survival. The effect spreads across an entire organization. If the reduction is expected to include managers, then it will permeate all levels of the organization. As morale declines, it is often replaced by anger. Over time, organizational chaos will occur.

Even when a layoff is far-reaching in terms of numbers, usually far more people remain working than were released. Prolonged layoffs take their toll on the morale and attitudes of those who remain. The time required for healing is proportional to the magnitude of the staff reduction. Layoffs that are prolonged and that inflict pain require more time for recovery. Phased-in layoffs are easier to administer in that operating managers have more time to adjust layoff schedules. However, from an employee perspective, they produce more stress and anxiety than a single mass layoff.

Other Layoff Considerations

Most organizations apply some form of severance policy in conjunction with layoffs that are considered permanent. These are reductions in which employees have no realistic possibility of being recalled to work within a reasonable period. Severance pay is ordinarily based on an individual's final salary in combination with length of service and is usually capped at a stated maximum number of years. A common example of severance pay determination is 1 or 2 weeks' pay for every year of service. An alternative is to provide 2 weeks' pay per year of service to a maximum of, for example, 15 years. On average, healthcare organizations tend to offer less generous severance pay than can be found in other industries.

In exchange for a severance pay arrangement and possible outplacement assistance, the organization may ask a departing employee to sign a waiver of the right to sue. In doing so, an employee agrees not to bring charges related to the termination in trade for what is likely to be a more generous severance arrangement than would otherwise be obtainable. However, employees often successfully challenge such waivers after the fact. In reality, waivers provide no guarantee that legal complications will be avoided.

When a layoff is coming, all employees should be given the reasons for the action. The approach should be as straightforward as possible and accompanied by as much detail as is available and should be readily understood. Economic issues are the basis for most layoffs. While some employees will choose not to believe the reasons provided, if no explanations are forthcoming, employees will likely feel they are being treated unfairly. Ideally, employees should be kept advised of the organization's financial health on a regular basis. Reminders that layoffs are possible may be useful; surprises should be avoided. The reality of a layoff is sufficiently shocking when it is announced even when the employees have been led to expect it.

No Easy Time

From the perspective of management and HR, nothing is easy about implementing a reduction in force. However, managers and HR have a far easier time than do the employees who are being laid off. The initial impact is invariably stressful for both laid-off employees and those who remain.

Feelings of anger and betrayal are normal among employees who are laid off. Terminated employees face psychological stress and economic hardship. Personal routines are disrupted, as are relationships that may have existed for years. For all practical purposes, lives are turned inside out as individuals are thrown into a mode that some of them may never have experienced. Those who have experienced employment displacement will not look forward to repeating the experience.

For many individuals, the loss of a job is nearly as traumatic as a death in the family. The grieving process is proportional to the degree of loss. Employee assistance programs and other resources may be used to help ease the transition for both laid-off staff and stressed-out survivors. The overall impact of a reduction in force is eventually healed with the passage of time. This occurs more rapidly if a measure of employment stability returns to the organization.

▶ Related Dimensions of Termination

Unemployment Compensation

As noted earlier, an employee who is discharged for cause is technically not eligible for unemployment compensation. One who is dismissed for reasons related to performance or laid off for lack of work or for economic reasons is considered eligible for unemployment. However, regardless of the reasons behind any particular termination, any discharged employee is free to apply for unemployment. It costs only the time to complete an application. Many claims receive favorable determinations even though the organization considered them ineligible.

Consider an example. The organization, following its own procedures for progressive discipline, provides counseling sessions and warnings before discharging an individual for chronic tardiness. As long as policy is followed and applied in a consistent manner, the organization has every right to release such an employee for not meeting the expectation of being on the job when needed. This individual is technically not eligible for unemployment. This person applies for unemployment compensation and pleads hardship due to an inability to get to work on time. The stated reason may involve a supposedly regular ride that has been erratic, a constantly changing bus schedule, child care arrangements in a state of flux, or some other issue why the starting-time expectation has not been met. If the unemployment office determines that the discharged employee is eligible for benefits, the former employer will be notified. If the employer protests the determination and the employee chooses not to accept the employer's decision, a hearing is held. Discharged employees claiming hardship are frequently granted unemployment compensation benefits.

Human resources, acting on the organization's behalf, initially responds to every claim for unemployment compensation, making an initial determination as to which claims to contest and which to concede. Some HR departments have taken the authoritarian stance of automatically contesting every unemployment claim. This practice accomplishes little more than consuming time and energy while generating ill will. The HR assessment of each unemployment claim should involve an honest judgment of the merits and validity of the claim. Only those claims that appear invalid or questionable should be contested.

When a contested claim results in a hearing before an administrative law judge, the department manager and an HR representative usually attend the session. The former employee typically attends. The information provided by the attendees will be used to make the determination. An unemployment hearing can consume several hours when travel and waiting time are included. A conscientious HR manager will be mindful of the impact on managers and will contest only those claims that honestly appear to be unwarranted.

Employee Privacy

Any termination, regardless of the reasons behind it, should be accomplished in private and in a place where the interchange is neither visible nor audible to other employees. Terminations should be scheduled near the end of the workday so an individual who has just been let go can leave the premises without being forced to give an explanation or answer employee questions about what has happened.

Terminated employees should be allowed as much dignity as possible. Managers must weigh considerations of trust and caution. Many organizations have policies that require dismissed employees to be accompanied when they return to their workstations or offices. This precaution is taken to deter the possibility of damage to computer files or other property. Human resources personnel ordinarily have the responsibility to recover keys, employee identification cards, and other organizational property. Security generally has the responsibility to delete electronic access codes given to former employees.

Discharged employees should be escorted from the building. However, not all experts agree on this practice. Angry former employees may commit acts of vandalism or sabotage. In contrast, employees who were terminated and then escorted out have sued because of the humiliation experienced in the manner of departure. Juries are frequently sympathetic to allegations that defamation can result from actions as well as from words. Terminations occasionally require the presence of security personnel. A security officer's presence should be discreet, not especially visible but readily available.

Outplacement

When significant numbers of employees are being released during the same reduction, an organization often provides access to some form of outplacement service. Individual outplacement services may be extended as part of the severance arrangement made with a manager or professional employee. These are individualized services intended to assist the person in preparing a résumé, initiating a job search, and securing future employment. Group outplacement activities are often provided for rank-and-file employees. Direct contact with organizations known to be recruiting may be arranged. Any assistance toward new employment that can be provided will lessen the feelings of betrayal or abandonment that employees experience when they are laid off.

▶ Human Resources Follow-Up

For all terminations, HR representatives should discuss issues related to benefits with departing employees. An important topic is continuation of insurance coverage under the Consolidated Omnibus Budget Reconciliation Act (COBRA). Options should be discussed and employees should be shown how to apply for coverage.

Other options should be explained. Unemployment compensation benefits, if applicable, should be discussed. Human resources may request a signed release allowing them to give out reference information. Human resources will ordinarily explain how remaining vacation or sick time and applicable severance will be paid and who the departing employee should contact with questions.

▶ The Survivors of Reduction

Before, during, and immediately after a reduction in force, people who have been laid off receive a great deal of attention. Those who have been terminated receive so much attention that individuals who remain often feel forgotten. However, employees who remain must not only keep the organization running but also pick up the slack created by the loss of those who were dismissed. They often think of themselves as survivors rather than as regular employees.

Survivors commonly feel overworked, if not overwhelmed. This is most acute in the days immediately following the reduction when the shortfall created by the absence of some staff is most pronounced. Survivors experience guilt over having avoided the reduction while so many others lost their employment. They distrust management for terminating so many of their coworkers and wonder about the security of their own employment, fearing they may be next to depart. Survivors experience an overall decrease in morale, productivity, and employee loyalty. They feel less compelled to be at work on time or at all. This contributes to a general increase in absenteeism and tardiness. In some extreme instances, they may carry out acts of sabotage or violence or engage in other disruptive behavior.

Inevitably some survivors of a reduction react by looking for new employment. In this way, critically needed staff may be lost because of a feeling of insecurity in the post-layoff environment. Skilled technical and professional employees often feel more loyalty to their occupations than to the organization. Organizational loyalty has eroded with the reduction in force, and employees are ripe for offers of more secure employment. A job market favorable to highly skilled professionals can cause an organization to lose staff members they worked so hard to recruit or retain.

The attitude among the survivors of a reduction can be particularly grim if the organization had implemented a total quality management (TQM) or other motivational program during recent years. These programs, launched and pursued with much promotional activity and a strong emphasis on the value of employee participation, deliver a strong message: All employees are important, their contributions are essential for the organization's continued success, and they are needed. When layoffs follow, the message is changed and the organization is now perceived as saying that employees have become less important. When a significant reduction in force follows a motivational program, the cumulative effect is more demoralizing than if employees had never heard about the original program.

Following a significant layoff, top management must be openly supportive of those who remain and must be visibly active in efforts to help all survivors adjust to changes and return to normal operations. Reassurance about continuing employment without additional layoffs is helpful. However, it is useful only if it is true. A second round of layoffs made after a message of employment assurance is often catastrophic to the morale of remaining employees. Decreased morale is again followed by decreases in productivity. This cycle is vicious and highly detrimental to an organization.

Human resources and management at all levels can provide valuable support to the survivors of a reduction in force by stressing training and education as employees attempt to adjust to new or altered roles. Specifically, this is an appropriate time to provide training in time management and coping with change or managing stress. Any action that promotes a sense of business-as-usual or allays fear among workers has value. The overarching goal is to allay fear and change the focus of employees from survival and security to service and productivity.

During the recovery period following a reduction in force, managers must maintain close communication with their employees. Employees will have questions, many of which cannot be answered. Employees will be stressed out, worried, and demoralized. As employees, managers are subject to the same negative influences as their subordinates. However, as managers they must keep their employees upbeat and willing to produce in spite of what is occurring around them. This often requires great effort in the face of potential discouragement. It also requires support from executive management. The outlook, morale, and productivity of an entire group of people often hinge on the attitude of a single person: the department manager.

▶ Conclusion

Involuntary terminations include layoffs and firing. The former are usually triggered by economic considerations, while the latter are due to problems meeting organizational expectations or observing policies. Allowing a person to resign instead of being fired has great potential for creating future problems. Persons who are involuntarily terminated may be eligible for unemployment compensation benefits. Human resources provides essential services whenever an employee leaves an organization. Survivors of any reduction in force have special needs; ignoring these has the potential to cause losses in employee morale and productivity.

🔍 CASE STUDY: Resolution

The case of Joan von Willebrand demonstrates the importance of following policies and procedures faithfully and consistently applying all rules during an involuntary termination.

Joan should be discharged. However, unnecessary information will have to be collected and reviewed. Extra time and unnecessary aggravation will result from George's off-and-on, lax application of the tardiness policy. At present, enough information is available to document the fact that Joan was given an opportunity to correct her offending behavior but did not do so. All of the provisions in the organization's progressive disciplinary policy must be followed. George should be reprimanded for inconsistent application of his supervisory responsibilities. In all involuntary terminations, it is essential that an organization has clear, comprehensive policies and procedures and that these are applied consistently and in a strict, nondiscriminatory fashion.

SPOTLIGHT ON CUSTOMER SERVICE

Customer Service and Terminating Employees

At first glance, customer service and terminating employees are, in the language of geometry, nonintersecting sets. Some reflection may provide useful insights. Common reasons for terminating employees include consistently poor job performance, violation of organizational policies, and endangering the health or well-being of other employees.

A common denominator of these infractions is disregard toward others and ignoring their safety or personal needs. Stated simply, it is selfish behavior. Others can include people as well as organizations such as an employer.

It should not be surprising to learn that people who are terminated rarely provide customer service. They have difficulty leaving their own worlds that are defined by selfish behaviors and are unable to put others ahead of themselves.

While it may seem tempting to use nonparticipation in an organizational customer service program as an early predictor of future difficulties, such a leap would be foolish because it overlooks other explanations for not providing customer service. Lack of awareness of an organization-wide customer service program or a lack of training may be the reason. These are easily remedied. Only after ruling out all other reasons for nonparticipation should customer service inactivity be considered as a harbinger of future problems.

Modified from Advisory Board. (2013). Hospital mass layoffs on the rise. Retrieved from https://www.advisory.com/daily-briefing/2011/09/30/hospital-mass-layoffs-on-the-rise; Bureau of Labor Statistics. (2013). Workforce statistics. Retrieved from http://www.bls.gov/iag/tgs/iag622.htm; Serb, C. (1998). Is remaking the hospital making money? *Hospitals and Health Networks, 72*(14), 32–35.

Questions for Review and Discussion

1. What are the differences between dismissal and discharge?
2. In your opinion, should a general layoff be implemented at one time, or over a period of weeks or months? Why?
3. What steps would you advise a department supervisor to take before laying off employees? Why?
4. What are the principal advantages and disadvantages to an organization in implementing a voluntary early retirement program?
5. What is a constructive discharge? Provide an example of a constructive discharge.
6. Why should some form of seniority be used as a criterion in identifying employees for layoff?
7. Why is it necessary to pay particular attention to the employees that are retained following a reduction in force? What is the basis for concern, recognizing that these survivors still have their jobs?
8. When should employees who are laid off be expected to leave? Why? What are the advantages and disadvantages of leaving at the time that they are notified? What are the advantages and disadvantages of being allowed to work out a reasonable period of notice?
9. Why do mergers and other affiliations often lead to the consolidation of positions and reduction of the workforce?

10. Should a manager be able to use a reduction in workforce to rid the department of its less effective employees? Why or why not?
11. Once all employees have been designated for layoff, what should HR do before the layoff is implemented? Why?
12. What steps can an employer take to minimize the possibility of terminations being overturned by legal action? Why?
13. Assuming that a significant number of skilled employees are designated for layoff, how can an organization assist these workers following dismissal? Can an organization protect selected skilled workers in a layoff? Why or why not?
14. Why is it advisable that human resources provide individual meetings with each employee who is terminated in a workforce reduction?
15. Should an employee who is about to be discharged for cause be allowed to resign? Why or why not?

References

Advisory Board. (2013). Hospital mass layoffs on the rise. Retrieved from https://www.advisory.com/daily-briefing/2011/09/30/hospital-mass-layoffs-on-the-rise

Bureau of Labor Statistics. (2013). Workforce statistics. Retrieved from http://www.bls.gov/iag/tgs/iag622.htm

Serb, C. (1998). Is remaking the hospital making money? *Hospitals and Health Networks, 72*(14), 32–35.

Resources

Books

Fleischer, C. H. (2004). *The complete hiring and firing handbook: Every manager's guide to working with employees—Legally*. Naperville, IL: Sourcebooks.

MacKay, I. (2005). *35 checklists for human resource management*. London, UK: Ashgate.

McConnell, C. R. (2019). *The effective health care supervisor* (9th ed.). Burlington, MA: Jones & Bartlett Learning.

Niles, N. J. (2013). *Basic concepts of health care human resource management*. Burlington, MA: Jones & Bartlett Learning.

Riccucci, N. (2005). *Public personnel management: Current concerns, future challenges*. New York, NY: Longman.

Periodicals

Blackman, M. C., & Funder, D. C. (2002). Effective interview practices for accurately assessing counterproductive traits. *International Journal of Selection and Assessment, 10*, 109–116.

Caramela, S. (2016). How to fire and employee the right way. *Business News Daily*. Retrieved from https://www.businessnewsdaily.com/7963-how-to-fire-employee.html

Galle, W. R., & Koen, C. M. (2001). Reducing post-termination disputes: A national survey of contract clauses used in employment contracts. *Journal of Individual Employment Rights, 9*, 227–241.

Kappel, M. (2017). 5 Tips on how to fire an employee gracefully. *Forbes*. Retrieved from https://www.forbes.com/sites/mikekappel/2017/04/05/5-tips-on-how-to-fire-an-employee-gracefully/

Lansbury, R., & Baird, M. (2004). Broadening the horizons of HRM: Lessons for Australia from experience of the United States. *Asia Pacific Journal of Human Resources, 42*(2), 147–155.

Roberts, R., & Hirsch, P. (2005). Evolution and revolution in the twenty-first century: Rules for organizations and managing human resources. *Human Resources Management, 44*(2), 171–176.

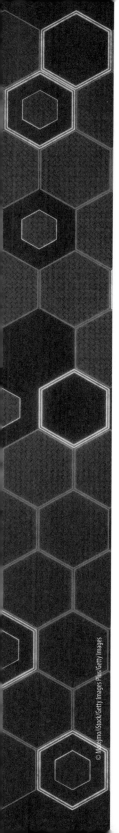

SECTION V

Special Situations

Under some conditions, human resources (HR) may be called upon to provide services to address problems or situations not universally encountered. In certain other instances, the organization may elect to employ outside HR experts for a brief period of time. Chapter 17 (Documentation) covers the creation and retention of documentation of all kinds, Chapter 18 (Ethics and Ethical Behavior) addresses ethics for managers and others at all organizational levels, Chapter 19 (The Impact and Effects of Social Media) examines the advantages and drawbacks of social media in the workplace, Chapter 20 (Relations with Labor Unions) discusses a department manager's essential role during union organizing and addresses the changes that must occur when a union represents all or a portion of an organization's employees, Chapter 21 (Special Support: Human Resources Arbitration and Human Resources Consultants) addresses the place of these two special services in HR functioning, and Chapter 22 (Maintaining an Effective Human Resources Department) looks at the ways in which managers can make better use of the HR services available to them.

CHAPTER 17

Documentation

CHAPTER OBJECTIVES

After studying this chapter, readers will be able to:

- Differentiate required formal documentation and informal documentation.
- Know the legal implications of employment documentation.
- Understand the role of human resources in maintaining and safeguarding personnel files.
- Recognize an individual manager's responsibilities relating to employment documentation.
- Know how and when to create, maintain, and purge anecdotal note files.
- Appreciate the importance of complete, properly executed, appropriately retained documentation.
- Understand the individual department manager's role in ensuring document security.

▶ Chapter Summary

Paper records are essential. The human resources (HR) department has an important responsibility concerning employee personnel files. Managers at all levels share in documentation responsibilities. Relevant documents include personnel files, job descriptions, employee handbooks, and policy and procedure manuals. Departmental files are important, but many are temporary. Human resources maintains long-term files. Paperwork is necessary and should be completed in a timely fashion. Without proper and complete records, an important matter, issue, or event can be considered never to have occurred. Also an important part of every manager's area of responsibility as well as an essential aspect of the organizational mission of human resources is document security and the all-important task of safeguarding employee privacy and confidentiality.

Although this chapter emphasizes several forms of documentation, patient medical records are excluded. Two general classes of employment documents are addressed. The first encompasses formal documentation resulting primarily from adherence to laws, regulatory requirements, or policies. This includes the majority of items found in an employee's personnel file. The second class is informal documentation. Such documentation is not required by law or regulation but is helpful in running the organization. Examples include internal reports, statistics, meeting minutes, anecdotal notes, and personal reminders.

🔍 CASE STUDY: "Relax, It's Only a Little Paperwork"

Middle manager Kathy Mason was talking to a colleague. "I have a great supervisor in charge of the evening shift housekeeping crew, Julius Newton. He's probably better at keeping a diverse crew happy and productive than any other first-line manager we've got. But he drives me absolutely nuts with his casual attitude toward documentation." Kathy slapped the file in front of her and added, "Honestly, Julius is a good person and a strict but fair supervisor. Still, a lot of my time and attention are needed to keep him out of trouble."

Employee relations manager Dan Howland asked, "How can he be so good if he causes you so much aggravation?"

"Because everything else is great. He has a tough group to run. They're all entry-level personnel, and he puts up with plenty of employee changes. Despite these challenges, he's successful. The problem is that I'm always getting stung by a lack of critical documentation when it's needed."

"Can you give me an example?"

"Sure," Kathy said, slapping a file folder on Dan's desk. "He submitted a discharge notice for an employee. The reason was excessive absenteeism. For months, he worked with the guy, counseling, offering assistance, you name it. Eventually, he gave up, decided he'd spent enough time and discharged the employee."

Kathy tapped the folder and continued, "Now I've got a legal complaint claiming unjust discharge. The guy says he never knew his absences were a problem until he got fired."

Dan said, "But he did really know? And where is the proof?"

"Right. Where we should have Julius's counseling notes and a record of three or four warnings under the progressive discipline policy, all we have is the dismissal–discharge notice. Julius *had* to provide the discharge notice to let the guy receive his final check and get him out the door."

Kathy went on. "This isn't the first time this sort of thing has occurred. And don't even mention performance evaluations. If Julius gets them done at all, they're months late and consist of a few generalizations dashed off in a hurry."

Dan asked, "Have you talked about this with Julius?"

"Yes. Multiple times."

"Then why not replace him?"

"I'd rather salvage him. When it comes to guiding people one on one, he's a natural manager. But he worries me. Whenever I bring up the subject of documentation, he brushes me off. Just yesterday I tried, and his reaction was, 'Relax, it's only a little paperwork.' I'm afraid we will be really stuck if anything involving him goes to court and we find the personnel files practically empty."

Dan nodded. "Agreed. You know the attitude of the courts and the advocacy agencies. Their approach is that if it's not on paper, it never happened."

What advice would you offer to Kathy Mason? If you were in her position, what actions would you undertake or recommend for supervisor Julius? What options does Kathy Mason have regarding required employee documentation?

▶ Paper Remains Important

Although computers and electronic records have become increasingly important in recent decades, paper has not been totally replaced. More to the point, paper still dominates in many respects. It is required in many legal settings. Computer output is often printed and retained in paper files.

Many documents are created for simple record-keeping reasons. Indexes and other records ensure that particular documents are available for reference or other ordinary business purposes when needed. In recent decades, however, an increasing amount of documentation has been created and maintained largely as protection against legal challenges.

Documentation can be troublesome for a department manager in two ways. The first is when it is not available and appears never to have existed. The other is when documents do exist but are weak, inaccurate, or incomplete.

▶ Legal Implications of Employment Documentation

The Legal Importance of Paper

Every piece of paper ever generated concerning an employee is a potential key in resolving a legal complaint involving an organization or a manager. Evidence of discrimination or its absence is often inferred from the contents of documentation relating to employees. The most common kind of discrimination charge involves disparate treatment. These are allegations claiming violations of the Civil Rights Act and other pertinent employment laws. This legislation requires that all individuals be treated equally concerning terms and conditions of employment. Another common basis for a charge of discrimination involves allegations of disparate impact. These result from job requirements imposed or actions taken by an employer that have a discriminatory effect on members of a protected group. When either type of charge is investigated, existing documentation concerning all affected employees may be requested.

Employment documentation is always important when responding to charges of discrimination. If requested documentation cannot be produced, the worst is often assumed.

Documents related to employment in any way can be requested in a legal action. Under a legal order known as a *notice to produce,* an organization can be required to produce, for copying and inspection, any documents that may be possibly or even remotely related to the charge. A notice to produce can ask for a considerable variety of material, including the personnel files of persons involved in an action. This can be extensive and can encompass many personnel files. For example, in an action involving three employees alleging a history of discriminatory behavior that followed them from their former departments to their present situation, the personnel files of all employees in all involved departments were requested. Overall, the complete personnel files of more than 100 people were requested, filling six or seven document boxes.

An organization's personnel policy and procedure manual, including all policies applicable to the complaining employees' employment, may be requested. While this may seem straightforward, changes and revisions to a document can complicate the request. Two comments are in order. First, every page of every document should have a unique page number and an identifying title. All documents should be identified with the date they become effective or the date when they will expire if of a limited lifetime. Second, HR should retain complete copies of all versions or revisions of all organizational documents that affect employees. These provide a document trail for future use. Prudent organizations retain copies of additional documents, including work rules, job postings, and employment advertisements. No information that cannot legally be used as the basis for a personnel decision should ever enter an employee's personnel file and should never be retained in a manager's anecdotal or personal files.

Records Retention

Some records are retained on the basis of common sense; there may be legitimate needs to retrieve the information they contain at some time in the future. Other records are retained because of external or legal requirements. All federal laws that address aspects of employment include requirements for record retention. In most organizations, retaining the majority of records related to employment is a continuing responsibility of HR; however, records of a financial nature are usually the responsibility of the organization's finance division.

Regulatory agencies that administer employment legislation specify the minimum length of time pertinent records must be retained. The lengths of retention time differ. For example, under the Fair Labor Standards Act, payroll records and supporting information such as time cards and time sheets must be retained for 3 years. Other related information, such as job evaluations, merit system descriptions and records, and payroll deduction records, must be kept for at least 2 years.

Under the Age Discrimination in Employment Act, all employment-related records must be retained for no less than a single year. This is consistent with the provision that a charge of age discrimination must be filed within 1 year after the alleged act occurred. The Occupational Safety and Health Act requires that all records related to employee injuries or illnesses be retained for 5 years. The Civil Rights Act requires that all records of personnel transactions be retained for at least 6 months unless charges are filed. In that case, the records must be retained until the final disposition of all charges.

The Joint Commission (TJC) requires retention of a number of types of documents so they can be reviewed during periodic accreditation surveys. The affected papers include all documents demonstrating compliance with federal laws, all licenses held by the organization and its individual employees, records related to employee training, detailed records of safety practices, copies of organizational policies and procedures, job descriptions, and employee performance appraisals. (TJC is a voluntary organization, not a government agency.)

In its periodic surveys, the health department of the state in which an organization is located may elect to review much of the same documentation. States having right-to-know laws concerning toxic substances are always interested in related records.

Hazardous materials and toxic substances present some of the most rigid record retention requirements. Under the rules of the Occupational Safety and Health Administration, records of personal or environmental monitoring of exposure to hazardous materials must be retained for 30 years. The same requirements apply to records retained when complying with the Toxic Substances Control Act. In New York State, records of exposure associated with the New York State Right-to-Know Law must be kept for 40 years.

The threshold for retaining most employment documentation is 6 years. This is the statutory limit for filing most employment-related charges arising from violations of the Civil Rights Act.

Because there is such a broad range of necessary retention periods for various personnel-related documents, many organizations simply assume that all personnel files should be permanently retained. Employees come and go and in the process generate files that eventually become inactive. Employees who remain for many years often generate thick files over the course of their employment. The net result is that HR has a considerable records retention challenge.

Personnel files of former employees must be accessed when responding to reference requests and other legitimate external requests for information. Occasionally, former employees return, requiring the retrieval of stored records. For these reasons, files of recent former employees must remain accessible. Because it is generally true that older files are less likely to be needed, many HR departments have implemented systems for document storage and retrieval. Old files are often stored on microfilm. Newer systems save documents in electronic form; paper files are scanned and then stored as electronic images. While this approach saves space, it requires that records be periodically re-saved on different media to maintain accessibility as equipment and processes change.

▶ Human Resources and Personnel Files

The responsibility for employee documentation resides primarily in the HR department. This department must ensure that all required documents in each personnel file are in fact there and complete. A department manager's role in supporting personnel files consists primarily of ensuring that departmental inputs to each personnel file get to HR properly completed and in a timely fashion. Foremost among the documents coming from a department manager are performance appraisals and disciplinary actions. Other information provided includes routine employee information such as changes of address or other contact information for employees.

A department manager may expect to hear from HR when documentation is not forthcoming. Performance appraisals and disciplinary actions are most likely to require additional input or revision. Depending on organizational policy, licensure information may be an HR retention responsibility. Department managers may have the responsibility to ensure that caregivers renew their licenses in a timely fashion and submit copies for their personnel files. Organizations occasionally maintain a separate central license repository.

Regarding disciplinary actions, organizational personnel policies usually include guidelines governing disciplinary actions. Written warnings in employee files are often allowed to expire after a period of time if subsequent related infractions do not occur. To comply with such a policy, HR must monitor written warnings and invalidate them as needed. Human resources staff may not be required to review all personnel files to remove expired warnings. However, when expired warnings are encountered, they should be removed and placed in a separate file.

EXHIBIT 17-1 Guidelines for Confidentiality of Employee Information

- Employees must know of the existence of all systems that retain personal information; no such systems should be kept secret from employees.
- A procedure must be established for individuals to determine what information exists about them and how it is to be used.
- Personal information obtained for one purpose cannot be used for another purpose without the consent of the individual to whom the information pertains.
- A process must allow individuals to correct or amend records of personal information pertaining to them.
- Any organization that creates, maintains, and uses or disseminates identifiable personal information must ensure that the information is reliable for the intended use and must take steps to prevent misuse of the information.

The objective of a warning is correction of behavior. The point of invalidating and removing older warnings is to prevent an infraction from permanently harming an employee. Documents that are removed should not be destroyed in case they are needed in future legal actions. Documents removed from employee files should be re-filed in a separate, central location.

The HR department must control access to personnel files. Internal access to personnel files is ordinarily limited to designated HR staff who must have access to files to complete their work. An employee's immediate supervisor and the department manager often have limited access to employee files. An organization's legal counsel has access to pertinent files as required when addressing specific legal matters. Certain managers may have limited access to specific employee files when considering those employees for promotion or transfer. All employees have the right to review their own personnel files, although this is permitted only under HR supervision, and removing any documents is prohibited.

Access to personnel files by interests external to the organization is strictly limited. Such requests are typically limited to furnishing copies of documents only upon receipt of a written release signed by the affected employees giving permission to release specific information. Documents specifically requested via subpoena or other court order must be furnished as requested without employee permission. **EXHIBIT 17-1** contains guidelines related to the confidentiality of employee records. These guidelines are based on principles developed by a governmental task force.

▶ The Department Manager's Responsibilities

Job Descriptions

Job descriptions have several uses in an organization. They provide day-to-day guidance for workers. Supervisors use them when evaluating their subordinates' performance. Human resources uses them when recruiting. However, they are occasionally nonexistent and if existing are ignored until needed. Thus, organizations have a vested interest in creating accurate job descriptions and maintaining them in an up-to-date fashion.

Department managers and HR staff are often required to work together to create or update job descriptions. Ordinarily, the content comes from managers, while HR provides the format, arrangement, and items that must be contained in every position description in the organization. Employees should participate in revisions of existing job descriptions. Workers should be involved in an annual review and update of their own job descriptions.

Different versions of job descriptions contain different information. This can create confusion. An easy way to avoid problems is to date each job description when it is modified in any way. A message to destroy all previous versions should accompany the distribution of revised job description. Human resources must issue all revisions and retain a copy of every description in a master job description file. This reduces confusion and provides a resource for determining that the most current document is being used.

Employee Handbook

Every organization should have an employee handbook, and all department managers and supervisors should be familiar with its contents. Two reasons support this suggestion. The first is for personal knowledge and use, because managers are employees as well as supervisors. The second is to answer employee questions. Managers must be able to handle general questions about the handbook's contents and must know how and where to secure clarification of any of the book's contents.

Managers must ensure that all employees in their departments have copies of the handbook or have ready access to the current handbook. Employee handbooks are not revised as often as policy and procedure manuals, but new editions are periodically issued. When the handbook is reissued and circulated or made available to all employees, managers must ensure not only that all employees receive one but also that they sign and submit the receipt, acknowledging that they have received and read the handbook. Handbooks include work rules as well as general information about the organization. They often include information concerning key personnel policies.

A signed handbook receipt is retained as evidence that an employee has received and reviewed the handbook. The receipt is kept in the employee's personnel file. This can be extremely important to an organization should an employee attempt to deny knowledge of a particular rule or policy as an excuse for a rule violation or similar problem. Also, many handbooks carry a prominently displayed disclaimer to the effect that the employee handbook is not a contract of employment. However, on numerous occasions, at times even when a disclaimer has been present, courts have ruled a handbook to indeed be a contract of employment. Therefore, employee handbooks must be carefully written to avoid conveying the impression of promises or guarantees. For example, it is best to refer to one who has completed and passed a probationary period as a "regular" employee, because past references to one who has passed probation as a "permanent" employee have been interpreted as rendering the employee immune from termination.

Policy and Procedure Manuals

An organization's personnel policy and procedure manual is ordinarily issued and maintained by HR. Most policies are prepared by HR directly or by using input from other organizational units and distributed by HR. In most organizations, every department has a copy of the manual. Larger departments may have multiple copies.

Department managers or the person in each department delegated to maintain a policy and procedure manual should file updates as soon as they are received without allowing them to accumulate. Rapid references to specific policy information are often required. If a manual has not been kept up to date, then it is not possible to know whether or not a given policy is current. A manual that has been allowed to go out of date has the potential to be damaging if a wrong reference is taken as applicable.

A departmental policy and procedure manual is not the exclusive property of the manager and should not be kept in the manager's office. A policy and procedure manual must be stored where employees can access it and make reference to it as needed, without having to ask for it. When the manual is retained in an office and cannot be readily accessed, employees are left feeling that it is being kept from them and that it contains information management does not want them to see. Because personnel policies exist for every worker, all employees must have equal access to the manual.

Releasing Employee Information

Sometimes department managers directly receive requests for information about particular employees, requests from outsiders who have—usually deliberately—bypassed human resources or other channels such as administration. Requests for employee information from outside of the organization should not be honored. The people requesting the information should be referred to the appropriate person or department, usually HR. The HR policy governing external release of employee information should be the entire organization's policy on this matter—no information will be released to an outside party without signed consent from the affected employee or a subpoena or other court order.

Requests from within the organization should be honored on a need-to-know basis. When responding, opinions and subjective assessments must never be offered. Organizations should provide only objective information that can be supported or verified by an official record such as a performance appraisal, attendance record, or other documentation.

▶ The Department Manager's Employee Files

A department manager will have occasion to create and retain records, both formal and informal, concerning each employee. Employee records maintained in a department are not considered permanent. Only one permanent record of employment exists—the personnel file maintained by HR.

The files maintained by a department manager should not be approached or maintained in a careless or casual manner. Employee files maintained by a manager are not the manager's personal property. Like all other files, employee information created by the department manager and kept in the department must be appropriately maintained, although the manager may feel that notes personally created and kept in a private file, say in the manager's desk, can in some circumstances be made public.

Regardless of the amount of information contained, the manager should maintain a separate file folder for each employee of the department. Doing so can potentially avoid charges of favoritism or discrimination by denying any individual employee reason to claim that notes were kept on just a select few, that some employees were watched or "written up" while others were allowed to go their own way.

A manager's file for each employee ordinarily includes copies of the most recent one or two performance appraisals; permanent records of previous performance appraisals are retained in HR files. Notes regarding both positive and negative items to include in the next performance appraisal are useful. Copies of warnings, reprimands, or other disciplinary information concerning an employee should be retained. Depending on the disciplinary system guidelines, records of oral warnings may remain with the manager instead of going to HR. These should be forwarded to HR along with subsequent written warnings for similar offenses that may occur.

First-line managers are busy people, and they often tend to skimp on informal documentation. Negative comments seem to get written up more often than positive comments; these are supposedly "important" in that they may lead eventually to larger problems or counseling or disciplinary action. Too often, positive comments do not get entered for employees who do something commendable. However, positives can be just as important as negatives—even more important to the employees themselves—to capture in a manager's anecdotal note file.

Accurate records of performance improvement activities undertaken, including all reminders for follow-up and notes indicating that problems are being resolved, should be retained. Copies of complaints or compliments received should be discussed with the employees at the time these are received. Notes of counseling sessions should be kept. Any other information relevant to an individual's employment or performance in the department that is not customarily included in the formal documentation required of a personnel file should be retained. Everything that managers write for employee files must be expressed in accurate, objective language without name-calling or insupportable opinions. Avoid writing anything that can be personally or organizationally embarrassing.

The manager's employee files should be periodically reviewed and purged. Notes that have been incorporated into formal appraisals are no longer needed. Old counseling notes can be discarded if the problems prompting the intervention have not recurred. With a single exception, personal files related to employees can be purged at any time. The exception: Once a legal action is started and notice is served on an organization, files in any way pertaining to the legal issue cannot be destroyed; to do so is a violation of federal law. Restating this in a different way, routinely discarding files is permissible as long as no legal action is being threatened or under way. Should a discarded document be requested at some time in the future, it cannot be produced if it does not exist.

Always be cautious in choosing what to say about an employee in an anecdotal note file. Some managers have been careless with their comments, believing that what they express in an anecdotal note is theirs and theirs alone. One might reason, *it's my note, kept in my desk drawer, and no one else sees it; it's my personal property.* Not strictly true; when a legal issue arises, all a complaining employee needs to do is convey the belief that this manager keeps a file of notes about employees, and suddenly the manager's "personal" files are subject to a notice to produce. Anything in the file that includes name-calling or unsubstantiated negative commentary suddenly becomes visible to all. Avoid this sort of potential trouble by following one simple rule: never make a note about an employee that you would find embarrassing to you if it suddenly appeared in the daily news. In brief, write nothing that cannot be shown to be objective and factual.

302 **Chapter 17** Documentation

▶ Do the Paperwork

Attending to necessary documentation is a task that is frequently put aside until spare time becomes available. Typically, documentation that is left until time becomes available is not completed thoroughly, if it is completed at all. Documentation should be completed on a timely basis. Even in the immediate presence of pressures on a manager, it is best to address documentation right away. This is the time that facts and data are freshest and when the most accurate recording of information is possible.

Many problems occur after the fact because of documentation that is missing or incomplete. Instances of incomplete documentation are common in every organization. These include forms that are not completely filled out, papers that are not signed, and information that is illegible or incomplete. An ongoing and recurring problem exists with documents that lack dates. Always enter a date on any paper before adding any words; this simple act can prevent many problems associated with documentation.

▶ Document Security

On the Way to the Shredder

At a hospital employing more than 3000 people a listing referred to as the "employee alpha" was generated along with each biweekly payroll. This listing, including all employees and their home addresses and telephone numbers, was produced in a single reference copy to be maintained by human resources. Procedure called for each outdated listing to be given to a building services supervisor who would assure it was shredded.

After following the procedure for a few months, the building services manager independently decided shredding was inefficient because it took too long, so this manager decided to incinerate the outdated employee listing. After personally overseeing the incineration of several reports, the building services manager left this task to a trusted senior employee. Eventually, however, the assigned employee drifted away from immediate destruction and instead began simply dumping it into the "burn-bin" to await destruction.

Some months later, the hospital came under union organizing pressure and an alert building services worker, sympathetic to the union, rescued the most recently discarded alpha from incineration and gave it to the union organizers. In this one simple move, the union acquired a complete listing of the hospital's employees with addresses, telephone numbers, job titles, and department designations. In this one instance in which the confidential nature of certain material was ignored, a union was able to secure information it could have otherwise acquired only through the expenditure of large amounts of time and effort.

Trash-Can Raiding

In another instance involving a union, the leaders of an employer team engaged in stressful contract negotiations were frustrated with what seemed to be the union team's ability to second-guess the employer's strategy at every turn. Each day when the management team sat down with the union to negotiate, it seemed the union had accurately predicted management's strategy. The answer was in the trash; a night-shift custodian was simply taking the trash from management's meeting room and turning it over to a union representative. The trash, containing rough notes and jottings and occasional first drafts, gave the union solid information about management's intentions.

We can cite numerous instances in which managers, reviewing personnel files to learn about potential transfer candidates, have decided against particular candidates because of information they should not have had access to: short-term disability records, Workers' Compensation records, and other medically related correspondence. Some managers have decided against particular transfer candidates because this legally forbidden information caused them to bypass employees who might present performance or attendance problems.

No Longer Just Paper

Today, it is essential to fully recognize the importance of ensuring the security of documentation in the healthcare organization. However, in addressing document security, one is inevitably reminded of the constant clash of opposing rights and needs—on one hand the right to privacy of any individual and on the other hand the often-cited "need to know" or business need for certain information.

The security of documentation is inextricably linked to the security of information created and maintained electronically. However, this section focuses primarily on the security of documents created and maintained in paper form. Technology has created some significant information security concerns that lie well beyond the scope of this brief treatment. When business systems were largely paper based and the few existing automated systems were limited to single applications, all files were essentially separated from each other according to use. With modern systems integration, however, large data repositories became the rule, and increasingly large databases created greater security issues. Electronics aside, however, the focus herein remains on the security of paper documentation.

All functioning organizations, whether for-profit or not-for-profit, have particular concerns for the security of information. For some organizations, proprietary information is one of their most valuable assets. Document security in health care may not be nearly as formal as, for example, that in government, but it will always be apparent that some documents are more sensitive than others and thus require closer safeguards.

In health care in general, and within the realm of concern of the department manager in particular, the primary concerns are privacy and confidentiality, which are overlapping if not essentially congruent concerns, as they apply to patients and employees.

Privacy and Confidentiality

For several recent decades, as the amount of information collected about individuals has increased, there has been growing concern about encroachments on individual privacy. To a considerable extent, this concern has been reflected in an increasing number of guidelines for the collection and use of personal information.

Some years ago (1973, to be precise), the Department of Health, Education, and Welfare (the forerunner of the Department of Health and Human Services [DHHA]) set forth some principles of fair information handling with regard for an individual's right to privacy. These principles called for the following:

- Individuals must be able to learn what information is kept about them and how it is used.
- Information gathered for one stated purpose must not be used for other purposes without the consent of the individuals concerned.
- Individuals must be able to correct or amend records of information about them.
- There can be no system of personal data the existence of which is kept secret.
- The organization is responsible to assure the reliability of the data for its intended use and must take reasonable precautions to prevent misuse of the data.

The Privacy Act of 1974 outlined privacy principles similar to those summarized previously. These principles legally applied only to government entities, but they served as the foundation for state privacy laws affecting the private sector. The Privacy Protection Study Commission Report (1977) recommended voluntary private-sector compliance with guidelines similar to those of the Privacy Act. A number of additional laws, among them the Fair Credit Reporting Act, the Freedom of Information Act, the Employee Polygraph Protection Act, the Immigration Reform and Control Act, the Occupational Safety and Health Act, and various individual state laws all included additional protections for the privacy of the individual.

The work organization's role in the protection of personal information has broadened to encompass all aspects of the collection, possession, use, and disposition of information concerning employees and former employees. No longer is it sufficient to ensure that personal information is simply safeguarded from theft or destruction; it is now necessary to justify the reasons for its collection and to ensure that it is used for only the purposes stated and that it will not be accessed by anyone who does not have a legitimate business need for the information.

Is "Big Brother" Watching?

Continuing advances in information technology have spurred many improvements in methods of collecting and storing and accessing information. Along the way, there have been many blatant abuses of personal information; consider the dramatic increases of recent years in the kinds of crime involving identity theft. Such problems have contributed to uneasiness in the population about the availability of personal information and its likely uses. With the feeling of many that "Big Brother is watching," it is reasonable to conclude that:

- The majority of people believe most organizations that collect personal information request more than is necessary;
- A growing number of people are worried about how the government uses personal information collected about them;
- There is concern about the increasing difficulty of keeping aspects of people's lives private from the government;
- Many people worry whether business organizations properly use the personal information collected about them.

Nothing has occurred to alleviate any of the foregoing worries and beliefs. Rather, these have intensified considerably with recent revelations concerning the amount of information gathering that goes on: spying on email transmissions, capturing cell phone records, looking into financial records and transactions, and gathering citizens' personal information from various sources. Regardless of the possible validity of some of the reasons for this deepening intrusion into the lives of people, it is increasingly clear that personal privacy is a dwindling reality.

Addressing Employee Concerns

What can and is being done in many organizations to alleviate employee concerns about the use of personal information is summarized in these few brief guidelines:

- Always explain *why* the requested information is being collected and what is to be done with it, limiting its utilization to specific business uses.
- Inform employees of what kinds of information are retained concerning them.
- Permit employees to review what is retained concerning them and allow them to amend or correct it as necessary.
- Retain particularly sensitive personal information, such as records bearing on health or credit matters, separate from other records of employment.
- Limit the use of employee information to absolute necessities. For example, the organization's benefits administrator will have a legitimate need for information about an employee's family status, but line management has no such need.
- Release employee information to outsiders only upon written employee permission or receipt of a subpoena or other legal order.

Kinds of Documentation

There are two general categories of documentation to address: *formal documentation* and *informal documentation*.

Formal documentation consists of anything that becomes part of some official record or file. Most of what eventually comes to rest in an individual's personnel file is formal documentation, as is most of what comprises a patient chart or other medical record. Formal documentation may be created and maintained to serve a business need or to serve a patient care need. Formal documentation also includes letters, memos, reports, meeting minutes, schedules, and numerous other documents generated in the course of business. Formal documentation also includes any documentation retained because doing so is required by law, regulation, or conditions of accreditation.

Informal documentation is essentially any documentation not falling within the formal definition. Generally, informal documentation can be expected to consist of anecdotal notes, rough meeting notes, notes written to one's self, jottings on a desk calendar, rough drafts of letters and memos, and such. With informal documentation, there is often little thought given to matters of security, most likely because so much informal documentation is temporary in nature.

Within formal documentation, along with and often inclusive of the many forms utilized in delivering health care, the organization is concerned largely with patient medical records and employee personnel files. Within informal documentation, the primary concern of the healthcare department manager is that for anecdotal notes and their creation and retention and use as addressed in an earlier section.

Patient Documentation and the Manager

The responsibilities of the healthcare department manager for the security of patient information can be summarized in the following guidelines:

- Leave no documentation pertinent to a patient in a place where it can be seen or read by parties who do not have a legitimate need for the information. For the most part, those who have the need to know will be those participating in the care of the patient.
- Strictly limit access to patient information to caregivers addressing the needs of specific patients.
- Observe all existing filing and document security practices, taking every reasonable step to ensure patient records are not left unattended or unsecured.
- Protect appointment books and schedules and such so the names of patients cannot be read by other patients, visitors, and staff not involved in the patients' care.

Personnel Files

In creating, maintaining, and using personnel files, the organization is constantly in a position of having to balance various perceived needs for information against every employee's right to privacy. The human resources department is the custodian of personnel files and usually the primary user of these files. In addition, however, individual department managers are frequently legitimate users of employee personnel files, but it falls to human resources to provide security against unauthorized access, disclosure, modification, or destruction of employee records.

Access to employee personnel files should be limited to persons who have a legitimate need for the information contained therein. Some persons within human resources will have to access personnel information for different purposes, various department managers may at times need to examine personnel records in their evaluation of potential transfer candidates, and on occasion the organization's legal counsel may need personnel file information. Concerning employees' personnel files:

- Access should be controlled. Although HR is responsible for maintaining the files, not all HR staff should be permitted file access. Rather, only those who need file information for specific purposes should be permitted access. A department manager considering an employee as a transfer candidate may be entitled to access certain work-related information in the file.
- Although the information it contains is undeniably the employee's, the physical personnel file itself is the property of the organization. The responsibility for safeguarding the file belongs to human resources.
- An employee should be entitled to review the contents of his or her personnel file if desired. The employee should be permitted to amend or otherwise clarify anything in the file but should not be allowed to remove anything from the file. (Employee review of the personnel file is ordinarily accomplished only under HR supervision.)

- Policy and practice should require that no information from a personnel file will be supplied to anyone outside of the organization without the employee's signed permission to do so. The only reasonable exception to this rule occurs when the organization must comply with a subpoena or other proper legal order.
- Certain kinds of information about employees should be maintained separate from personnel files. Any documentation having to do with an employee's physical or mental well-being should be maintained separately (usually by the employee health office). Records of periods of disability, Workers' Compensation, and the like are to be considered medical records and thus held to a stricter standard of security.

Nothing, Too Little, or Too Much

Only marginally related to document security but having a direct bearing on the usefulness of information retained and retrieved are the problems presented by documents that are incomplete, missing altogether, or just plain unnecessary. In addition to having numerous practical implications, incomplete, missing, or unnecessary documents often have legal significance as well. Documents, often by the hundreds and even thousands, are central to almost every legal action involving charges of discrimination or disparate treatment in the workplace.

At some point when plaintiff's counsel is preparing a case, usually early in the process, the organization may be served with a legal demand known as a *notice to produce*. This order will name certain documentation either known to exist or thought "on information and belief" to exist and will demand that it be produced for "examination and copying." Legally, the organization has little choice; if the demanded documents exist, they must be produced.

When Documents Are Missing

A document that does not exist cannot be produced. It may occur to some who have received a notice to produce that this might be a good time to clean out certain files, especially those that might contain something questionable. However, there is a significant problem with the timing of such a file purge: once a notice to produce has been received, it becomes a violation of federal law to destroy any requested documentation.

In some legal actions, an organization can be harmed by the contents of its own documentation. However, it is still usually preferable to have the documentation and be able to produce it. When documentation is missing, it is usually assumed that the organization has either destroyed or otherwise failed to turn over material damaging to the organization's position. When the documents are missing the worst is assumed.

When Documents Are Incomplete

A problem usually encountered more often than missing documentation is incomplete documentation. A form that gets filled out and finds its way into some file can be lacking almost any kind of information, but the two greatest categories of incomplete information are dates and signatures. As well as causing occasional confusion and delay in the normal course of business, missing dates and missing signatures can both be especially troublesome in legal proceedings. Often of critical importance is *when* some particular event occurred or *who* was involved. In many legal proceedings, it is essential to establish a clear chronology of events and a clear record of who was or was not involved, so dates and signatures are essential to the completeness of documentation.

Unnecessary Documentation

In many work organizations, unnecessary documentation exists in large amounts. And often a legal notice to produce will result in an in-depth "fishing expedition" for anything that might even remotely relate to a particular complaint. If there is no organizational requirement to retain, for example, material such as outdated job code listings, revised job descriptions, outdated procedure manuals, or in general anything not needed for current purposes or "aged out" beyond legal retention requirements, get rid of it. Unnecessary documentation takes up valuable space, its accumulation often causes difficulty in locating stored documents that *are* necessary, and it can conceivably cause needless work and expense if called upon via a notice to produce.

The Manager and Anecdotal Notes

The issue of anecdotal notes and the department manager's "personal" files was addressed in an earlier section. It is likely that your informal notes will never be accessed by anyone other than yourself, but there is no absolute guarantee that your personal notes will never be made public. No manager's anecdotal note files or employee files are as private as one might think upon originating them.

A manager's personal files surely have their uses. One important purpose of such files is to accumulate information relevant to coming performance evaluations. Another is to keep track of informal counseling and discussions having to do with possible disciplinary issues. However, in creating and utilizing anecdotal note files or files on each employee:

■ Avoid duplicating the official personnel file. It is fine to keep copies of recent evaluations or other pertinent information in an employee file, but clean these out on a regular basis.

■ Remember that such files can sometimes become public, so keep the material in them as factual and objective as possible, free from name-calling and subjective judgments.

■ Periodically purge these files, getting rid of anything that has been folded into an evaluation or other record and in general disposing of informal notes that have outlived their usefulness.

■ Never create a file note, even the simplest, briefest of informal notes, without dating the page and either signing or initialing it. Documentation that does not indicate who created it and when it was created is of greatly diminished usefulness.

Document Security Considerations

In addition to exercising responsibility for document security within one's own area of responsibility, each department manager should also act to safeguard documentation on an organization-wide basis. As an individual department manager:

- Do not misuse accidently acquired information you know you should not be seeing.
- Report apparent lapses or laxities in document security you observe.
- Ensure that documents used in your department are not left out in the open during breaks, lunch times, meetings, and such. This may also include ensuring your offices themselves are secured when not in use and sensitive documents are always put away when unattended.
- Ensure that sensitive documentation is stored reasonably protected from fire and water and theft.
- Periodically, survey disposal practices to ensure that confidential material cannot be accessed.
- Pay attention to the disposition of the unused parts of some multipart forms, ensuring that extras are properly disposed of and not allowed to accumulate (and suggest redesign of those forms for which all parts are no longer necessary).
- Limit the photocopying of sensitive material to as few individuals as practical.
- If periodically committing some records to microfilm, ensure that the originals, once filmed, are either committed to secure storage or destroyed as appropriate.
- Within the department, have a procedure for accessing sensitive documents and for loaning them out to authorized individuals such that some responsible individual always knows where every document is at any given time.

▶ Conclusion

The importance of complete and accurate documentation cannot be exaggerated or overstated. Records should always be completed in a timely manner and must be transmitted or retained according to applicable rules. Electronic storage formats have eased the burden of retaining large volumes of paper. Although not the most popular task of a manager, record keeping is an absolute organizational necessity.

🔎 *CASE STUDY: Resolution*

Returning to the initial case situation, a reasonable question is Julius Newton's overall use to his employer. Is he an asset to his employer when he neglects a significant part of the job? By ignoring a component of his job description, he is technically guilty of insubordination and of potentially placing the organization in legal jeopardy. Julius must be made to appreciate the importance of employee documentation. Although he deserves praise for his successful one-on-one supervisory style, he must be reprimanded for neglecting to complete and file documents. Any lawsuit has the potential to harm his employer. His reprimand should be written, and it should specify what he is to do and when his expected compliance will be reviewed. In any event, the warning or reprimand must be noted in writing and included in his personnel file. There is no such thing as "only a little paperwork."

SPOTLIGHT ON CUSTOMER SERVICE

Customer Service and Documentation

Documentation is essential in the contemporary world. Words on paper or pictures on a page provide proof that an event occurred. Not only is documentation expected, it is essential in situations involving components of the legal system. When disciplining employees, managers are advised to document the process as required by the organization's personnel policies. Most experts agree that unless actions are documented, they are presumed not to have occurred.

Providing good customer service requires documentation only infrequently. A kind word, going out of one's way to assist a customer, or simply smiling requires only a conscious commitment to the concept. In an organization that promotes customer service, these actions often become automatic for employees. Rest assured that acts of kindness or assistance are rarely overlooked or become automatic for customers. Good customer service is always appreciated.

Questions for Review and Discussion

1. Describe several implications of the statement, "If it isn't in the personnel file, it never happened or does not exist."
2. Why have many organizations adopted the practice of permanently retaining the personnel files of past employees? What events have led to the creation of such a policy?
3. Why should an organization retain all documentation that is required by law but periodically clean out and dispose of unneeded records?
4. Under what circumstances are employees permitted to add items to their personnel files? Under what circumstances are employees permitted to remove items?
5. What problems most frequently occur when organizations create and retain working documents? How can these be addressed?
6. Why should a department manager make an organizational personnel policy and procedure manual readily available to employees?
7. How do you handle a written request for reference information concerning a past employee that is addressed to you personally and includes the former employee's written permission to release information? Why?
8. Why should a manager always remain objective, factual, and nonjudgmental in private anecdotal notes concerning employees when no other persons are intended to see them?
9. Why should a manager's anecdotal note files be periodically purged of all but currently essential information?
10. How and why can some documentation be more damaging to an organization in a legal matter by being missing and unattainable rather than readily available?

Resources
Books

Atkinson, F., & Fathers, D. (2005). *Training workshop for supervisors: Building the essential skills*. London, England: Ashgate.

Bruce, A. (2005). *Perfect phrases for documenting employee performance problems: Hundreds of ready-to-use phrases for addressing all performance issues*. New York, NY: McGraw-Hill.

Bucknall, H. (2005). *Magic numbers for human resource management*. New York, NY: John Wiley.

McConnell, C. R. (2011). *The health care manager's legal guide*. Burlington, MA: Jones & Bartlett Learning.

McConnell, J. H. (2004). *How to develop essential HR policies and procedures*. Chicago, IL: American Management Association.

Periodicals

Grandey, A. A. (2003). When "the show must go on": Surface acting and deep acting as determinants of emotional exhaustion and peer-rated service delivery. *Academy of Management Journal, 46,* 86–96.

Heathfield, S. M. (2018). The importance of documentation in human resources. *The Balance Careers*. Retrieved from https://www.thebalancecareers.com/documentation-1918096

Nakhinikian, E. (2005). Breaking the turnover cycle. *Health Progress, 86*(6), 21–24.

Robie, C., Zickar, M. J., & Schmit, M. J. (2001). Measurement equivalence between applicant and incumbent groups: An IRT analysis of personality scales. *Human Performance, 14,* 187–207.

CHAPTER 18

Ethics and Ethical Behavior

CHAPTER OBJECTIVES

After studying this chapter, readers will be able to:

- Define ethics within the context of the modern healthcare organization.
- Introduce the major areas of concern in medical ethics.
- Introduce business ethics within the specific context of the manager's work environment.
- Describe the areas of ethical concern having the greatest impact on the role of the individual manager.
- Outline possible ethical standards of conduct for the organization.
- Review the manager's responsibility for modeling ethical behavior for the employees.

▶ Chapter Summary

Ethics may be defined as the system or code of morals of an individual or a particular group, such as an organization, profession, religion, or other collective. Ethics may also be simply described as *moral code.* Every person or organization has standards of conduct, though these may be unwritten and thus inferred from behavior. Doing business of any kind always presents a manager with the need to address ethical issues. In healthcare operations, there are a number of ethical lapses that fall under the heading of fraud and abuse; a department manager must be able to recognize these, conscientiously guard against their likelihood, and work toward the elimination of all such ethical breaches that occur. Above all, the individual manager must be a model of ethical behavior; as the employees see the manager behave, so too will they be encouraged to conduct themselves.

🔍 CASE: Should These Holiday Gifts Be Accepted?

Christmas was swiftly approaching, and Central Hospital was busier than ever as staff did their best to keep up with a greater-than-average census while preparing for the holiday. Francine Murphy, Vice President for Human Resources, was in her office when a heavy package addressed to her was delivered by a building services employee. Inside a plain shipping box was a holiday-decorated wooden wine crate containing a dozen bottles of high-quality wine. An attached note said, "A little something for you and your capable assistant Ms. Bowman." It was signed by a benefits provider who handled a small amount of the hospital's insurance business and regularly submitted proposals to take on more. Later this same day, one of the hospital's medical chiefs, Dr. Weston, dropped in on Ms. Murphy's office to wish her Merry Christmas and leave a beribboned bottle of champagne as he was doing for every department head in the hospital. With these gifts arrayed on her conference table, Francine wondered what to do with them. The champagne was no surprise; Dr. Weston had done the same—a bottle to every department head—for several years, but the case of fine wine from the benefits broker bothered Francine; she felt at a loss as to what to do about it.

▶ Ethics and the Healthcare Manager

For purposes of this chapter and within the context of the work organization, ethics is defined as follows: *the system or code of morals of an individual or a particular group such as an organization, profession, religion, or collective.* There is of course a broader definition describing ethics as a particular field of study—that is, the study of standards of conduct and moral judgment, or moral philosophy. The first definition, placing ethics in the context of the work organization, is the one under consideration here; however, whether we adhere to this definition or another, we will find that all definitions of ethics focus on morals or morality. One of the briefest but most useful descriptions of ethics is *moral code.*

Whether published or unwritten, every organization has a system or code of morals based on how its leaders want to relate to customers and others and thus governing how the organization's employees should behave as well. An increasing number of organizations, both inside and outside of health care, have established formal ethical standards of conduct for their employees.

Many specific occupations, including the healthcare professions, have also published ethical standards that proscribe the conduct required of their practitioners. In most instances, people admitted to membership in a profession are called upon to agree to adopt these ethical standards of conduct as a condition of entry.

Whether they realize it or not, most individuals also have "standards of conduct," although for most people these standards must be inferred from their behavior. (And as far as individual standards are concerned, one's observable behavior is usually a far more accurate indication of true ethical standards than one's own words might be in attempting to articulate these standards.)

Whether exhibited by an individual or by an organization, behavior is generally governed by these ethical standards of conduct plus legal requirements in the form of applicable laws and regulations.

Within the healthcare organization and from the average department manager's perspective, one might find it convenient to consider medical ethics and business ethics worthy of separate consideration. The medical ethics arena is complicated and growing more complex each year, presenting many more thorny and emotionally charged issues than business ethics. Fortunately, many medical ethics issues are addressed at administrative and board levels and are embodied in policies governing behavior; it also is fortunate that medical ethics concerns do not impact all employees. Issues of business ethics, on the other hand, although less complex and less emotionally charged than medical ethics issues, are of concern—or should be of concern—to all employees at all organizational levels.

▶ Brief Overview of Medical Ethics

Today's medical ethics issues are complex, often many-sided, and generally emotionally charged. They include the following:

- Genetic testing, with the primary concern being that information acquired through such testing could be used to discriminate in hiring and insuring, enabling employers and insurers to weed out prospects that exhibit certain genetic predispositions.
- Genetic manipulation, with supporting arguments citing the ability to correct or prevent potentially serious conditions and opposing arguments questioning the morality of such manipulation.
- Cloning, with claims of human cloning eventually becoming practical countered with arguments concerning the perceived dangers, and again, the issues of morality.
- Reproductive freedom, including all facets of the abortion issue fraught with moral and religious arguments and pitting individual rights against the rights of the unborn, plus consideration of sterilization and birth control methods as well as prenatal diagnosis of fetal disorders.
- Patient self-determination, addressing the right of an individual to designate the extent to which he or she will be cared for under certain extreme circumstances and generally to accept or refuse treatment, and the right to complete an advance directive as permitted by state law.
- Since acquired immunodeficiency syndrome (AIDS) first emerged, disclosure of one's positive status for human immunodeficiency virus (HIV) infection has been a significant ethical issue. There is on one side the desire to protect the general population, and on the other side are the rights of the individual to privacy and confidentiality.

Fortunately for the healthcare department manager, the known and anticipated medical ethics issues will, in many instances, be addressed by policies established by the institution's board of directors. To address medical ethics issues that may not be clearly covered by policy and those that would appear to involve exceptions or extraordinary circumstances, governing boards of larger healthcare organizations ordinarily have ethics committees.

▶ When Medicine and Business Meet

During the 1960s when concern over escalating healthcare costs first emerged and healthcare organizations (mostly hospitals) were urged to adopt cost-control practices, managers frequently heard statements such as, "A hospital should be run like a business."

Think about that statement. Should a hospital be run as a business is run? No doubt many sound business practices belong in a healthcare organization as well as any other enterprise. Consider, however, that running a healthcare entity of any size, from a solo medical practice to a major medical center, as a business has raised—or at least made more prominent—a number of ethical issues, such as the following:

- There is the issue of who gets service and who does not. Many say that all deserve service according to their needs, but when there are more apparent needs than service capacity, who determines who is served and how shall this be determined? Since a business must remain solvent to continue in business, who gets service may at times be determined by the ability to pay. The ethical and moral issues involved in the apportionment of services have long been with the industry and remain so whenever a decision to provide service is based on ability to pay via either one's personal resources or insurance plan.

- As the incomes of some providers, specifically physicians, have risen over the recent four decades, questions concerning compensation have arisen. How much compensation is legitimate? In defense of high fees and high earnings, some will point out the long, difficult, and costly education involved in becoming a physician. Those who defend high physician incomes will frown on those who question high medical fees, suggesting these people are "putting a price on their health." Yet others will claim that one's health, precious indeed, is being held hostage to the ability to pay.

- Not too many decades ago, it was generally considered unethical for professionals, especially physicians, dentists, and attorneys, to advertise. We hardly need to point out that today healthcare organizations from individual practitioners to multihospital systems advertise regularly. Few people find this practice unethical, any more than they find competition among providers to be unethical. Occurring gradually over a few decades, this change in practice illustrates perfectly how a set of ethical standards can change with the times.

- Considerably more pertinent to the individual healthcare supervisor, however, are the business ethics governing the situations the supervisor encounters on virtually a daily basis.

▶ Business Ethics and the Healthcare Organization

Regulatory Compliance

An organizational commitment to integrity is often expressed in the form of a regulatory compliance program. As the name implies, the purpose of such a program is to ensure compliance with all applicable laws and regulations. However, the emphasis of a regulatory compliance program usually concerns primarily compliance in billing and reimbursement from Medicare, Medicaid, other government programs, and private insurers. Many such programs are directed toward achieving thorough and accurate compliance with areas of concern that the Office of Inspector General of the Department of Health and Human Services (DHHS) has identified as receiving insufficient care and attention—that is, areas that are susceptible to fraud and abuse as well as error.

Among the areas of concern identified by DHHS are the following:

- Duplicate billing, or billing for services not actually rendered
- "Unbundling," the practice of submitting bills piecemeal to maximize payment for services or tests that would ordinarily be billed together
- "Upcoding" to provide a higher rate than the code that reflects the actual service
- Using a diagnosis-related group (DRG) code that provides a higher rate than the code that most accurately describes the service rendered (known as "DRG creep")
- Rendering outpatient services in conjunction with inpatient stays
- Filing false or erroneous cost reports
- Billing for discharge in lieu of transfer
- Limiting a patient's freedom of choice
- Failing to refund credit balances
- Utilizing incentives that violate antikickback regulations or other similar statutes
- Engaging in questionable financial arrangements between hospital and hospital-based physicians
- Participating in violations of the Stark physician self-referral law
- Violating patient antidumping regulations
- Knowingly failing to provide covered services or necessary care to health maintenance organization (HMO) members

The elimination and continuing prevention of fraud, abuse, and waste in healthcare billing and accounting are the goals of any sound regulatory compliance program, and the department manager is ethically obligated to support all personally applicable aspects of the program to the best of his or her ability. All employees are responsible for understanding and complying with all laws and regulations applicable to their jobs, and the manager is responsible for ensuring that employees have all the information they need to enable them to do so.

Conflict of Interest

An organization's employees have the right to engage in outside financial, business, or other activities as long as these do not interfere with the conscientious performance of their duties. Nevertheless, it is necessary to avoid both actual conflict of interest and any behavior that creates the *appearance* of conflict of interest; a merely perceived conflict of interest is genuine to the perceiver.

Conflicts of interest exist when employee loyalty is divided between an individual's organizational responsibilities and some outside interest. A potential conflict of interest is present whenever an objective observer of one's actions would have cause to wonder whether the observed actions are motivated solely by organizational concerns or personal or external concerns.

Conflict of interest is the area of ethical concern likely to emerge most frequently in the healthcare manager's management of a department or group. Some of the following guidelines apply to all employees at all levels. Some are most pertinent to specific employees, such as those responsible for purchasing. A great many of them are of concern to every department manager as they affect employee behavior.

- Avoid placing business with any firm in which you or your family or close business or personal associates have a direct or indirect interest (usually financial).
- Derive no personal financial gain from transactions involving the organization unless the organization is advised of—and approves of—your potential benefit.
- Conduct all aspects of a personal business venture outside of the organizational environment and on nonwork time. This is an area of significant concern as it is an ethical principle regularly violated and often implicitly condoned by department management through failure to address the offending behavior. For example, the employee who solicits orders at work for cosmetics, food containers, or whatever is in active violation of ethical standards; the person who makes photocopies for a part-time activity on work time using the organization's equipment is similarly in violation.
- Do not employ a relative in any situation where you have hiring authority or supervisory responsibility.
- Avoid soliciting, offering, accepting, or providing any consideration that could be construed as conflicting with the organization's business interests, such as meals, gifts, loans, entertainment, or transportation.
- Do not accept gifts exceeding the maximum value established by the organization (limits may exist in amounts up to perhaps $50 but are commonly lower); never accept gifts of cash of any amount.
- Safeguard patient and provider information against improper access or use for financial gain by unauthorized interests.
- Never charge, solicit, or accept any gift, donation, or other consideration as a precondition of admission, expedited admission, or continued stay.
- Require vendors and contractors to abide by your organization's ethical standards in their business relationships with the organization, and maintain impartial relationships with all actual and potential vendors and contractors.
- Do not endorse any product or outside service on behalf of the organization.
- Abstain from any discussion or decision affecting your employing organization and make clear your reasons for abstaining when serving as a member of an external organization or board of directors or in a public office.

If in doubt, always disclose the situation and seek resolution of an actual or potential conflict of interest before taking what might later be deemed an improper action. Questions concerning a potential conflict of interest can usually be addressed with the organization's human resources department.

Finally, in many organizations, department managers are asked to sign a conflict-of-interest statement indicating the presence of potential conflicts or the absence of such. This statement is usually renewed annually; ordinarily, it is the same conflict-of-interest statement executed by members of the board of directors.

Use of Organizational Assets and Information

It is the responsibility of all employees to protect the assets of the organization against loss, theft, and misuse. The organization's property may neither be used for personal benefit nor be loaned, sold, given away, or disposed of in any manner without appropriate authorization. Material that is declared surplus, obsolete, or scrap must be disposed of according to specific organizational policies.

An organization's assets are intended for use for business purposes only during legitimate employment. Improper use ordinarily includes unauthorized personal appropriation or use of tangible assets such as computers and copiers and other office equipment, medical equipment, vehicles, supplies, reports and records, computer software and data, and facilities. Intangible assets such as intellectual property, trademarks and copyrights, proprietary information including computer programs, confidential data, business plans, and such must be protected as vigorously as tangible property.

It also is necessary to protect patient property and information in accordance with established policies requiring that patient information is to be shared only with those who are authorized to receive such information and have a legitimate need for it.

The responsibility for protection also extends to proprietary information entrusted to the organization by vendors, both actual and potential, referral sources, contractors, service providers, and others. This standard invariably includes the requirement to use only legally licensed computer software, with the use of bootleg or pirated software considered unethical—not to mention illegal.

Concerning information, an organization's ethical standards of conduct may set forth the following principles:

- It is prohibited to disclose business secrets or proprietary information to anyone external to the organization, whether during or after employment, except as specifically authorized.
- All organizational property and information in one's possession must be surrendered upon termination of employment.
- It is prohibited to use, either directly or indirectly, inside information (i.e., information acquired through employment with the organization) for personal gain or the gain of others.

Referral Practices

The laws governing Medicare, Medicaid, and other federally sponsored programs prohibit the payment of any form of remuneration in return for the referral of patients. It also is illegal to induce the purchase of goods or services by Medicare or Medicaid for such referrals. The federal antikickback statute imposes criminal penalties on individuals and organizations that knowingly and willfully seek or receive compensation in return for referring patients or arranging for the provision of services for which payment may be made under a federal healthcare program. The kinds of payments prohibited by the statute include kickbacks, bribes, and rebates.

The Self-Referral Law (Stark law) prohibits a physician with a financial relationship with an entity providing any designated health service from referring Medicare and Medicaid patients to that entity unless the service or relationship falls within the Stark law's statutory exemption. The law also prohibits an entity from billing federal healthcare programs for items or services ordered by a physician who has a financial relationship with that entity. The Stark law, in other words, sought to eradicate the practice of some physicians of referring or sending patients to other provider organizations (e.g., clinical laboratories, radiological services, pharmacies, medical supply firms, etc.) in which they had an ownership interest.

The foregoing may be incorporated in an organization's ethical standards of conduct in the following manner:

- No employee shall solicit, receive, offer to pay, or pay remuneration of any kind in exchange for referring or recommending referral of any individual to another person, department, or division of the organization for services or in return for the purchase of goods or services to be paid for by a federal program.
- No employee shall offer or grant any benefits to a referring physician or other referral source to secure the referral of patients or patient business.
- No physician shall make referrals for designated health services to entities in which the physician has a financial interest through either ownership or a compensation arrangement.
- No physician shall bill for services rendered as a result of an illegal referral.

Political Activity

It is not unusual to find in an organization's code of conduct an expectation that employees who participate in government through political activity will ensure that they are not seen as representing the organization. There is a legal prohibition against political activity by not-for-profit hospitals and nursing homes and such; participating in political activity can jeopardize the employer's tax-exempt status. Specifics in the code of conduct may include the following:

- An employee speaking out on public issues must avoid the impression or appearance of speaking for the organization.
- Employees who hold public office must do so as individuals, not as representatives of the organization; they must pursue the duties of such office in a manner that does not conflict with organizational responsibilities.
- No organizational funds may be used to support any political activity, and no one may make political contributions on behalf of the organization.
- No employee may be reimbursed in any manner for political activity.
- No organizational facilities may be used for political activity.

▶ Privacy and Confidentiality

Employee Privacy

Although personnel files will ordinarily remain the property of the employer, the organization having a privacy policy in place will strictly limit access to personnel files to those having a legitimate need for the information. Such policy will usually state that personnel information will be released externally only upon employee authorization or to satisfy legitimate legal requirements (court orders, subpoenas, etc.).

Patient Confidentiality

Patient records, results of tests, diagnoses, and other information relating to or concerning individuals to whom the organization is providing or has provided service should be held in the strictest confidence. It is considered a violation of the ethical code of conduct to reveal patient information to anyone outside of the organization without the express written authorization of the patient (or the patient's legal representative), or a court order or other appropriate legal instrument.

Internal to the organization, patient information is to be retained in confidence. It is to be revealed on a need-to-know basis only.

Admission and Care of Patients

A health facility's ethical code of conduct will customarily require the organization and its employees to:

- Admit and care for persons without regard to their race, color, creed, national origin, or economic status, accepting and treating all with a caring response to their needs.
- Provide each patient (for hospitals) or resident (for nursing homes or other long-term setting) with a patient's bill of rights.
- Treat all patients or residents in a manner that fosters trust, extending every reasonable consideration to diversity of background, culture, religion, and heritage.
- Involve patients, whenever possible, in decisions regarding their treatment, and assist them in understanding proposed treatments and potential risks and outcomes.
- Respect the privacy and individuality of all who come to the organization for service.

Employee Relationships

The following is a suggested model for the section of an organization's ethical standards of conduct that addresses relationships with employees:

1. (The organization) recognizes people as valued resources. Employee relationships built on mutual respect are essential to maintaining a high level of integrity in our work.
2. Every employee will be treated and judged as an individual on the basis of individual qualifications without regard to race, sex, sexual orientation, religion, national origin, age, disability, veteran status, or other characteristic protected by law. This pledge extends to all areas of the employment relationship including hiring, promotion, benefits, training, and discipline.
3. (The organization) will conscientiously observe all federal, state, and local laws and regulations applicable in any way to the employment relationship.
4. (The organization) is committed to providing a work environment in which employees are free from harassment, sexual or otherwise. No employee will be made to feel uncomfortable in the work environment through exposure to coarse, profane, or derogatory comments or sexual language.
5. Employees are encouraged to express themselves freely and responsibly through established channels and procedures. Complaints will be treated as confidential information and will be revealed only to those

who need to know as part of a process of investigation or resolution. (The organization) will not tolerate any interference, retaliation, or coercion by any employee against an employee who registers a concern or complaint.

6. We will observe the standards of our profession and exercise judgment and objectivity at all times. Significant differences of professional opinion should be referred to the appropriate management for prompt resolution.
7. We shall show respect and consideration for one another regardless of position, status, or relationship.
8. (The organization) will promote its ethical standards of conduct among all physicians who practice in our facilities and encourage their observance and support of these standards.

▶ Addressing Ethical Issues

Ideally, an organization should publish its ethical standards of conduct and disseminate them to all employees. These standards also should be distributed externally as appropriate to vendors, contractors, third-party agents, and others as necessary to advise these entities of what to expect in business dealings with the organization.

It also is advisable to establish a system for reporting alleged or potential violations of the organization's ethical standards. Each employee is urged to report what he or she believes may be a violation of these standards. Reports should be immediate, thorough, and directed to either the individual's immediate supervisor or the chief human resources officer. For potential violations that might appear especially sensitive and for those of such a nature that direct reporting might compromise the reporting employee, it would be advisable for the organization to establish an "employee ethics hotline" number. An employee may use this number to make an anonymous report or to request guidance in describing or addressing a potential violation.

As mentioned earlier in the chapter, most larger healthcare organizations operating today have formal ethics committees to address ethical questions as needed. A typical committee might include the organization's:

- Patient care services executive
- Human resource executive
- Finance executive
- Medical director
- Corporate compliance officer
- Managers from specific functional areas as needed

▶ Management's Responsibilities: A Top-Down Obligation

One need not look far or long to appreciate the presence of a crisis of ethics in American business and government. Much of the highly publicized unethical behavior is unconscionable and greed driven, but perhaps some unethical conduct evident in business is also owing to the increasingly competitive nature of business. With competition attaining cutthroat dimensions in some industries and with other pressures increasing, some organizations, including many healthcare providers, are fighting for their very existence. Many employees—including managers at all levels—see themselves as fighting for their jobs or careers or at least struggling to get ahead on an uphill playing field.

A great deal has been published concerning high-profile ethical breaches. Hardly a week passes without news of alleged wrongdoings in high places as CEOs, elected officials, and other leaders apparently seek to enrich themselves by questionable means at the expense of employees, taxpayers, and other stakeholders. In classrooms, students of business and the professions hear that ethics should be a vital concern, but outside of school they see that it does not receive a great deal of serious attention in the workplace and in the halls of government.

What are employees to think when they see the kinds of behavior typified by the high-profile cases of recent years? Major scandals have tended to undercut worker trust and whatever loyalty employees might have extended to their employers during these volatile times. Also, scandals at high levels in the government serve to further feed worker distrust.

But the majority of today's ethics problems are not those presented by high-profile cases. The prominent cases simply feed attitudes that prevail at lower-management and rank-and-file levels. Consider just a few of the numerous ethical decisions many people face from day to day:

- Am I justified in calling in sick when I'm really not ill? Doing so can cause the loss of the value of the output that was not realized because you were not there, or it can cost the organization out-of-pocket for a replacement to cover your job.
- Do I work the full 8 hours, or do I start late, leave early, spend time socializing, or amuse myself surfing the Web or playing computer games? Some employees waste 25% or more of the workday by giving in to such practices.
- What's the harm if I take care of personal business during work time? The harm of course is that doing so costs your employer the value of the time taken away from the organization's work.
- Is it really up to me to point out the error being made by the sales clerk who is giving me too much change? It is indeed up to you; to knowingly accept the incorrect change is essentially stealing the amount of the excess.
- Surely, it must be all right for me to punch a friend's time card because I've been asked to do so? After all, lots of others do it. This practice is actually falsification of business records, an infraction described in many personnel policy manuals and in some instances punishable by discharge.

The foregoing are but a few of the ethical breaches occurring regularly in the majority of organizations. These might even be called the smaller breaches; beyond these there are outright theft, the acceptance of bribes or kickbacks, sexual harassment, deliberate discrimination, the practice of favoritism in matters of hiring and promotion, violations of confidentiality, and cutting corners and jeopardizing safety or quality for the sake of meeting deadlines, schedules, or budgets.

One might reason that taking an unwarranted day off once in a while or fudging a few dollars on an expense report are insignificant compared with what some highly placed "leaders" seem to be doing regularly. Up and down the line the reasoning becomes: They're doing it—why shouldn't I?

Recall the definition of ethics as a system or code of morals. Perhaps this broad definition is itself part of the problem, since moral principles and values differ among people, often significantly. Often the dilemma is a rules-based perspective dictated in laws and policies versus a values-based perspective, that is, one's personal beliefs and individual sense of right or wrong.

It is clear that the strongest examples of unethical behavior are those visible breaches that occur at high organizational levels. The problem is not a lack of rules; most of the larger organizations have a published code of conduct or ethical standards. The problem is in the lack of observance of the code and especially in the absence of modeling behavior.

Every business should have a code of ethics actively modeled by top management. It is critical that the people at the top be visible models of ethical behavior. Whether they realize it or not—and if they fail to realize it, perhaps they are unsuited for their elevated positions—top management's behavior sets the tone for the rest of the organization.

A business's ethical standards should be written in positive, constructive terms, laying out practical guidelines for ethical practice. This is no place for legalese that can be variously interpreted or ignored as some might choose. All employees should be aware of this code and share an understanding of appropriate conduct. Also, every such system needs features that protect those who report unethical conduct. Ethics has to be taught, actively communicated to employees without assuming that all in the company automatically share an understanding of ethical behavior.

The creation and maintenance of a dedicated and motivated workforce begins with the ethics and character of its leaders. The latter-day catch-phrase "walking the talk" has never been as true as it is concerning management's ethical behavior.

▶ The Department Manager's Key Role

It falls to the individual manager to ensure that all employees receive, review, and understand the organization's ethical standards of conduct. The ethical standards of conduct should be a regular subject of both new employee orientation and continuing education.

In managing a department or group, the manager should strive to model ethical behavior in all aspects of job performance. Thorough orientation and education notwithstanding, there is probably no more effective influence in shaping employee behavior than the manager's visible behavior. If the manager visibly observes and conscientiously adheres to the ethical standards of conduct, the employees are more likely to do the same. The manager's continued demonstration of ethical behavior is one of the most important dimensions of successful management in the modern healthcare organization.

▶ It Remains Everyone's Job

All employees at all levels have the continuing responsibility to display complete integrity in all aspects of their work activity. Integrity influences the reputations of people as individuals, and individual reputations together ultimately determine the reputation of the organization. Indeed, no set of ethical standards can ever replace a balanced combination of sound judgment, common sense, and personal integrity.

CASE STUDY: Resolution

What About Those Holiday Gifts?

In the majority of organizations, there would be no significant issue arising from Dr. Weston's annual bottle of champagne for every department head. Dr. Weston has done this regularly, and if the organization has a value limit on gifts accepted as many organizations do, as long as the value of the gift falls within the specified limit there is no problem. And since this gift was given to every department head, there is likely to be no perception of an attempt to curry favor with any specific department head.

The case of expensive wine is a different matter. Ms. Murphy should not accept the wine as a gift for Ms. Bowman and herself. To do so would be to play into the perception that the benefits provider was seeking favorable treatment in the placement of some of the hospital's benefits business. Ms. Murphy knew this benefits provider well enough to believe that it would be difficult to refuse the gift without possibly damaging a long-standing relationship. Ms. Murphy's solution was to give the case of wine to the hospital's volunteer association where it was welcomed as a contribution to the volunteer group's next fundraiser and ensured that a gracious letter was sent to the benefits provider expressing thanks for the generous gift to the volunteer association.

Note 1: Portions of this chapter were adapted from Chapter 18, "Case Study: Balancing Needs," *Human Resource Management in Health Care: Principles and Practice* (2nd ed.), Fleming Fallon, L., Jr., & McConnell, C. R. Burlington, MA: Jones & Bartlett Learning (2014); and Chapter 16, "Ethics and Ethical Standards," *The Effective Health Care Supervisor* (9th ed.), McConnell, C. R. Burlington, MA: Jones & Bartlett Learning (2019).

🔊 SPOTLIGHT ON CUSTOMER SERVICE

Customer service is commonly interpreted as dealing with customers external to an organization. However, a more inclusive definition takes into account internal customers, people who are employees of the organization. Good customer service involves treating people with kindness and honesty; it encompasses both external and internal customers.

The brief example cited in the chapter serves to demonstrate the modeling of ethical behavior in relations with an external customer (the benefits broker) and an internal customer (the volunteer organization).

The power of customer service becomes even more apparent when it is viewed as a process rather than as a discrete program. For essentially every job in the healthcare organization, there are always both internal and external customers, and neither is more important than the other.

Questions for Review and Discussion

Provide an example of how ethical standards can change over a period of time.

1. Why is it necessary for a healthcare institution to have official written policies for addressing issues of medical ethics?
2. What is ordinarily the function of an institution's ethics committee?
3. What is self-referral, and why is it considered unethical as well as illegal?

4. What is the single ethical issue that is—or should be—of broadest concern among health institution employees? That is, which one concern affects more employees than any other?
5. Why is it important for the department supervisor to be a model of ethical behavior?
6. Is it both legally and ethically correct to hire the family member of a friend over other applicants as long as no involved parties belong to a protected class (i.e., there is no discrimination)?
7. What ethical breach might a supervisor commit that will likely pave the way for similar breaches by the employees?
8. Is it an ethical violation for a clerk in human resources to read parts of a few personnel files while putting them away? Why, or why not?
9. What should be the principal guiding rule for determining who is allowed to see confidential information?

Resources

Books

Hammaker, D. K., & Knadig, T. M. (2017). *Health care ethics and the law*. Burlington, MA: Jones & Bartlett Learning.

Morrison, E. E. (2016). *Ethics in health administration*. Burlington, MA: Jones & Bartlett Learning.

Morrison, E. F., & Furlong, B. (2019). *Health care ethics: Critical issues for the 21st century*. Burlington, MA: Jones & Bartlett Learning.

Pozgar, G. D. (2019). *Legal aspects of health care administration* (13th ed.). Burlington, MA: Jones & Bartlett Learning.

Periodicals

Skeet, A. (2017). *A model for exploring an ethical leadership practice*. Santa Clara, CA: Markula Center for Applied Ethics at Santa Clara University.

Wright, E., Marvel, J. E., & DesMarteau, K. (2014). Exploring millennials: A surprising inconsistency in making ethical decisions. *Journal of Academic and Business Ethics, 9*, 1–14.

CHAPTER 19

Impacts and Effects of Social Media

CHAPTER OBJECTIVES

After studying this chapter, readers will be able to:

- Recognize the growth of social media use in business settings.
- Discuss the impact of using social networking sites for hiring decisions.
- List three ways in which organizations can use social media to their advantage.
- Articulate the need for organizations to craft a clear social media use policy.

▶ Chapter Summary

There are both challenges and opportunities when it comes to social media use in healthcare organizations' human resource departments. Social media can be used effectively in the personnel recruitment and hiring processes, although it is not without its pitfalls. Beyond hiring, human resource professionals must balance their focus on employee performance with promoting and protecting an organization's image. Social media offers some effective tools to do so. The number one task facing human resource personnel is to ensure they have crafted a clear social media use policy for their organization.

▶ Hiring and Networking

Several years ago, a job applicant might send a letter of inquiry to a company about job openings. As jobs were available, these letters and accompanying resumes were batch processed until the position was filled. Progress in technology allowed companies to create electronic job boards for employment postings, many of which still exist on internal and external company sites. The landscape has changed again, and

CASE STUDY

Miranda Greggs is new to the human resource (HR) department at New Health Memorial Hospital (NHMH). She was hired in the past 30 days due to NHMH's anticipated expansion via a new wing, three satellite health centers, a community outreach health program, and a teen peer-to-peer health outcomes research study that NHMH is leading. The demand for recruiting and hiring personnel to accommodate this level of growth meant an increase in the HR department staff.

Miranda noted during her first week at NHMH that the current personnel recruitment methods for nonexecutive positions include internal electronic job boards, postings on NHMH's public website, job announcements on employment websites like Monster.com, and an employee referral bonus program to encourage current employees to recruit qualified candidates they know. With the level of staffing needed for the new programs and to meet her weekly new-hire target goals, Miranda knows she will need to implement new strategies to attract more job applicants.

What are some ideas for how Miranda can reach a wider audience in her recruitment efforts? How can she differentiate her message and its delivery for different staffing levels (e.g., nurses, community outreach workers, teens, facilities management staff)?

While reviewing the current list of applicants in her inbox, Miranda opens her browser and starts looking up the first few names on Facebook. One applicant in particular is very qualified for the nurse manager position at one of the new community health clinics. Miranda has already arranged for her to come in and interview the following day. The lead physician at that clinic is a religiously conservative man who has lobbied hard publicly for taxpayers to pick up more of NHMH's healthcare costs. As Miranda scans the applicant's Facebook profile, her heart sinks. Her family photos clearly show that she is gay and that she strongly supports the gubernatorial candidate who wants to end taxpayer subsidies to all healthcare organizations. Despite being qualified for the job, Miranda wonders if she should cancel the interview as it seems like it will not be a good match.

organizations may now use online job sites, such as Indeed.com, iHire, Monster, SimplyHired, and Glassdoor, as well as other social media avenues, for posting open positions.

There are important differences in these websites and how both employers and potential employees use them. While Monster.com is truly a job and résumé posting site, Indeed acts almost as an intermediary—the first step in the employment screening process, if you will. Employers and applicants can decide online if they are a good match before either party moves forward. Platforms such as LinkedIn are considered social networking sites (SNS). Using Boyd and Ellison's 2007 definition of SNS, these are "web-based services that allow individuals to (a) construct a public or semi-public profile within a bounded system, (b) articulate a list of other users with whom they share a connection, and (c) view and traverse their list of connections and those made by others within the system." In practice, the platform is not limited to individuals, such that both companies and applicants engage in self-branding through building a profile and creating a network. LinkedIn also offers algorithms to indicate to an applicant what the current competition is for a given job, which might encourage them to apply (e.g., "You're in the top 25% of 42 applicants"). Sites such as Glassdoor reflect today's viral marketing and social input; companies are anonymously rated and reviewed by current and former employees, salaries are shared, and perceptions about work environments are confirmed.

This online transparency and scrutiny allow workers to make savvy choices about where to apply. Many are looking less for just a job and more for the "right fit." They want to know if the company (healthcare or otherwise) pays employees fair market wages. Do they offer a broad array of benefits? Are there "perks" to working there? Is it a socially conscious company? Do current employees seem satisfied?

What about the company perspective? While applicants can now screen potential employers just as they screen potential dates, how can healthcare organizations benefit from these social media and online job-hunting forums? For many organizations, social media now plays a much bigger role in the hiring process than ever before. In fact, the results of a 2013 white paper found "64% of employers…used social media to inform hiring decisions, with one quarter using the information gained from these sites at the interview stage and 35% when assessing new applications" (HR review). Some surveys have shown that up to 80% of businesses use social media in human resources decision-making (Burgdorf, 2018), a process referred to as cyber-vetting. LinkedIn allows employers (and third-party recruiters) to see an enhanced résumé as well as business contacts, volunteer work, current interests, and degree of influence. Because HR personnel are tasked with finding top talent, they may notice any of the following when looking at an applicant's online profile:

- Is this a healthcare executive who posts or comments frequently on payer reform and who has a wide network of followers?
- Do his or her comments align with the company's mission statement?
- Is this a nurse who volunteers part-time in rural clinics and has led healthcare access initiatives?

Some of these attributes that might make a candidate more attractive to an organization are not easily conveyed through a traditional paper résumé.

LinkedIn and Indeed are business and job-posting platforms, and as such, one can expect that résumés or profiles displayed on those sites are intended to be seen by potential employers. But there are other forms of social media, such as Facebook, Twitter, Instagram, or YouTube, that have become part of today's job search. These are some of the most-used social media sites (Sözbilir & Dursun, 2017), and while they have each experienced growth in business usage, they are still dominated by personal users. Lest one think this use is limited to Millennials, the fastest-growing demographic on Google+ is 45- to 54-year-olds and on Twitter, 55- to 64-year-olds (Meister, 2014). Using some of these social networking sites as part of the employment screening process may benefit the applicant or the organization, depending on how the site is used and the outcome of the process (Elias, Honda, Kimmel, & Chung, 2016).

Applicants who present well on social media (by whatever criteria the business decides on) will find it advantageous for a human resources (HR) recruiter to view their Facebook profile or follow their Twitter feed. In fact, a social media profile can positively influence a potential employee's standing in the recruitment queue (Cooley & Parks-Yancy, 2016), as HR professionals may use those sites to evaluate an applicant's professionalism and writing skills (Schwabel, 2012), or to determine from reviewing profile pictures and other posted photographs that they possess traits of maturity and extroversion (Caers & Castelyns, 2010). In the world of college football recruiting, Bigsby, Ohlmann, and Zhao (2019) found a positive correlation between high school athletes' level of engagement on Twitter and the number of college recruitment offers received. Engagement was analyzed for both self-promotion, defined as posting positive content about one's own athletic prowess and academic abilities, and ingratiation, defined as posting positive comments about other athletes and teams.

Due to the pressure to find and retain talent, some recruiting firms monitor social media to identify top candidates even before they apply for a job. Take, for example, the websites Entelo and TalentBin. These companies use search tools to "consider the experience and history mentioned in users' profiles, but also their use of social networks. These companies can pinpoint users who have updated their bios lately or often, to determine which candidates are getting ready to enter the job market" (Meister, 2014). Community sites like Dribble encourage design professionals to showcase their best work, and Github provides software developers a collaborative forum for building open-source software or working as teams to respond to client-based requests. Recruiters can monitor these sites to see who is most active or most in demand and cultivate a network of top talent.

What about applicants who do not present well on social media? Who tweet offensive comments or have content on their Facebook or Instagram accounts that runs counter to the values or culture of the employing organization? Just as some profile photographs are determined to show traits like maturity, others may negatively influence a hiring decision. A candidate who posts "provocative" photos may not be hired (Broughton, Foley, Ledermaier, & Cox, 2015), and those with alcohol-oriented profiles were rated lower in an experimental study than those with family- or professional-oriented profiles (Bohnert & Ross, 2010). Overall, nonprofessional content on SNS is found to be detrimental to an applicant's opportunities for recruitment (Alarcon, Villarreal, Waller, Degrassi, & Staples, 2018). Even email addresses may affect a recruiter's impression of a candidate, with an informal address having the same impact as spelling errors on a résumé (van Toorenburg, Oostrom, & Pollet, 2015).

Human resource professionals are expected to know and follow laws pertaining to discrimination when it comes to hiring decisions. Moving back to our case study, how can Melinda Greggs show that the qualified was not hired based on something other than her Facebook posts? Or that she was denied an interview after her social media accounts were viewed? Can HR professionals guarantee that lack of access to an interview was based on not having proper credentials or experience rather than ethnicity, age, or political leanings?

Cyber-vetting is still an emerging business practice, and there is much theoretical research underway on job seekers' perceived respect for privacy, self-disclosure, and social media content effects during the job recruitment or selection process. To combat potential accusations of bias, the Society of Human Resource Management recommends that HR managers "create policies to protect themselves and their organizations from allegations of discrimination by assigning a third-party person to screen applicants based on specific criteria for jobs" (Human Resources MBA, n.d.; ManagerSkills, n.d.). This allows an HR manager to make decisions and extend interview invitations based only on qualifications, as they would be blind to potential discriminatory factors such as age, race, gender, national origin, or sexual orientation.

▶ Social Media Use for Business

To date, there is still a relatively small—though growing—body of research on how social media use impacts individuals and organizations. Human resource managers might consider following this research as it develops to note the potential impact of social media on organizational behavior (e.g., through social exchange or social network theory), both at a theoretical and a practical level.

Beyond personnel recruitment, organizations use social media sites and apps to conduct business. It is not unusual for a business to have a Facebook page and Instagram and Twitter accounts. Marketing can be enhanced by YouTube videos. Networking is broadened through LinkedIn. Communication with colleagues, customers, and subject matter experts is made easier through Facebook Messenger and WhatsApp. Organizations can use any and all of these sites or apps to promote new products, introduce logo changes, announce successful revenue results, or reveal new ad campaigns.

Organizations—most often through the HR department—can also use social media to announce changes or dispel rumors. There may be news of an impending merger between two healthcare organizations. Addressing rumors or confirming breaking news via social media allows for organizational transparency and timely response to concerns. When combined with or followed by an online question and answer forum (facilitated by HR personnel), employee concerns, fears, and speculation can be managed effectively and in real time. There may still be a place for company-wide memos, but a timelier approach to announcements is via a video-based "town hall," allowing even remote employees to be as up to date and informed as those onsite.

Social networking sites can be used to communicate with employees about upcoming open enrollment deadlines, wellness program registrations, volunteer opportunities, or policy changes. SNS can also be used as beneficial training tools for organizations. Training is more collaborative in nature when online social platforms are used and employees can discuss and brainstorm via live chat. Organizations can leverage tools like Yammer or Google Hangout to facilitate peer-to-peer interactions. Montefiore Hospital in New York introduced social learning to build a "shared mental model of leadership." As part of a leadership development program, employees used Yammer to co-create a new behavioral interview guide (Meister, 2014).

Computer-based learning modules can be deployed online for organizations with offsite employees, or even for those inhouse. Companies have found that by accessing MOOCs (massive, open, online courses), their education and training budgets have decreased, whether through using external MOOCs like Coursera, or by building their own.

When one states that organizations use social media as a business tool, it overlooks the fact that it is individuals within those organizations who go online to create, deliver, and monitor the social media messages. Thus, (some) employees are explicitly authorized to use social media at work. And so, every business must determine what policies and boundaries they want to set regarding employee social media use. A seemingly easy fix is to ban social media use in the workplace and set up firewalls blocking social media sites such as Facebook. Such bans can be difficult to enforce, as restrictions need to balance the organization's legitimate business interests with employees' rights to use social media for labor-related activities. Pryme Group (2018) notes:

> By blocking access to social media by employees, an employer may run the risk of violating federal labor laws. In the United States, under Section 7 of the NLRA, any monitoring of social media use (and related policies) must account for the rights of workers to engage in protected concerted activities. Any prohibition against the use of social networks must avoid infringing the rights of employees to engage in those protected concerted activities.

Even if company computers have built-in firewalls, what about apps on smartphones? Or employees who must go on social networking sites to promote the business? Many employees request to bring their personal tablets or smartphones to work and use their apps for business, and some employers have a "bring-your-own-device" policy. A *Forbes* article commenting on social human resources noted a Microsoft survey of 9000 workers over 31 countries, which found that "31% would be willing to spend their own money on a new social tool if it made them more efficient at work" (Meister, 2014). Millennials, who will comprise 50% of the 2020 workplace, see the business value of technology in the workplace (Meister, 2014).

Even employees who work remotely and can have their personal Facebook page open while simultaneously working on company documents, and with more options for employees to work off-site, it is increasingly difficult for companies to monitor social media use. Human resource departments are tasked with creating organizational policies that are based on the needs and culture of the organization. No one policy will work for every business, as each has unique needs. Larger organizations with corporate counsel should bring together HR and counsel to consult on relevant labor laws when crafting a social media policy. Without such policies, both employees and employers are open to risk. Further, HR departments may wish to add cyberbullying and appropriate social media use to the current suite of mandatory employee trainings.

For those employers who do use social media to support work-related activities, it is easy for the lines between personal and business to become blurred with regard to access, content, and privacy. Employees' rights to personal privacy extend to not sharing personal social media passwords with an employer and to having protection from social media monitoring without explicit consent. HR professionals must understand employee privacy laws, especially when creating and enforcing organizational social media use policy. We will look at the complexity of balancing employee rights with the protection of employer liability.

▶ Employee Use of Social Media

Employee Rights

Employees in the United States have strong personal privacy and labor rights, as personal privacy is arguably tied to one's Constitutional right to free speech. There are industry-specific regulations that can impact and curb this free speech, such as those for finance, healthcare, and insurance organizations. Nonetheless, according to Pryme Group (2018), a successful social media policy should consider the following:

- Employment discrimination
- Free speech

- Labor- or union-related activities
- Account/password access and management
- Prohibition of social media use in the workplace
- Monitoring employee use of social media
- Regional privacy laws

Employment Discrimination

While employment discrimination may be difficult to prove if a company has a clear social media or other related policy, without such protection in place, a company can be liable for hiring decisions made. In the case of *Gaskell v. University of Kentucky*, an astronomer, C. Martin Gaskell, applied for the position of Observatory Director of the University of Kentucky's (UK) MacAdam Observatory. Gaskell was denied the position and filed a discrimination claim based on his religious beliefs. Gaskell had been a leading candidate for the position, and the UK agreed that he had more education and experience than the candidate who was ultimately hired. In fact, following phone interviews with the top seven candidates, the Search Committee ranked Gaskell first on the list, according to an objective scale in which a number score was assigned to each of five job criteria.

However, during the selection process, a committee member conducted an Internet search for more information about Gaskell and found a link to his personal website, which contained an article titled, "Modern Astronomy, the Bible, and Creation." The article was circulated to the entire committee, members of whom were concerned about whether they should consider Gaskell's statements in the article during the selection process, as they believed these statements to blend religious thought with scientific theory. Previous public lectures given by Gaskell were interpreted to uphold a "creationist" viewpoint, even though Gaskell denied being a creationist.

Ultimately, a lesser candidate (based on the objective ranking criteria of the search committee) was chosen and Gaskell's case was settled, with the university paying him $125,000. Arguably, a more objective approach might have landed Gaskell the job.

Free Speech and Labor- or Union-Related Activities

Employees do indeed have the right to free speech and to publicly express dissent, whether that be political dissent or dissatisfaction with their employer. Relatedly, employees have the right to express support for labor- or union-related activities. In *NLRB v. Pier Sixty, LLC*, the court sided with the National Labor Relations Board, which argued for the wrongful firing of an employee at a catering company. In 2011, several of Pier Sixty, LLC's employees were frustrated and began to seek union representation. This move was not supported by the company, and management inferred that employees might be disciplined for union activities. Two days prior to a vote to unionize, an employee posted negative comments about his supervisor, calling him a "loser" in a profanity-laced post. Although the post was deleted 3 days later, it came to the attention of Pier Sixty management and the employee was fired. An Administrative Law Judge found, and a Second Circuit court upheld, that the employee was protected under the National Labor Relations Act, which protects employee speech until the point that it is so "opprobrious" as to lose that protection.

Monitoring Employee Use of Social Media

If companies are going to monitor employee use of social media—during work hours or after—they need to ensure that their social media use policy is carefully worded and consistently enforced. In the case of *Jones v. Gulf Coast Health Care*, an employee who needed rotator cuff surgery was granted leave through the Family Medical Leave Act (FMLA). At the end of his approved leave, the employee's doctor indicated that he was not fit to return to work. The employee requested a return to work with "light duty" but failed to produce a certification that he was fit for either light or full duty. His employer granted him an additional month of non-FMLA leave. During this additional leave, the employee vacationed with his family and posted photos of the vacation on Facebook, including photos of him swimming in the ocean. These photos were shared with coworkers, and upon his return to work, the employee was confronted with them by his supervisor who noted that the employee was well enough to have returned to work without the extended 30-day leave. He was terminated after investigation.

The employee claimed interference with his FMLA rights. The defendant—the company that fired him—argued, in part, that the employee's conduct violated its social media policy, which allowed for employee termination if the social media posts had "an adverse effect on co-workers." Not only had the company not mentioned the social media policy at the time of the employee's termination, but the company could not produce evidence that any employee was adversely affected by the vacation photos. Further, the Eleventh Circuit argued that the purpose of the social media policy, as employees were trained to understand, was to prevent employees from posting harmful or negative comments about the company, the staff, or the facilities. Vacation photos posted by the employee while on leave were not found to violate the company's social media policy.

▶ Employer Rights to Limit Social Media Use

Firing an Employee

As noted, a company's HR department should create a social media policy that clearly outlines employer expectations. A "well-established and well-articulated social media policy" will generally be supported by the courts if used as a basis to fire an employee (Burgdorf, 2018). Instances in which organizations were supported by the court based on established policies follow.

Rodriquez v. Wal-Mart, Inc.

The plaintiff, a manager at a Wal-Mart store, noticed that employees who had called out sick for the day nonetheless posted on Facebook photos of themselves at a Fourth of July party. The plaintiff, who was their supervisor, commented on those photos via Facebook, "publicly chastising the employees by name." As this was a second company policy violation by the plaintiff, who was already on disciplinary status, she was terminated. She filed a discrimination suit on the basis of her age group (over 40 years) and national origin (Hispanic). The Court found that the "Plaintiff publicly—rather than privately—chastised employees under her management on a social media website," and that the "Defendant has satisfied its burden of producing evidence of a legitimate, nondiscriminatory reason for its decision to terminate Plaintiff in that she violated company policy" (*Rodriquez v. Wal-Mart, Inc.*).

The Matter of the Tenure Hearing of Jennifer O'Brien

In the Matter of the Tenure Hearing of Jennifer O'Brien, a New Jersey school district (City of Paterson) successfully fired a schoolteacher who had posted to Facebook derogatory comments about her students (all of whom were Latino or African American and were first graders). While a clear social media policy was not the cornerstone for the district's case, there was a clause in their employment policy regarding "conduct unbecoming a teacher." The case was referred to an Administrative Law Judge (ALJ) who dismissed O'Brien's claims that her Facebook comments were protected by the First Amendment to the U.S. Constitution and found the evidence supported the charge of conduct unbecoming a teacher. In regard to the teacher's claim that she had a right to express her views, the ALJ wrote:

> An internet social-networking site such as Facebook is a questionable place to begin an earnest conversation about an important school issue such as classroom discipline. More to the point, a description of first-grade children as criminals with their teacher as their warden is intemperate and vituperative. It becomes impossible for parents to cooperate with or have faith in a teacher who insults their children and trivializes legitimate educational concerns on the internet.

Thus, social media use is not always protected when it can be shown to clearly violate standards by which a company (in this case, a school district) has articulated how it expects its employees to act.

▶ Harassment

Organizations are within their rights to prohibit employee harassment conducted through social media, smartphone apps (including text messaging), and other Internet usage, even if it occurs outside of work hours. In the case of *Isenhour v. Outsourcing of Millersburg*, the Court ruled that an employee was subject to harassment and a hostile work environment after being sent sexually suggestive and explicit texts from a supervisor. An employer can be found liable for such behavior if the harassment can be traced back to the workplace and especially if the employer had any knowledge of the harassment (Burgdorf, 2018).

▶ Other Protections

A well-crafted social media policy should cover the following concerns:

- Disclosure of confidential business information
- Complaints about business customers/clients
- Disparaging comments about the business or how it is operated
- Harassment, intimidation, or other criticism of fellow employees.

There is very little guidance for HR personnel on how to create a social media policy that protects the interests of both the company and the employees. The U.S. Equal Employment Opportunity Commission (EEOC) has its own social media policy statement, but beyond a 2014 press release acknowledging the scope of the issue (EEOC, 2014), it has not provided employers with clear guidelines for how to word such policies or for social media business use in general. Likewise, the National Labor Relations Board has attempted to provide guidance for employers by issuing reports that detail the outcomes of social media cases brought to the NLRB Office of General Counsel but leave employers to craft their own policies based on the activities and policies reviewed in each of these cases. The NLRB notes that the cases underscore two important points related to social media:

- Employer policies should not be so sweeping that they prohibit the kinds of activity protected by federal labor law, such as the discussion of wages or working conditions among employees.
- An employee's comments on social media are generally not protected if they are mere gripes not made in relation to group activity among employees (NLRB, n.d.).

In addition to crafting social media policies, a business would do well to have the HR department prepare strategies for responding to negative publicity, employee dissent, and customer attacks. Any one of these social media activities may damage a company's reputation (Horn et al., 2015), and organizations should be prepared for the increasing use of social media across the spectrum of employee, customer, and business use.

▶ Conclusion

Human resource departments are challenged by the current state of social media use. Social media and social networking sites are accessed with increasing frequency to tap into pools of potential employees, yet there are any number of pitfalls when these sites are used without clear, written guidance or by third-party recruiters. Research continues to be conducted to look at whether the use of social media in hiring practices benefits the employer or the employee. Businesses have a number of legitimate uses for social media, and employees will use social media to express themselves whether during work hours or after. Human resource personnel must be prepared to respond to social media use across this spectrum by creating a clear, consistently enforced, widely distributed social media policy that neither violates employee privacy rights nor opens the business to potential litigation.

🔍 *CASE STUDY: Resolution*

Melinda Greggs decided to move forward with interviewing the qualified candidate for the nurse manager position, despite Facebook photos and posts that indicated it might be a poor social fit. Given the number of employees that must be hired to fill all the open positions the hospital's expansion plans created, she recommended to her supervisor that the department contract a third-party recruiter to post positions and screen applicants. Only those most qualified based on objective criteria would be passed to the HR department for interviews. Melinda also worked with her supervisor and the hospital's counsel to construct a clear social media policy that balanced employee rights with protection of the hospital.

Questions for Review and Discussion

1. What are the advantages to an organization using social networking sites to identify potential candidates for employment? What are the disadvantages?
2. Is it fair for organizations to view applicants on social networking sites without their knowledge? What are the legal ramifications for doing so? Does your answer change if the person being viewed is not yet an applicant for an open position?
3. Do you see a difference between employees using employer-owned laptops or cell phones to access social media versus using their own devices? Why or why not?
4. What further guidelines could the U.S. Equal Employment Opportunity Commission provide to employers regarding social media use?
5. What further guidelines could the U.S. National Labor Relations Board provide to employers regarding social media use?
6. In your opinion, do social networking sites have a role in employee performance reviews? Why or why not?

References

Alarcon, D., Villarreal, A., Waller, A., Degrassi, S., & Staples, H. (2018, March 7–10). *Follow me: The use of social media in recruitment*. Southwest Academy of Management Proceedings Annual Meeting, Albuquerque, NM.

Bigsby, K. G., Ohlmann, J. W., & Zhao, K. (2019). Keeping it 100: Social media and self-presentation in college football recruiting. *Big Data, 7*(1), 3–20. doi:10.1089/big.2018.0094

Bohnert, D., & Ross, W. H. (2010). The influence of social networking web sites on the evaluation of job candidates. *Cyberpsychology Behaviour and Social Networking, 13*, 341–347

Boyd, D. M., & Ellison, N. B. (2007). Social network sites: Definition, history and scholarship. *Journal of Computer Mediated Education, 13*(1), 210–230.

Broughton, A., Foley, B., Ledermaier, S., & Cox, A. for Institute for Employment Studies. (2013). *The use of social media in the recruitment process*. ACAS Research Paper. Retrieved from https://s3.amazonaws.com/academia.edu.documents/35744264/The-use-of-social-media -in-the-recruitment-process.pdf?response-content-disposition=inline%3B%20filename %3DSETA_survey_of_representatives_in_Tribun.pdf&X-Amz-Algorithm=AWS4-HMAC -SHA256&X-Amz-Credential=AKIAIWOWYYGZ2Y53UL3A%2F20190723%2Fus-east -1%2Fs3%2Faws4_request&X-Amz-Date=20190723T180131Z&X-Amz-Expires=3600&X -Amz-SignedHeaders=host&X-Amz-Signature=c022c9c92b8ab0a7635fb8d662db68d9e31aaa6 f4e3275d8f2055b1aa926ce7a

Burgdorf, B. (2018, September 18). Hiring, firing, and HR rewiring: Human resources in the age of social media. *Pillsbury—Internet and Social Media Law Blog*. Retrieved from https://www .jdsupra.com/legalnews/hiring-firing-and-hr-rewiring-human-70943/

Caers, R., & Castelyns, V. (2010). LinkedIn and Facebook in Belgium: The influences and biases of social network sites in recruitment and selection procedures. *Social Science Computer Review, 29*, 437–438.

Cooley, D., & Parks-Yancy, R. (2016). Impact of traditional and internet/social media screening mechanisms on employers' perceptions of job applicants. *The Journal of Social Media in Society, 5*(3), 151–186.

Elias, T., Honda, L. P., Kimmel, M., & Chung, J. (2016). A mixed methods examination of 21st century hiring processes, social networking sites, and implicit bias. *The Journal of Social Media in Society, 5*(1), 189–288.

Gaskell v. University of Kentucky, CIVIL ACTION NO. 09-244-KSF (E.D. Ky. Nov. 23, 2010).

Horn, I., Taros, T., Dirkes, S., Hüer, L., Rose, M., Tietmeyer, R., & Constantinides, E. (2015). Business reputation and social media: A primer on threats and responses. *Journal of Direct, Data and Digital Marketing Practice, 16*, 193. doi:10.1057/dddmp.2015.1

HRreview. (2013). 60% of job seekers do not like recruiters searching social media profiles. Retrieved from https://www.hrreview.co.uk/hr-news/recruitment/60-of-job-seekers-do-not-like-recruiters-searching-social-media-profiles/49324

Human Resources MBA. How does social media affect a human resources professional? Retrieved from https://www.humanresourcesmba.net/faq/social-media-affect-human-resources-professional/

Isenhour v. Outsourcing of Millersburg, Civil Action No. 1:14-CV-1170 (M.D. Pa. 2015)

Justia US Law. In the Matter of the Tenure Hearing of Jennifer O'Brien. (2013). Retrieved from https://law.justia.com/cases/new-jersey/appellate-division-unpublished/2013/a2452-11.html

ManagerSkills.org. How social media affects HR: 2017 guide. Retrieved from https://www.managerskills.org/hr/social-media-hr/

Meister, J. (2014, January 6). The future of work: Why social HR matters. *Forbes*. Retrieved from https://www.forbes.com/sites/jeannemeister/2014/01/06/the-future-of-work-why-social-hr-matters/#6590e15ed06a

National Labor Relations Board (NLRB). (n.d.). The NLRB and social media. Retrieved from https://www.nlrb.gov/rights-we-protect/rights/nlrb-and-social-media

NLRB v. Pier Sixty, LLC, CIVIL ACTION No. 15-1841 (2d Cir. 2017).

Pryme Group. (2018, January 25). 7 ways employee privacy laws impact social media in the workplace. Retrieved from https://allpryme.com/employee-privacy-laws/employee-privacy-laws/

Schwabel, D. (2012). How recruiters use social networks to make hiring decisions now. *Time*. Retrieved from http://business.time.com/2012/07/09/how-recruiters-use-social-networks-to-make-hiring-decisions-now/

Sözbilir, F., & Dursun, M. K. (2017). Does social media usage threaten future human resources by causing smartphone addiction? A study on students aged 9–12. *Addicta: The Turkish Journal on Addictions, 5*(2), 185–203.

U.S. Equal Employment Opportunity Commission. (2014). Social media is part of today's workplace but its use may raise employment discrimination concerns. *Press Release* 3-12-14. Retrieved from https://www.eeoc.gov/eeoc/newsroom/release/3-12-14.cfm

van Toorenburg, M., Oostrom, J. K., & Pollet, T. (2015). What a difference your e-mail makes: Effects of informal e-mail addresses in online resume screening. *Cyberpsychology, Behavior, and Social Networking, 18*(3), 135–140. doi:10.1089/cyber.2014.0542

Virginia C. Rodriquez, Plaintiff, v. Wal-Mart Stores, Inc., Defendant. Civil Action No. 3:11-CV-2129-B. 2013 U.S. Dist. LEXIS 3025.

Resources

Alexander, E., Mader, D., & Mader, F. (2017). Using social media during the hiring process: A comparison between recruiters and job seekers. *Journal of Global Scholars of Marketing Science, 29*. doi:10.1080/21639159.2018.1552530

Jeske, D., & Shultz, K. S. (2019). Social media screening and content effects: Implications for job applicant reactions. *International Journal of Manpower, 40*(1), 73–86. doi:10.1108/IJM-06-2017-0138

Slovensky, R., & Ross, W. H. (2012). Should human resource managers use social media to screen job applicants? Managerial and legal issues in the USA. *Info, 14*(1), 55–69. doi:10.1108/14636691211196941

CHAPTER 20

Relations with Labor Unions

CHAPTER OBJECTIVES

After studying this chapter, readers will be able to:

- Overview the history of unionization.
- Know why many employees turn to unions.
- Appreciate why executive management prefers to remain union-free.
- Understand about health care's unique treatment under prevailing labor law.
- Identify the different bargaining units possible in a healthcare facility.
- Describe a department manager's role during union organizing.
- Identify visible signs of union organizing activities.
- Describe the process occurring after the arrival of a petition for a representation election.
- Understand what managers can and cannot legally do during a union organizing drive.
- Know how to coexist with a union on a day-to-day basis.

▶ Chapter Summary

Unions have considerable allure for workers who are dissatisfied with aspects of their jobs. Employees join unions when they believe doing so can improve their personal situations. Employers usually resist unionization because a union's presence is invariably seen as increasing costs and complicating operations. Interactions with employees are governed by a contract, also known as a collective bargaining agreement.

Unions and managers are both bound by laws. The National Labor Relations Act (NLRA) of 1935, commonly known as the Wagner Act, is the basis of most labor laws in the United States. Labor legislation provides rules of conduct for both employers and employees. Violations of said rules are defined as unfair labor practices. The rules also specify the steps that a union must take when seeking to represent workers. Unions can be removed through a legal process known as decertification.

🔍 *CASE STUDY: Is That a Union Forming?*

Jane Pinkerton was in a meeting with her supervisor, Chris Smith. "I wanted to share some observations with you," said Jane. "Some employees in my section have become distant. Over the past 6 months they have had progressively less to say to me."

"Do the employees have any problems you're aware of?" asked Chris.

"No," came the reply, "but they've become jumpier since the merger rumors started."

"I'll bet the two events are related," mused Chris. "See what you can find out. Try meeting with a couple of groups of employees."

"Do you think the employees might be thinking about forming a union?" asked Jane.

"Maybe. That's one of the things that I want you to find out," replied Chris.

What advice would you offer to Jane and Chris? Does the real possibility of a union's presence change your advice? Why?

▶ Unions: Health Care and Elsewhere

For years, many people working in health care behaved as though their industry was recession-proof and essentially layoff-proof. As demonstrated during the closing decades of the 1900s, nothing could be further from the truth. Financial pressures, mergers and other affiliations, and the proliferation of healthcare systems have changed health care from an arena in which employment could be considered relatively secure to one in which job security is fully as elusive as it is in many other businesses. When faced with insecurity and uncertainty in an environment they traditionally regarded as stable, some employees will turn to labor unions.

As viewed from an overall perspective, it may seem as though the labor movement in the United States is gradually dying out; for a number of years union membership has been steadily declining in the aggregate workforce. However, at the same time, union membership in the healthcare industry has been increasing. In 1945, American union membership reached its peak, accounting for some 36% of the workforce. Late in the year 2000, union membership totaled about 13.9% of the workforce, the lowest level of union membership in the country since the NLRA was passed in 1935. According to the U.S. Bureau of Labor Statistics, by the end of 2009 the union percentage of the workforce had fallen to 12.3%, and by the end of 2010 it had dropped to 11.9%, representing a loss of 612,000 members during 1 year. Further, it has been estimated that organized labor must add 250,000–500,000 new members per year just to keep pace with the annual attrition in manufacturing jobs (Knight Ridder, 2000). As a consequence of such continuing losses and the perceived need to compensate for them, unions are listening carefully to healthcare workers and high-tech workers and in many instances are actively pursuing these groups of traditionally nonunionized employees.

Although union presence and influence overall may be diminishing, the unions are not going to quietly fade away. Many organizations, surely labor unions, government agencies, and various other entrenched bureaucracies, are self-perpetuating entities whose leaders and members will do everything possible to ensure their continued existence. This is simple human nature, the drive for self-preservation. So, the losses of membership in manufacturing have spurred unions on to redoubling their efforts to organize employees in other industries.

Especially susceptible to organizing pressure in health care are direct caregivers, particularly nurses. Dissatisfaction with pay and increasingly stressful working conditions, aggravated by a shortage of nurses at hospitals across the country, are spurring job actions and the formation of nurses' unions. The recently created National Nurses United, resulting from a combination of the California Nurses Association and several state nursing associations, is doing all it can to develop public support and convince nurses that they need representation, especially during this era of dramatic and often unpredictable change in health care.

The Department of Health and Human Services predicts a shortage of 400,000 nurses by the year 2020. Although the number of registered nurses has increased by approximately 40% since the last half of the 1990s, an increasing number are choosing not to work in hospitals or nursing homes. Rather, approximately two of every five new nurses are opting for easier, better-paying jobs with health maintenance organizations or pharmaceutical companies. The financial pressures holding down salaries and restricting staffing in hospitals are likely to continue for some time; according to the American Hospital Association, fully a third of all hospitals operate at a loss.

Why Workers Join Unions

When unions are organizing or when they are striking or threatening to strike, the public hears a great deal about monetary demands being made of employers. While economic issues are important, insecurity is usually a dominant factor in causing employees to seek union representation. Mounting healthcare costs, layoffs resulting from mergers and acquisitions, and fiscal belt-tightening all have caused many workers to seek protection from a union because they perceive threats to their job security.

Many factors compel employees to seek affiliation with a union. Often, senior managers make erroneous assumptions about their employees. One common error is to assume that the primary goals of most employees are always economic. Another error is to believe that employees are inherently lazy and must be constantly supervised to get them to produce.

If the basis of employee dissatisfaction is lack of trust, giving employees more money will not resolve the underlying problem. Insecurity and lack of communications are significant drivers of employee unrest. Employees want someone to listen to them. This need is strongest when conditions are unsettled and they feel threatened. If workers perceive that no one in their organization is willing to listen to them, they will turn elsewhere, seeking persons who demonstrate a willingness to listen and promise to help them. Union organizers are all too willing to be the ones who will listen.

Another classic error of top management is to assume that because they hear few negative comments, everything is fine among the ranks of employees. Information does not readily travel upward in an organizational structure; numerous obstacles inhibit the upward flow of information. If relationships are weakened by distrust or uncertainty, little of relevance will reach senior managers. Most senior managers know little about what is on the minds of the people at the bottom of the structure.

Another mistake top managers make is assuming that all first-line supervisors and middle managers are, by virtue of their positions, automatically on the side of management when a union beckons. Most lower-level managers started as rank-and-file employees, and some of them have never felt fully accepted by higher management. Senior managers may not realize they have ignored or mistreated supervisors and middle managers until they are threatened by unionization.

Another significant error is to ignore the potential contributions of lower levels of management when union organizing occurs. Top managers often fear the possibility that supervisors will inadvertently commit unfair labor practices or make other mistakes, and they give way to this fear by keeping first-line supervisors away from the organizing action. However, first-line supervisors are in a position to provide the strongest, most direct communication links between workers and higher management. Union organizing campaigns depend on communications. If first-line supervisors are isolated, then management may be stifling its best communication channels.

Economics are usually involved in union campaigns. If all other factors are satisfactory, however, economics alone will promote interest in a union only if the economic disparity is dramatic. Otherwise, employees may seek unionization if they feel insecure about their employment and their future prospects. Major changes in organizational structure, management, operating requirements, job content, and equipment made without notice or explanation invite the sort of unrest that can lead to unionization. If significant changes in upper management alter the prevailing style of organizational culture from being open to authoritarian or autocratic, then unions often follow. When employees are given little or no information about their organization's financial status or its plans and key decisions affecting jobs and careers are made in isolation, they often seek help from unions. Ignoring employee dissatisfaction promotes unionization. If employees rarely receive feedback from management in response to their questions, complaints, or concerns, and the comments they hear are negative, then they will seek unions that will listen to them.

Why Organizations Try to Avoid Unions

Executive management and the board of directors generally want the organization to remain union-free. A primary reason for wishing to remain union-free is to preserve greater latitude in operations and in managing employees. A union is more often than not thought of as an obstacle or hindrance that restricts management's freedom of operation. When a union is in place, the terms of a collective bargaining agreement (union contract) must be followed.

Unions usually increase the cost of doing business and thus increase the cost that must ultimately be borne by consumers. Increases in wages and benefits gained through negotiations are not the only costs attributable to a union. The cost of paying for labor counsel and maintaining a labor relations department or staff can be considerable. From the perspective of management, a union adds cost and effort to running an organization but does not provide tangible or revenue-producing benefits.

A union can significantly realign communicating relationships within an organization. Without a union, communication can flow directly between managers and employees. With a union in place, however, some information must flow through the union. This has the effect of interjecting a third party into an existing two-party relationship. Also, unions often have their own agendas that are not consistent with an organization's goals.

Once established, a major objective of a union is remaining in place. A union can remain and continue to collect its dues and assessments for a prolonged period only by providing value to its members (the organization's employees). One way in which some unions attempt to establish value is by encouraging distrust between employees and management. If relations between employees and management are completely open, cordial, and satisfactory in all respects, then the union is not needed. From the perspective of management, therefore, a union is an extraneous element that increases expenses and aggravation. Unions also make operations more difficult because they are self-perpetuating entities with their own long-range goals.

Management is often late in coming to appreciate the value of positive labor relations. Some senior executives understand some basic truths only after a union has become entrenched. If employees are treated fairly, dealt with openly and honestly, and provided with salaries and benefits that are comparable to those offered throughout the local community, employees are unlikely to turn to a union.

The Legal Framework of Unions

The NLRA of 1935, commonly known as the Wagner Act, is the basis of most of the labor laws in the United States. This act guarantees the right of employees to join unions and engage in collective bargaining, as well as the right to refuse to do so. The NLRA was amended in 1947 by the Taft–Hartley Act. The NLRA established the National Labor Relations Board (NLRB), a government agency created to enforce the provisions of the NLRA.

The Wagner Act originally put clout in the hands of the unions and ended many practices of employers. After a few years, however, it began to appear that too much power had been given to unions. Steps were taken to achieve a better balance between labor and management. The Taft–Hartley Act was an attempt to level the playing field by returning some options to employers and making unions more accountable.

From passage of Taft–Hartley in 1947 until 1975, not-for-profit healthcare institutions were exempt from all provisions of federal labor laws. During that period, only state labor laws applied to such organizations. In 1975, the Taft–Hartley Act was amended to include not-for-profit healthcare organizations as covered employers. The 1975 amendments broadly defined healthcare institutions to include any hospital, convalescent facility, health maintenance organization, clinic, nursing home, extended care facility, or any other institution devoted to the sick, infirm, or aged. They superseded all existing state labor laws that applied to nongovernmental healthcare provider organizations.

The amendments established a 90-day legal notification period for intended negotiations for renewals or modifications of contracts. In all other industries, this period is 60 days. The new law required that the Federal Mediation and Conciliation Service be notified 60 days before a contract expires. In all other industries, the requirement for advance notification is 30 days.

The amendments stated that unions could be required to participate in mediation as necessary for both initial contracts and renewals. No such requirement applies in other industries. Unions must provide 10-day advance notification of a strike, picketing, or any other concerted refusal to work. No such requirement pertains to unions in other industries. In the event of a work stoppage that can disrupt patient care delivery, the Federal Mediation and Conciliation Service can order an impartial board of inquiry to investigate the dispute and report its findings. This provision is unique to the healthcare industry. Finally, the legislation exempted employees belonging to any religion, sect, or other group that conscientiously objected to participation in or support of labor organizations from being required to join or financially support a union as a condition of employment.

Congress intended the 1975 Taft–Hartley amendments to have the NLRB focus on labor disputes and charges of unfair labor practices in health care. It wanted to ensure that patients could be transferred to other institutions without the risk of secondary strikes or boycotts while preserving the right of healthcare employees to strike. It reaffirmed NLRB definitions of supervisors in healthcare institutions being considered as professional employees. It tried to minimize the number of different unions representing employees in a single institution.

Essentially ignoring the intent of the 1975 amendments, the NLRB moved to increase the number of bargaining units in the late 1980s. The Board's rule-making authority came under legal challenge. In April 1991, the U.S. Supreme Court found in favor of the NLRB and the new unit designations. The court allowed up to eight different unions in any acute care facility regardless of its size. The eight units can represent registered nurses, physicians, other professionals, technical employees, skilled maintenance employees, business office clerical employees, security personnel, and other nonprofessional employees.

The Ever-Changing Organizing Environment

As union presence and influence decline in many settings, organized labor and pro-union elements in government are striving to reinvigorate the union movement in the United States. On March 10, 2009, a bill titled the Employee Free Choice Act was introduced into both chambers of Congress. The purpose of this proposed legislation was to establish what was referred to as an "efficient system" to enable employees to form, join, or assist labor organizations; to provide for mandatory injunctions for unfair labor practices; and to serve other purposes. The Employee Free Choice Act was meant to amend the NLRA in three significant ways:

- Eliminate the need for an election to require an employer to accept a union if a majority of employees had already signed cards expressing interest in a union
- Require an employer to negotiate a collective bargaining agreement within 90 days or face compulsory mediation and binding arbitration if mediation fails
- Increase penalties on employers who commit unfair labor practices
- In other words, under the Employee Free Choice Act, a union could become certified without having to win a secret-ballot election.

Reaction to the possibility of the Employee Free Choice Act becoming law was strong from both proponents and opponents. Those who favored it and most likely saw it as an opportunity to revitalize the labor movement claimed that the process that had existed for years was skewed in favor of those who opposed unions, and that workers must literally risk losing their jobs to form a union. Opponents contended that the act would strip workers of the right to a secret ballot, would permit organizers to intimidate workers into accepting a union they might not otherwise choose, and generally would lead to overt coercion by organizers.

As of this writing, the bill advocating the Employee Free Choice Act has gone nowhere, having last been acted upon on April 29, 2009, when it was referred to the House Subcommittee on Health, Employment, Labor, and Pensions. For all practical purposes, this proposed legislation is dead for the time being; there undoubtedly remains among some in Congress the desire to reinvigorate the union movement by making successful organizing easier.

NLRB Involvement

Since the Employee Free Choice Act is currently perceived as a nonissue, the NLRB, which includes in its membership several strongly pro-union activists, is using its substantial ability to shape labor organizing activity through its rule-making authority. The NLRB seems to decide most of the cases that come before it in a manner that makes it easier for unions to coerce and persuade employees and makes it more difficult for union-free employers to oppose organizing. NLRB activity would currently seem to represent the path along which organized labor proponents will work to stimulate increased union organizing.

The Department Manager's Role

If a union is not present and there is no immediate prospect of one being formed, most department managers will have little concern for them. However, employees can seek union representation at any time. Supervisors should have basic knowledge about how unions form and how they operate.

Before a Union Is Formed

The most effective way to prevent union organizing is to create and maintain a work environment in which employees do not feel the need for such representation. Such a work environment includes caring managers who believe that satisfied employees are the best producers, that thorough and open communication is essential, and that one of the most important attributes of supervisors is a willingness to listen to employees. Astute department managers are aware of one fact of organizational life upon which every union organizer counts: If no one in an organization is listening to them, employees will turn to someone else who *will* listen.

Unions are uncommon in organizations having clear, reasonable, and well-communicated work rules and personnel policies consistently applied to all employees. When senior management treats first-line supervisors and middle managers as full-fledged members of management, unions are rarely encountered. Executives make a serious error when they assume that all supervisors are automatically pro-management and anti-union. Union-free organizations implement major changes only after giving ample notice and providing thorough explanations to all employees. Such employers have ongoing and open communication channels to keep employees advised of the organization's status and its financial position. They convey an honest belief that employees and management together can do a better job of serving the organization's customers without the intervention of an outside third party.

Early Organizing Signs and Concerns

Organizing drives are costly for unions. Unions deciding to organize the employees of a particular organization may undertake their activities without fanfare. Unions commonly test their appeal and potential to organize by talking with employees. They quietly estimate their chances of success before becoming a visible presence.

Unions sometimes plan to organize employees in a particular geographic area. They may undertake unionization because a number of employees have asked the union to do so. However, before seeking a representation election, a union will still analyze a facility in an attempt to assess whether the overall climate is favorable.

First-line managers are the first line of defense in union organizing situations. They are in the best position to be the eyes and ears of management before and during an organizing campaign. They are best positioned to serve as effective liaisons between employees and upper management. In general, employees typically view an entire organization in a way similar to how they view their own managers. If a supervisor, the member of management that a group's employees know best, is seen as cold, indifferent, or uncaring, this is how the entire organization is likely to be viewed by those employees.

The importance of security increases when a union is attempting to organize employees. Healthcare organizations are busy places. Without proper and visible means of identifying and controlling visitors, a healthcare organization is only as "secure" as any public gathering place.

When a union is investigating a facility, organizers commonly enter and mingle with employees in public spaces such as a cafeteria or snack bar. As outsiders who have no legitimate business in a facility, external organizers can legally be kept out of the building and off the grounds. When internal access is denied, organizers will often visit external locations frequented by employees. On occasion, they will host off-site informational meetings to which employees are invited.

Organizers look and listen for indications of employee unrest. They are especially interested in identifying problem departments, areas of high turnover and employee dissatisfaction, and managers who are disliked for their harsh, authoritarian, or arbitrary treatment of employees. Organizers often look for martyrs or so-called victims of the system who feel that they have been unjustly treated.

Wages, benefits, and other tangibles receive mention from the very beginning of unionization activity, but rarely are these the real issues that push employees toward forming a union. However, bargaining invariably includes economic issues. Although a union can demand pay and benefits, issues such as respect, inclusion, and open and honest communication are sufficiently intangible that they cannot be acquired by contract.

It is common for many first-line managers to believe that the first indication of union organizing activity consists of people passing out literature on sidewalks around their facility and at employee parking entrances. In addition to containing information about the union and what it claims to be able to do for employees, distributed material usually includes a postcard that employees can use to request additional information or arrange for a personal visit. However, before leaflets appear, a union will most likely have already spent several weeks reviewing a facility and assessing its chances for success. Union representatives may have been quietly meeting with groups of interested employees and have spent time circulating within the targeted facility.

Often a department manager has no way of determining the basis for apparent union interest. However, when there is active interest in organizing, managers may notice changes in employee behavior. Specifically, they may observe new or unusual groupings of employees. When people who have never before associated with each other seem close or secretive, it can mean they share a common interest in a union. Employees from other departments visiting workers during breaks or other personal time are often internal organizers promoting union representation.

Small groups of conversing employees who disband and scatter as a member of management approaches can be an indicator of union organizing activity. An increase in detailed questions about specific employee benefits and other conditions of employment, especially demands to know why some benefits are not more generous or why others are not provided, often herald an organizing campaign.

Other signs of union activity include specific disciplinary actions being openly and vocally challenged and a tendency for departmental employees to question decisions of management. Employees know that to be loyal to the employer or openly opposed to unions can get them ostracized when a union attempts to organize. Employees who are perceived as openly pro-management are kept out of organizing meetings. Some employees who would ordinarily talk with a manager often become silent during union organizing because they do not want to compromise themselves by being seen conversing with management.

After an Election Petition Arrives

After an election petition arrives, managers often work with their legal counsel and human resources to develop a strategy for coping with the organizing campaign. Supervisors must actively campaign against union representation for their employees. All customary methods of employee communication are used, including meetings, individual discussions, question-and-answer sessions, and a significant number of memos, letters, and other written materials.

Managers will be informed of the legal limitations on their actions during an organizing campaign. Inappropriate management conduct can have serious consequences up to and including negating the results of an election. A provision of the NLRA defines an *unfair labor practice* as a threat of reprisal or force or promise of benefits. The NLRA guarantees employers and unions the right to campaign actively during an organizing drive but within specified limits. A union has the right to explain its advantages to employees and convince them to vote for union representation. The employer has the right to try to convince employees that they are better off without the union's presence.

Many unions are not known for full and frank disclosure of all implications of unionization. They often neglect to mention some of the perceived disadvantages of membership.

Actions Managers Can Take

During union organizing efforts, managers are permitted to express opinions or present arguments to employees. They may discuss what is known about the particular union, and they may—and most assuredly should—describe the perceived advantages of remaining union-free. Managers are permitted to compare existing wages and benefits with those of unionized facilities. They may advise employees of the cost of dues, the losses of income during strikes and other work stoppages, and the possibility of fines and special assessments or of being required to serve on picket lines. Managers may note that a union contract may forbid employees from discussing certain kinds of problems directly with managers. They may point out that in some states, a union may demand union membership as a condition of continued employment (a condition referred to as a "closed shop," usually one of the first items demanded when contract negotiations are undertaken), and a strike may disrupt services and endanger health and safety for workers, managers, and the people they serve.

Before a union election occurs, managers are allowed to inform employees that signing a union authorization card is not a vote for the union and doing so does not obligate an employee to vote for the union. Representation elections are conducted by secret ballot so that no one will know how an individual votes. The outcome of a representation election is determined by the majority of employees who actually vote, not by a majority of all eligible voters. This fact alone makes it critically important that people opposing union representation should be sure to vote because it is a certainty that those who are in favor of having the union will vote.

A local union is subject to the governance of its international organization. In this way, considerable control over a facility can be exerted from a distance. Labor laws allow an organization to replace any employee who goes on strike for economic reasons. Such replacements are permanent. Despite any promises organizers may make, no union can force an employer to pay more than it is willing or able to pay in wages or benefits.

Actions Managers Cannot Take

During union organizing, managers cannot threaten or interrogate employees, make promises, or spy on employees for the sake of learning about union activity. A communication is not protected by the free-speech provisions of the NLRA if it contains any of the foregoing prohibited activities. In particular, when unions are trying to organize, management is restrained from promising that wages and benefits will be improved if the union loses its representation election. Supervisors cannot make promises of pay increases, promotions, or other special favors to individual employees in exchange for opposing the union. Department managers are not allowed to threaten employees with job losses, demotions, pay cuts, or reductions in benefits if the union wins.

Promises made by either side during an organizing campaign are regarded differently under organizing rules. As noted previously, the employer, usually speaking through its managers, is legally forbidden to promise rewards of any kind to employees for opposing the union. But while management can make no promises, the union's leadership and its organizers may promise anything they wish to promise. Why the difference? The critical difference lies in the fact that management has the power to deliver on its promises, while the union is powerless to deliver on its promises unless employees vote the union into power. Concerning a union's promises, many employee groups have discovered that after voting a union into the workplace, the union was unable to deliver much of what it promised.

Transferring employees and changing assignments to isolate union support-ers or break up concentrations of pro-union employees is an unfair labor practice and is illegal. Organizations cannot threaten to terminate operations if the union is successful. Managers cannot ask employees any specific questions about union relationships, how people intend to vote, what they think about the union, or who is or is not supporting the union. Questioning prospective employees about past or present union affiliations is illegal. Spying on union meetings or attempting to determine who is attending is an unfair labor practice. Using a third party to threaten, intimidate, or coerce employees is not allowed. Managers may not visit the homes of employees to campaign against a union, although union organizers may do so.

One Extremely Important "Can-Do" for Managers

From the foregoing descriptions of the many restrictions on a manager's behavior during organizing, one might conclude there is little a first-line manager can do other than dispensing prepared information about the benefits of remaining non-union. However, there is one extremely important "can-do" that arises from consid-eration of all of the stated prohibitions on managerial behavior: managers can *listen*.

Managers cannot legally question employees about any aspect of their interest or involvement with unions, but they can receive information that employees pro-vide voluntarily, and use knowledge gained in this manner to assist management's counter-organizing efforts. That is, supervisors are not permitted to ask employees if there is union activity going on, but if employees come to their managers and volunteer that or any other pertinent information, supervisors may listen and use it accordingly.

The implications of the foregoing can be significant. Ordinarily not all employ-ees in a given group will automatically favor the union; many will sign cards just to get the organizers to stop bothering them. If managers maintain honest, open communicating relationships with most of their employees, some of them will vol-unteer information that may be helpful to efforts to remain union-free. Again, there is essentially nothing that supervisors can legally ask their employees about possi-ble union involvement, but prudent managers can always remain available to their employees and listen to them.

Leading Up to the Election

After a union has made its organizing intentions known, it sometimes provides management with a list of internal organizers. These are usually employees in spe-cifically targeted departments. Once such individuals have been identified, their supervisors must become extremely careful in their dealings with them. The status of internal organizer gives them no special privileges. However, because they have declared their organizing status, they will be intentionally sensitive to any discrim-inatory treatment. By officially identifying internal organizers, a union often hopes to trap management into committing unfair labor practices.

Challenges concerning a union and the eligibility of employees to vote usually occur before an election. Managers are technically not included in union member-ship, although exceptions are made in some governmental institutions where repre-sentation is provided by public employer unions.

The activity leading up to a representation election can be frantic and time consuming for those who are working to keep a facility union-free. Although both sides must observe numerous rules, management and a union share the same overriding concern: winning. Each side carefully watches the other for signs of irregularities. Charges of improper conduct are common.

When election day arrives, the rules change. Managers may continue to speak individually with employees and pass out printed information but must avoid holding group meetings during work time at which employees are obligated to hear anti-union messages. The NLRB feels that the day before votes are cast should belong to employees and should be as free from interference as possible. The safest approach for management is to refrain from active campaigning on the day of the election. Managers often simply avoid any discussion of unions and only respond to employee questions.

After voting occurs, the NLRB will certify the results of the election and make them official. This process requires a number of days even though the vote count is immediately known. A simple majority of those voting determines the outcome unless a sufficient number of votes are challenged to question the results. Elections are monitored by employees on behalf of both sides. Individual votes may be challenged if the person voting is deemed to be ineligible. Challenged votes become important in close elections.

A union that loses an election may not try with the same employer again for a full year; NLRB rules require a lapse of at least 1 year before another election can be held involving the same unit of employees. Unions may lose repeatedly, while management can only lose once. In other words, management could conceivably have to win once a year for many years to stay union-free, but a union that wins once is in, usually for good because decertification elections are not especially common. Regardless of the outcome, however, managers must reestablish their working environments after an election is held.

Interacting with a Union

If employees have chosen union representation, all existing channels of employee communication must be kept open to the fullest extent possible. Managers must not back off simply because union representatives are regularly talking with employees. Department managers must understand the legal issues involved in interacting with a union. They must develop a complete understanding of the negotiated and approved collective bargaining agreement.

A common contract provision requires union membership as a condition of continued employment. This provision, resulting in the "closed shop" mentioned earlier, is extremely important to unions because their leadership wants to collect dues from all persons who will benefit from their negotiations.

Department managers often find that a union brings predictability to relationships with employees. Rules govern many activities that formerly depended on a first-line manager's decisions. For example, a formal grievance procedure may eliminate the need to argue with employees about some issues. Complaints are routinely processed rather than negotiated. Managers may not like the process or its outcomes, but the need to generate solutions is removed. For example, union contracts usually contain specific protocols for assigning overtime; these relieve managers of responsibility for many decisions about overtime because the provisions of the contract dictate overtime assignments.

Department managers must adjust to the presence of a union. Unions change normal patterns and often lend a measure of predictability to operations that some managers and employees alike may regard as beneficial even though additional channels of communication must be maintained. However, managers must never forget that a union has its own agenda that largely differs from meeting the needs of its members and the objectives of management.

Decertification

As initially enacted, the NLRA strongly favored unions and took numerous steps to protect employees from abuse by employers. In amending the NLRA, the Labor Management Relations Act (Taft–Hartley) took a more balanced approach to protecting the rights of individual employees from abuse by both employers and unions. Taft–Hartley made it possible for employees to get out from under a union that no longer seemed to serve their purposes or be acting in their best interests. This change allowed employees to remove a union when its leaders failed to meet membership expectations through a process called *decertification.*

A petition for decertification cannot be filed within a union's first year, that period legally described as its "certification year." A newly chosen union is given this period to negotiate a contract and demonstrate what it can do for its members. A bargaining unit is allowed to have only one election—whether for representation or decertification—within any 12-month period.

Management cannot be involved in initiating a move toward decertification. In particular, managers cannot volunteer information to employees about how decertification can be accomplished. Management cannot tell employees that they would be treated better without the union, nor can they suggest that employees generate a petition to decertify a union. Finally, managers must avoid behaving in ways that are intended to encourage employees to seek decertification.

During the initiation stage, management is legally permitted only to respond to employee questions about decertification. Managers cannot provide encouragement to pursue decertification or offer unsolicited advice on how to go about doing so.

Should a decertification effort reach the petition stage, the employer can still do little more than respond to employee questions. At this stage, however, some responses can be more specific and helpful. For instance, management can direct employees to appropriate authorities at the NLRB and can provide additional information about the decertification process as long as doing so is in direct response to employee inquiries. However, this is assistance at a minimal level because management is still forbidden to help with the wording of a petition, or allow the petition to be transmitted on the organization's letterhead. Managers cannot allow employees to solicit petition signatures during working hours or provide space for signing to occur. Management cannot provide time off for an employee to file the petition.

Once a decertification petition is filed and a decertification election campaign officially begins, management has options for its activities. Management is allowed to express its views about the presence of a union. However, these views cannot include direct or implied threats of reprisals for retaining the union or promises of rewards for removing it. At this stage of a decertification campaign, management may communicate its views to employees by letter or give comparisons of wages and benefits of union and nonunion workers to employees. Management may hold meetings with employees, provided that attendance is voluntary.

Two important limitations exist: Management may not interfere with the right of employees to choose between decertification or not; and management must avoid making promises or threats that could upset the conditions under which employees must make their choice.

The Future

The future of unionization in the United States is uncertain. Union membership peaked in the middle of the 1900s. It has gradually declined since that time. Experts do not agree on all of the causes for the decline, although most agree that unions have lost members as the basis of much of the American economy has changed from manufacturing to service. President Reagan's dismissal of the air traffic controllers in 1981, which effectively broke the Professional Air Traffic Controllers union, was a pivotal event. Trade agreements have led to the further loss of manufacturing jobs. The losses of auto manufacturers such as General Motors, Ford, and Chrysler and their suppliers have also led to decreases in union membership. Healthcare workers have become attractive targets for unionization, being courted not only by those unions that have traditionally sought the participation of healthcare workers but also by unions such as the United Auto Workers, Teamsters, and other unions not previously associated with health care. The future of labor unions will be interesting for workers, employers, and society.

▶ Conclusion

Unionization is attractive to workers who are frustrated. Historically, unions have offered what they claim to be a more attractive option to workers. Employers and employees have different opinions about unions. The former generally feel that unions lead to an erosion of management autonomy; the latter feel that unions provide a voice that will advocate for them. Collectively, bargained contracts govern the interactions between unionized workers and their employers.

Legislation governs the interactions and activities of unions and managers. The NLRA of 1935, commonly known as the Wagner Act, and its amendments remain the basis of most of labor law in the United States. These statutes provide guidelines for the conduct of both employees and employers as they interact with each other. Violations of these guidelines are known as unfair labor practices. The guidelines specify the steps a union must take when seeking to be accepted as the representative of workers as well as the steps necessary for the union to be discharged through a process called decertification.

🔎 CASE STUDY: Resolution

Returning to the conversation between Jane Pinkerton and Chris Smith, the two managers, Chris's instructions to Jane were not in the best interests of their employer. In fact, they could be interpreted as an unfair labor practice. Managers must follow established rules when union formation is involved. The Wagner Act and its legislative modifications delineate steps that employers can and cannot legally take. Managers must give union organizers reasonable courtesy and ensure that they are treated in a fair manner.

SPOTLIGHT ON CUSTOMER SERVICE

Customer Service and Relations with Labor Unions

The presence of a labor union in an organization usually adds an additional layer of responsibility to a human resources department. Federal laws require regular reports from the management of organizations in which employees are unionized.

A collective bargaining agreement (union contract) provides guidance as to how workers and managers must interact with each other, guidelines for how disputes will be resolved, and information on working conditions, pay bands, and benefits. Frequently, a union contract establishes formal channels of communication between workers and managers.

Despite the absence of formal references to customer service in most union contracts, the practice manages to survive (at worst) and flourish (at best). Managers and workers usually find common ground on the topic of customer service.

Questions for Review and Discussion

1. Why do unions target healthcare workers?
2. Why is unionization among healthcare providers increasing when union membership in the total workforce is declining?
3. Define an unfair labor practice, and provide three or four examples of unfair labor practices.
4. Why is it sometimes claimed that the majority of union elections are won or lost by management long before a union ever appears?
5. If noneconomic issues drive employees to become organized, why are nearly all bargaining table demands economic in nature?
6. Why is it advisable to have a comprehensive policy governing solicitation and the posting of information on the premises in place before any signs of active union organizing appear?
7. Why it is considerably more difficult to decertify a union than to elect one?
8. Provide two specific examples of behavior that represent each of the four prohibitions on management conduct during union organizing: threatening, interrogating, promising, and spying.
9. If two employees said, "We want to talk to you about this union stuff that's going around," how would you respond?
10. As a supervisor, would you prefer to interact with one or several unions? Why?
11. What are the advantages and disadvantages of working with a union contract on a day-to-day basis?
12. Why is distributing union literature to employees arriving to or departing from work frequently assumed to be the first stage of active union organizing?
13. What would you say to employees in a meeting if your organization was experiencing a union organizing campaign? Would you encourage them to think carefully about favoring union membership? Why or why not?
14. What help can you legally provide to a small number of employees who ask for your help in getting their union decertified?
15. What are the key differences between healthcare and non-health industries in the manner in which work stoppages may be conducted?

Resources
Books

Holley, W. H., Jr., Ross, W. H., & Wolters, R. S. (2017). *The labor relations process* (11th ed.). Boston, MA: Cengage Learning.

Huzzard, T., Scott, R., & Gregory, D. (2005). *Strategic unionism and partnership: Boxing or dancing?* New York, NY: Palgrave Macmillan.

Pozgar, G. D. (2019). *Legal aspects of health care administration* (13th ed.). Burlington, MA: Jones & Bartlett Learning.

Rowley, C. (2005). *The management of people: Human resource management in context.* London, England: Spiro.

Periodicals

Associated Press. (2001, June 1). Stressed nurses striking more. *Democrat & Chronicle*, Rochester, NY.

Colvin, A. J. (2003). Institutional pressures, human resource strategies, and the rise of nonunion dispute resolution procedures. *Industrial and Labor Relations Review, 56*, 375–392.

Knight Ridder News Service. (2000, September 20). Unions set sights on high-tech workers. *Democrat & Chronicle*, Rochester, NY.

Kristof, N. (2015, February 19). The cost of a decline in unions. *New York Times*, New York, NY.

Mishak, M. J., & York, A. (2011, October 11). Governor Jerry Brown is giving unions most of what they seek. *Los Angeles Times*, Los Angeles, CA.

Radcliffe, B. (2009, June 28). Unions: Do they help or hurt workers? Investopedia (Website).

CHAPTER 21

Special Support: Human Resources Arbitration and the Use of Consultants

CHAPTER OBJECTIVES

After studying this chapter, readers will be able to:

- Understand the process of arbitration and its advantages.
- Know the different variations of arbitration in use.
- Differentiate arbitration and mediation.
- Understand how arbitrators are credentialed and selected.
- Know about the different kinds of consultants and the services they provide.
- Understand the reasons for engaging consultants.
- Know how to locate and engage a consultant.

▶ Chapter Summary

This chapter discusses how and why outside consultants and arbitrators are used to resolve issues and complete projects within organizations.

Arbitration is a cost-saving alternative to litigation in which individuals present their positions to a neutral third party for resolution. Arbitration usually involves seeking resolution by consensus or compromise. Arbitration is becoming more common in human resources disputes; its use is frequently embedded in progressive disciplinary policies and ordinarily provided for in collective bargaining agreements (union contracts). Arbitration has far more flexible rules than courts. Critics argue that arbitration favors large organizations and is unfair to individuals. The lack of involvement by legal counsel is seen by some as a shortcoming of the process. Arbitrators usually have relevant credentials to the issue at hand.

$\mathcal{P}$ CASE STUDY: Ever Consider Arbitration?

Mike Stephens has been late for work five times in the last 3 months. Janice Brooks, his supervisor at Lakeview Medical Center, claims that Mike's behavior is unacceptable and discharges him. Mike's union complains that the discharge was unfair because the hospital's progressive discipline policy was not followed. The union claims that Mike was not properly warned that being chronically late was considered sufficiently serious that discharge was possible. Union and management representatives argue over the case. In four meetings involving progressively higher-level personnel, no agreement is reached. The options are dwindling. Mike wants to file for unemployment. A review of the collective bargaining agreement provides little guidance but does mention arbitration. Arbitration has never been used. What recommendations would you offer to the various parties in this case? Why?

Consultants are hired to provide technical expertise and experience. Although involving a service from outside of the organization, using a consultant is not the same as outsourcing an activity. Outsourcing literally involves sending the organization's work out to be accomplished by other organizations; a consultant, however, is engaged to come into the hiring organization to aid in solving particular problems for which the organization, for a variety of reasons, lacks the appropriate expertise and independent viewpoint of the consultant. The services of this professional resource represent a temporary partnership with the organization.

▶ Arbitration

Under the law, arbitration is a legal alternative to litigation; it is often used to avoid clogging court calendars. In arbitration, the parties in a dispute present their positions to a neutral third party for resolution. The parties involved may agree to the arbitration or it may be required by a contract provision or statute. This neutral third party is referred to as an arbitrator. In *binding arbitration*, the decision of the arbitrator is final; it cannot be challenged.

The American Arbitration Association creates arbitration panels from among its members. Unless one party claims there was gross injustice, collusion, or fraud, arbitration specified by a contract can be converted into a legal judgment by petition to the appropriate court. Often states will require mandatory but nonbinding arbitration to give involved parties a clear preview of the result they may receive in an attempt to have them accept an arbitrator's decision.

Arbitration uses rules of evidence and procedures that are less formal than those followed in trial courts. This usually leads to a faster and less-expensive resolution of disagreements.

Many types of arbitration are in use. Binding arbitration is similar to a court proceeding in that an arbitrator has the power to impose a decision; binding arbitration may be limited by one or more agreements made in advance of a hearing. A common example involves setting minimum and maximum limits on a settlement. In nonbinding arbitration, an arbitrator has the power to recommend but not impose a decision. Many contracts require mandatory arbitration in the event of a dispute. This may be reasonable when an arbitrator is neutral; however, it is open to criticism with reason when an organization that writes a contract is able to influence the choice of arbitrator. Financial and healthcare organizations frequently impose such requirements.

Another method used to resolve conflict is *mediation*. A mediator is a third party who attempts to find points of agreement between disagreeing parties. Mediation is a method of resolution that is designed to help disagreeing parties resolve a dispute without going to court. A mediator's goal is to find a compromise that is fair and acceptable to both sides in a dispute. The process is less formal than arbitration, and a mediator has no power to impose a solution. A mediated agreement is not legally binding without a court order. Mediation has no formal rules of evidence or set procedures to follow. A mediator and the parties usually agree on informal ways to proceed. Mediators' goal is to help disagreeing parties to find common ground. However, mediation does not always result in a settlement, and when mediation fails, a court trial typically follows.

Occasionally, an arbitrator is required to choose between the proposals of the disagreeing parties. This is referred to as final-offer arbitration and is specified before the arbitration begins. This approach is designed to encourage the parties to moderate their initial positions.

The only real limitation on arbitrators is that they may not exceed the limits of their authority in granting an award. An example of exceeding authority might be awarding one party with a personal possession belonging to the other party when the case concerns a contract dispute related to business.

To ensure that arbitration is effective and to increase the credibility of the process, arbitrators sometimes work in groups. This is known as "sitting as a panel." The most typical panel size is three. Often one member of the panel is known to be sympathetic to one party, the second member is known to be sympathetic to the other party, and the third panel member is neutral. Another division may include two attorneys with expertise in different aspects of the dispute and an experienced, neutral arbitrator as the lead panelist.

Certification is more commonly encountered in mediation than in arbitration. Certification is based on specific and substantive knowledge related to the case at hand. The standards of membership for some specialized organizations for which membership is voluntary often serve as a proxy for certification. For example, the National Academy of Arbitrators restricts membership to labor arbitrators who have written a specified number of decisions within the preceding 5 years.

Rosters of arbitrators are normally assembled based on combinations of the criteria used for credentialing. The composition of different rosters relies heavily on educational qualifications and experience rather than on assessment of performance. When rosters are used to assemble a panel of potential arbitrators, a short list of names is created. Each side is alternatively allowed to strike names until a single arbitrator is selected. An alternative approach is to apply a similar procedure to a prescreened roster of members.

Advantages of Arbitration

Arbitration permits all participating parties and the arbitrator to observe the total problem and related issues for themselves. This is especially useful in determining fault regarding issues surrounding adequate disclosure. Arbitration resolves problems rather than simply stating or restating opinions. It often prevents future conflicts from occurring by resolving present problems. Instead of creating adversarial positions, arbitration promotes relationships that can be constructive and helpful. In situations involving customers, goodwill is not damaged because existing customer relationships are not destroyed. Arbitration saves time. Hearings can be scheduled in a matter of weeks rather than the months typically required for a court hearing. Arbitration is flexible; parties to arbitration have the option of being represented by an attorney. Arbitration is an attractive alternative because of its flexibility and because its cost is usually far less than the cost of a court proceeding.

Arbitration can usually be conducted in a private setting, so others will not be aware of the proceedings. Arbitrators are chosen for their expertise in the area of conflict; they are typically attorneys or other experienced professionals with a specific background in the type of case involved. In consumer and other small-scale disputes, arbitrators may simply be local citizens who are willing to serve in this capacity.

Unlike attorneys and courts of law, arbitrators are not bound by precedent. They enjoy significant latitude in matters such as accepting evidence, participating in the proceedings, questioning witnesses, and reaching conclusions. Arbitrators may visit sites outside of a hearing room, seek additional evidence, or call on expert witnesses. They have the autonomy to decide whether the parties may be represented by legal counsel. They are not bound by the rules of procedure that guide court proceedings.

In labor–management cases and similar disputes, an arbitrator normally renders a decision in writing. This is accompanied by as much detail as a full written opinion handed down by a court. In other settings, awards may be delivered with no written or oral explanation. In general, full-length written awards are used in situations in which parties expect the case may provide guidance in similar situations in the future. A decision without a written explanation is generally used when the parties desire speed or economy. Unwritten decisions may be requested in situations where there is fear that a losing party might use an error in the decision to challenge the result in court.

Arbitration is appropriate when two parties know they will be unable to resolve a dispute by negotiation or mediation. The parties usually desire a decision that is likely to be both faster and more expert than they think they would be likely to receive in court. Arbitration is useful as a last resort embedded into a structured relationship in advance. It is typically the last step in negotiation because the prospect of compulsory and binding arbitration may help both parties to concentrate on achieving a settlement. Such a resolution may be less than ideal, but it is usually better than a court decision. It is usually less risky and costly than a trial. Arbitration is not useful in situations in which one party seeks a definitive answer that will provide public precedent for similar cases in the future.

Certification, credentialing, and rosters are different concepts that reflect levels of training or qualification for arbitrators. Certification is an official designation conferred on an arbitrator who has met particular standards. Credentialing is the process by which an official or semiofficial body determines the standards appropriate for practitioners of a particular profession or providers of a given service. Arbitrators may be credentialed by more than one group. Credentialing may be determined by philosophy, or it may be determined after reviewing the decisions of an arbitrator. Credentialing may refer to the act of obtaining particular credentials. Rosters are lists of professionals who have been determined to be appropriately credentialed. However, inclusion on a roster does not guarantee formal certification. Typical systems for credentialing, certification, and assembling rosters vary.

Establishing credentials for arbitrators usually involves educational qualifications and an assessment of prior experience and performance. Educational qualifications may include an advanced degree or other specialized education or evidence of having completed a particular course of training. Assessment of performance is accomplished by observing actual arbitration cases by an experienced arbitrator who rates the new arbitrator's performance on the basis of established performance criteria. Alternatively, similar observation and rating may be completed in a simulated setting. Unlike mediation, in which meetings provide the best opportunities for observation, most of an arbitrator's work is performed away from the disputing parties. A full written rationale usually accompanies every arbitration decision. Important criteria include fully understanding the facts in a case and interpreting conflicting facts in a sensible manner. An arbitrator must then decide the case according to standards, usually contractual, that actually apply to a given situation. Finally, an arbitrator must be able to explain the decision in a clear manner using language acceptable to a losing party.

Critics of arbitration argue that the process can be unfair to an individual in a dispute with a large organization. In such situations, the choice of an arbitrator may limit options of individuals. Arbitration panels may not be balanced. Some critics feel that an absence of legal representation is harmful to individuals; they also note that arbitration proceedings are rarely public events. These potential disadvantages increase the importance of professionalism and ethical standards among arbitrators.

Human Resources Arbitration

As human beings interact with each other in organizational situations, problems can and do arise. Many problems are resolved through conflict resolution processes and progressive discipline policies. Others are resolved using steps outlined in collective bargaining agreements. In recent years, arbitration has been introduced as another method. Managers and employees both generally appreciate the flexibility of arbitration. They also appreciate the opportunity to have a neutral third party listen and design a resolution that usually involves a measure of compromise. The element of compromise is often mentioned as a positive aspect of arbitration.

Organizations that have elected to incorporate arbitration usually specify it as a component or option of a progressive discipline process. Arbitration is directly specified in some collective bargaining agreements. The source of an arbitrator may also be specified. Successful organizations delineate a method for selecting an arbitrator.

Once an arbitrator is identified, a hearing date is agreed upon. The parties present their arguments and additional material they feel is needed. The arbitrator listens, asks questions as needed, and then dismisses the parties. A few weeks are typically allowed for the arbitrator to review the information of the case and search for other arbitration cases that may be relevant. The arbitrator usually renders a binding decision.

The majority of individuals and organizations having used arbitration with problems related to human resources have been satisfied with the process. Winning and losing parties both typically feel they have been treated in a reasonable manner. All parties appreciate the speed of binding arbitration, and they appreciate the common element of compromise. Each party gains something in most decisions, and allowing both parties to save face contributes to a more rapid restoration of normal relationships when compared with dispute resolution according to a set of inflexible rules.

🔍 *Ever Consider Arbitration? Case Study Resolution*

Returning to the matter of Mike Stephens, arbitration is the only remaining option. If the union requests arbitration, Lakeview Hospital has no choice but to agree. The union submits a form to the Federal Mediation and Conciliation Service requesting a panel of five potential arbitrators. The federal agency sends a list of five arbitrators and their biographies to both the union and the hospital. The names are chosen at random from the hundreds on file with the agency. Taking turns, each party strikes a name, alternating until only one name remains. This person becomes the arbitrator. The hospital and union agree to file informational briefs within 30 working days. A month later, the arbitrator issues a decision that is binding on all concerned. The arbitrator determined that the hospital acted improperly and ordered Mike to be reinstated. The hospital was also ordered to give him 75% of his back pay. At the same time and in accordance with the progressive discipline policy, the hospital may place a written warning in Mike's personnel file, bypassing the requirement for a verbal warning. This case illustrated one of the important features of arbitration: compromise.

▶ Human Resource Consultants

Expert advice and assistance are needed at various times in almost any business or organization. One source of such help is external consultants. Consultants are usually experts in their field with both experience and education that span years. They are often able to successfully address a particular problem or issue that persons within the organization cannot effectively deal with because they have failed to correct the situation themselves, they do not have the depth of knowledge required, they have vested interests in the status quo, or they are simply too close to the situation to see the possibilities for improvement. Consultants work with the organization's employees in seeking solutions to problems. The findings and recommendations of a consultant are turned over to the organization's management who will accept the recommendations in whole or in part, ask for more information, or reject the recommendations and go their own way in spite of consultants' best recommendations. (This latter state—rejection of a consultant's recommendation—occurs more often than one might think when a consultant's conclusions run contrary to certain parties' vested interest in the status quo or threaten a powerful individual's "territory.") Frequently, however, consultants' recommendations lead to positive change in the organization.

As noted earlier, engaging the services of a consultant does not constitute outsourcing. By conventional definition, outsourcing refers to a permanent or long-term arrangement between an organization and an outside party to provide specific services. Probably the most common example of outsourcing by a healthcare organization is the use of an outside payroll-processing service. Some experts in specific fields of interest provide both outsourcing and consulting services. The key difference is often the length of time for which services are engaged; outsourcing is more likely to be permanent or at least open ended, whereas consulting is temporary.

A consulting engagement may extend over months and once in a while years, but briefer engagements are more common. Typically, a consultant is engaged to address a particular problem or issue. When the objectives of the consulting project have been met, the consultants leave.

Senior managers often challenge the supposed necessity for the use of consultants. Consultants are often regarded as outsiders who lack knowledge of the managers' organization. Consultants are engaged for several common reasons: they have specialized knowledge, technical expertise, or experience that can be brought to bear on a particular problem. Outsiders are needed when no one present in the organization has the needed skills or knowledge.

Often making changes or altering the capability of a particular sector of the organization is facilitated when problems can be viewed from the perspective of an outsider. Although outsiders may lack organization-specific knowledge, they are not fettered by the traditions, experiences, and politics of existing relationships. The outside point of view is free from organizational bias; an experienced outsider arrives free of interpersonal entanglements or preconceived notions.

In addition to the foregoing reasons for using them, consultants are often used to do work for which regular employees do not have time. Consultants are also used to perform sensitive tasks; a consultant may be used when a scapegoat is needed to take the apparent responsibility for unpopular decisions. Some senior managers have been known to use a consultant to avoid making decisions that are likely to cause hard feelings. Examples include cases of reorganizing or downsizing that necessitate employee layoffs. Consultants in such roles do the "dirty work" for the organization and then leave. Remaining managers are then able to proceed without experiencing the ill feelings that might otherwise be attached to them for making unpopular decisions. An outside consultant may also be brought in to suggest changes when senior managers decide to reorganize a business unit. After the consultant makes the changes and leaves, the managers who remain are spared from responsibility for unpopular decisions made by the consultant.

Consultants are often cost efficient. Their services are specialized and usually needed for just relatively brief periods of time. Using a consultant avoids the costs associated with hiring someone into a specific position, and when a project is completed, the consultant departs, saving the organization the costs of termination. The organization does not have to be concerned with benefits because consultants are responsible for their own; consultants are contract employees, usually taken on for a specific project or task and paid what may be a negotiated fee or a fee based on the value of the estimated time the engagement will require.

Consultants provide an independent perspective, and they are usually immune to the political pressures or personality-based demands that may exist in the organization. They are free to provide expert opinions, opinions that are usually well grounded in experience or specialized knowledge. External funding sources may engage the services of a consultant to provide independent assurance of the viability of a project before investing in it.

Bankers and investors sometimes use outside consultants to provide additional expertise in investigating major potential transactions; there are some consultants who specialize in assessing the relative soundness of a proposed investment or transaction.

Consultants are sometimes used to provide training for key employees and are occasionally used to provide temporary leadership while an organization searches

🔍 CASE STUDY: Correcting Hodge-Podge Growth

Tom was appointed president of a community health system 18 months ago. In addition to a 350-bed hospital, the system had an outpatient facility, a rehabilitation center, and an occupational health clinic that served the workers of several industries in the surrounding area. Tom has come to know the senior managers and other supervisory personnel in the system. He appreciates how proudly the people in the community regard the health system.

The system had expanded over the years without any master plan for growth. This fact was becoming painfully obvious as Tom contemplated the organizational chart for the system. The outpatient clinic originally began as an independent practice started by three physicians. In a single month, the senior partner had become the hospital's medical director, another partner had died in a car accident, and the third had been recalled to naval duty. The hospital simply absorbed the practice.

The occupational medicine clinic began as a rehabilitation service for the clinic and was working to return local farmers to their fields. Several manufacturing facilities had located nearby, bringing jobs and more people to the community. None of the growth had been planned.

Tom wanted to reorganize the system. He discussed the idea with several senior managers. Each had different suggestions. He tried a second round of informal conversations that had yielded similar results—or as Tom preferred to think of them, nonresults. He was getting frustrated. Tom's classes in business school had not included training in organizational design or human resources. He decided to seek out the services of a consultant or consulting firm that specialized in human resources.

Why should Tom think about getting help from a consultant? What advice would you offer to Tom? Where could he find a consultant? How could he engage the services of a qualified consultant?

for a permanent successor to a key manager or a specialized employee who departed unexpectedly.

Consultants generally provide benefits to the organizations using their services. They bring their added expertise to strengthen and focus business plans; they introduce new expertise or skills into an organization or department. A consultant can usually focus attention in a sufficiently clear manner such that objectives are clarified and targets become more achievable.

Astute employees are able to learn from consultants. Often, the employees' ability to solve problems improves through their exposure to knowledgeable consultants. Even if the advice a consultant provides is not better than the advice of existing supervisors and managers, the consultant's advice is often perceived as superior because it comes from an outside source.

Types of Consultants

Based on the services they provide, consultants can be divided into two major categories: *process* and *expert*. Process consultants typically possess general knowledge about business or organizations; they are hired to address a variety of general issues.

Their experience has been acquired in a variety of settings, and this variety of experience is their strength. Process consultants draw upon their experience to solve problems in new situations. Because they are outsiders, they can provide a less biased perspective than can an employee.

In comparison, an expert consultant has specific training or experience in a particular field. An expert consultant is hired for that specialized knowledge. In human resource terms, experts are often hired to conduct training, create strategic plans, or provide focused advice.

Organizations often use process consultants when they decide to identify problem areas and make changes. Such a consultant may be used when no clear consensus exists among senior managers. Process consultants gather information by reviewing data and observing and talking with employees throughout an organization. During the conversations, process consultants often teach employees about alternative procedures or operations. Although employees usually appreciate such information, they must understand that the consultant is a helper and facilitator of change, not a permanent employee. At the conclusion of the fact-finding phase of an engagement, a process consultant meets with senior managers to discuss proposed changes and how best to introduce and implement them into the organization.

The services of an expert consultant are typically engaged to address a specific problem. Reorganizations are common tasks that are assigned to experts. They are also used to analyze problem areas or processes. Examples include recruitment, payroll, employee training, benefits administration, and creating retirement packages. Expert consultants usually have experience directly applicable to the problem. After gathering data and analyzing an organization's situation, they make recommendations to senior managers. Implementation of their recommendations may be continued by the expert consultant, coordinated by a different expert, or handled by the organization's employees who have the necessary knowledge and expertise.

Engaging a Consultant

Before contacting or interviewing potential consultants, it is essential to understand the need to be addressed by a consultant. Once the need has been specified and the type of consultant has been determined, prospective consultants can be identified. A package of information, often called a request for proposal (RFP), should be prepared before seeking an individual consultant or firm. The request should include an overview of the organization, its structure, its mission, and a short history. The request should outline the problem and why the organization considers it to be an area or topic of concern. The expectations of the consultant, an estimate of the time to be made available, and a starting date should be included. Finally, the request should identify the organization's contact person who will oversee the project. The RFP will be used by potential consultants to generate their proposals.

Consultants are identified by several processes. Experience or word of mouth is typically a reliable method. Professionals who provide services are usually able to recommend qualified consultants. Such referrals are reliable to the extent that the word of the person making the suggestions is trusted. Local universities and colleges may have faculty members with the desired expertise. The reliability of such contacts rests on the reputation of the educational institution and the person being asked for the referral. Most reputable consultants and consulting organizations belong to professional associations. These associations can provide leads for consultants. The reliability of the leads is proportional to the code of conduct that such associations have and the extent to which it is enforced. Telephone directories list consultants. This approach is appealing by its simplicity and ease of access; however, the directory publisher simply collects a fee for listing and does not screen or review any persons or firms that are listed. A local Better Business Bureau or Chamber of Commerce may be able to provide information about complaints received.

Two to four potential consultants are commonly identified, presented with the RFP, and asked to submit a proposal that responds to the request. Proposals from ethical firms or individual consultants should include a budget. A proposal forms the basis for negotiations. As negotiations progress, individuals or firms submitting noncompetitive proposals should be identified and notified that their proposals have been rejected. This is both polite and an appropriate business practice, and it retains the possibility of again sending RFPs to these firms at some time in the future. Issues of work and cost are discussed until a single consultant is identified and selected. All parties should clearly understand the nature of the services that will be provided, who will be performing the work, the nature of any products to be generated, who will own them, the cost, and the schedule for activities. A contract based on the proposal is created and signed. A sample consulting contract is found in Appendix 22-A at the conclusion of this chapter.

A consulting contract should include details of the work to be completed, products to be developed, and a means for evaluating progress. Fees should be delineated. Time and available money for each phase of a project should be clearly defined. The responsibilities of both the consulting team and the organization's personnel should be defined. A schedule for payment should be included. Finally, a means for terminating the contract should be agreed upon. Although contracts for consulting engagements are infrequently terminated early, agreeing upon a method before beginning work is appreciated if such a need arises.

Large engagements often require many individuals to perform the work. Personnel who will be performing the work should be understood and agreed upon. Ethical consultants discuss the qualifications and costs of proposed members for a consulting team. The person presenting the proposal may not be the individual supervising the activities of junior consultants on a day-to-day basis. Access and clearance for all members of a consulting team must be arranged prior to the beginning of a project.

On the first day of an engagement, members of the consulting team and organization managers should be introduced to one another. Organizational personnel to be included should reflect internal political protocols and the nature of the project to be addressed. The location for working should be agreed upon. Organizations usually provide space for consultants to do their work. This alternative is usually preferable to taking data and documents away from the premises of a client.

A consultant's progress should be monitored on a regular basis. Regular monitoring helps to prevent surprises for all concerned. Regular meetings provide an opportunity to learn and identify related or unanticipated issues. Potential solutions can be discussed. Consultants have an interest in monitoring the implementation of their proposed solutions to ensure that they are carried out as planned. The essentials of this section are summarized in **TABLE 21-1**.

TABLE 21-1 Rules or Guidelines for Using Consultants

1. Define the scope or boundaries of the problem or issue to be addressed
2. Investigate expertise of consultant
   - Previous clients
   - Previous work
   - Basis for expertise
     ○ Education
     ○ Experience
3. Know the fee and how it is calculated
   - Hourly
   - For the engagement
4. Establish responsibility for expenses
   - Who pays for what
   - What expenses are included
     ○ Food
     ○ Transportation
     ○ Lodging
     ○ Per diem
5. Payment schedule
   - What documentation is required
   - When are expense reimbursements due
   - What form should the payments be in
6. Set limits on service or length of engagement
7. Establish prior to signing a contract
   - Objectives
   - Timetable
   - Deliverables
   - Standards for evaluation
   - Exit strategy or conditions
8. Establish supervisory and reporting relationship in organization
9. Establish mechanism for dissolving contract

Summary: Why a Consultant?

Consultants are hired or engaged for a number of reasons. They are commonly used to resolve a particular problem. Expertise may or may not be available within an organization. An organization may have tried to resolve a problem and failed. A consultant provides a fresh start and opportunity for resolution. A consultant may represent a compromise when an organization's internal managers cannot reach a consensus. Time may be lacking.

Consultants should not be used when complete trust is lacking between an organization and a proposed consultant. They should not be used when questionable or illegal activities are contemplated. Finally, they should not be used when the qualifications of the consultant cannot stand up to external scrutiny.

In general, all parties should strive to minimize or eliminate surprises except in the nature of findings generated by a consultant. Trust is an essential component that must be present before a project begins. Remember that a consultant is an outside contractor who is usually engaged for a particular purpose or to achieve a specific objective.

🔍 *Correcting Hodge-Podge Growth— Case Study Resolution*

Returning to Tom, president of a community health system, his plan to hire a consultant specialized in human resources made sense. If carefully selected, the consultant had the potential to make up for an educational deficiency in Tom's professional training. Using a consultant also allowed Tom to avoid criticism when reorganization was announced. Unpopular changes could be attributed to the consultant, allowing Tom and the other managers to move forward.

Tom called several friends whose opinions he trusted. Their suggestions led to two different consulting firms. Tom checked out the reputations of each before making a personal contact. He also put together a request for proposal that outlined his goals for the hospital system, provided a bit of history, and included a general timetable. Both firms responded with proposals. Over the next 2 weeks, Tom discussed each proposal and chose the proposal that satisfied his goals. He let the other firm know that another consultant offered a proposal more appropriate to his organization's needs. The competitor thanked Tom and offered to stay in contact in case difficulties arose in the future.

Tom completed and signed a contract. Because of the work and level of detail that had gone into the plan, the consulting engagement and reorganization were successfully completed. The consultant helped affected managers adjust to different roles in the healthcare system. At their final meeting, the consultant asked Tom if he would be willing to provide a business reference in the future. Tom agreed, and the consulting engagement was brought to a successful conclusion.

▶ Conclusion

Arbitration and consultation offer attractive alternatives to internal problem-solving. Organizations can use the expertise and knowledge of a consultant or arbitrator to resolve a variety of issues. Consultants are becoming more commonly used by organizations throughout the United States in health care as well as in other industries. Managers in health care must understand the potential uses for consultants as well as how to establish trust and good working relationships, and communication of roles and responsibilities.

Arbitration is a useful way to resolve disputes while avoiding the impracticality and cost of the court system. A neutral third party, an arbitrator, hears the positions of two parties in a dispute. The arbitrator presents a solution to the problem. When compared with traditional court systems, arbitration uses different, more relaxed rules of operation. Arbitration usually results in faster and less expensive resolutions compared with courts. Arbitrators are typically credentialed by a professional organization or through other means. Many disputes related to human resources are being arbitrated rather than litigated. Guidelines for the use of arbitration are typically found in collective bargaining agreements or progressive disciplinary policies.

SPOTLIGHT ON CUSTOMER SERVICE

Customer Service and Consultants

Consultants are experts in a particular aspect of knowledge or operations. They are usually hired to perform a limited task. Consultants are typically short-term visitors in organizations. They are not employees of the organizations that hire them. Rather, they are employed by companies that rent out their services.

Most consultants provide excellent customer service. This is essential to their continued employment and long-term professional success. Many employees of organizations that hire consultants lack a commitment to providing good customer service. To a casual observer, this must seem strange because good customer service is always appreciated.

A crucial difference between "regular" employees and consultants is the length of time that they spend serving the organization that funds their paychecks. Consultants are short-timers compared with employees. Short-timers must constantly prove themselves, while long-timers have the luxury of stable, steady employment. If long-timers regarded their employment as a series of short-term engagements, they would be likely to have different attitudes toward their customers. They would also be likely to understand the importance of customer service if their continued employment depended on their treatment of users of the programs or services that their organizations produced.

Questions for Review and Discussion

1. Is arbitration an option for human resources problems? How do employees enter arbitration?
2. How are the processes or rules of arbitration different from those of courts?
3. What are the advantages and disadvantages of arbitration?
4. What is final offer arbitration? What are its advantages and disadvantages?
5. What advantages and disadvantages exist for using a panel of arbitrators?
6. Would you prefer arbitration or a court hearing to resolve an issue? Why?
7. List at least three advantages to using a consultant and three disadvantages to using a consultant.
8. What are the sources of a consultant's expertise? Why are these valid?
9. What information should be included in a request for a consulting proposal? Why is each component important?
10. How should a consultant be selected?
11. Briefly discuss three different situations in which a consultant can provide value to an organization.
12. Why should a consultant's progress be regularly monitored?

Resources

Books

Bradley, K. R. (2005). *Human resource management: People and performance*. London, UK: Ashgate.
Burke, R. J., & Cooper, C. L. (2005). *Reinventing HRM*. London, UK: Taylor & Francis.

Cook, M. F. (2004). *The complete do-it-yourself human resources department 2005*. Amsterdam, The Netherlands: Wolters Kluwer.

Dessler, G. (2004). *Human resource management* (10th ed.). London, UK: Pearson.

Heneman, R., Tansky, J., & Greenberger, D. B. (2005). *Human resource management in virtual organizations*. Greenwich, CT: Information Age.

Periodicals

Bingham, L. (1997). Employment arbitration: The repeat player effect. *Employee Rights and Employment Policy Journal, 1*, 189–220.

Brutus, S., London, M., & Martineau, J. (1999). The impact of 360-degree feedback on planning for career development. *Journal of Management Development, 18*, 676–693.

Budd, J., & Scoville, J. (2005). *The ethics of human resources and industrial relations*. Ithaca, NY: Cornell University Press.

Delery, J. E. (1998). Issues of fit in strategic human resource management: Implications for research. *Human Resource Management Review, 8*, 289–310.

DePaulo, B. M., Lindsay, J. L., Malone, B. E., Muhlenbruck, L., Charlton, K., & Cooper, H. (2003). Cues to deception. *Psychological Bulletin, 129*, 74–118.

Estreicher, S. (2001). Saturns for rickshaws: The stakes in the debate over pre-dispute employment arbitration agreements. *Ohio State Journal on Dispute Resolution, 16*, 559–570.

Gillespie, T. L. (2005). Internationalizing 360-degree feedback: Are subordinate ratings comparable? *Journal of Business and Psychology, 19*(3), 361–382.

Holman, D., Wall, T. D., Howard, A., Sparrow, P., & Clegg, C. W. (2004). *The essentials of the new workplace: A guide to the human impact of modern working practices*. New York, NY: John Wiley.

Hunter, I., & Sanders, J. (2005). *The future of HR and the need for change: New operating models to deliver increased value*. Princeton, NJ: Thorogood.

Kochan, T. (2004). Restoring trust in the human resource management profession. *Asia Pacific Journal of Human Resources, 42*(2), 132–146.

Lawler, E., Ulrich, D., Fitz-enz, J., & Madden, J. (2005). *Human resources business process outsourcing: Transforming how HR gets its work done*. Thousand Oaks, CA: Jossey-Bass.

Lawler, E. E., & Mohrman, S. A. (2003). HR as a strategic partner: What does it take to make it happen? *Human Resource Planning, 26*, 15–29.

Lepak, D. P., & Snell, S. A. (2002). Examining the human resource architecture: The relationships among human capital, employment, and human resource configurations. *Journal of Management, 28*, 517–543.

Mahony, D. M., Klaas, B. S., McClendon, J. A., & Varma, A. (2005). The effects of mandatory employment arbitration systems on applicants' attraction to organizations. *Human Resource Management, 44*(4), 449–470.

Moss, K., Swanson, J., Ullman, M., & Burris, S. (2002). Mediation of employment discrimination disputes involving persons with psychiatric disabilities. *Psychiatric Services, 53*(8), 988–994.

Paauwe, J., & Boselie, P. (2003). Challenging "strategic HRM" and the relevance of institutional setting. *Human Resource Management Journal, 13*(3), 56–70.

Richey, B., Bernardin, H. J., Tyler, C. L., & McKinney, N. (2001). The effect of arbitration program characteristics on applicants' intentions toward potential employers. *Journal of Applied Psychology, 86*, 1006–1013.

Siderman, M. N. (2001). Compulsory arbitration agreements worth saving: Reforming arbitration to accommodate Title VII protections. *UCLA Law Review, 47*, 1885–1894.

Torres-Coronas, T., & Arias-Oliva, M. (2004). *E-human resources management: Managing knowledge people*. Hershey, PA: Idea Group.

WetFeet. (2005). *Careers in specialized consulting: Health care, human resources, and information technology*. San Francisco, CA: WetFeet.

Wright, P. M., & Snell, S. A. (2005). Partner or guardian? HR's challenge in balancing value and values. *Human Resources Management, 44*(2), 177–182.

APPENDIX 21-A

Sample Contract Agreement for Consulting Services

This Agreement for Services, or Contract, is for a project [describe the services expected and objectives of the engagement].

1. [Identify the consultant or firm] (hereafter called Contractor) agrees to provide the following products and services to [Recipient or organization seeking advice and assistance] (hereafter called Client):

    A. Information gathering: Contractor will review the following information compiled by Client:
        1. Background information related to objectives
        2. Data related to objectives
        3. Samples of data available in organization (as needed)
        4. Financial information related to the project and its goal (as needed)
        5. Contractor will also inquire into the availability of [external data that have relevance for project, as needed].

        Contractor will also confer by phone with [relevant individuals or organizations, as needed].

    B. [Describe first phase of project in sufficient detail so that the tasks are clearly understood. Describe responsibilities of both Contractor and Client.]

    C. [Describe next phase of project in sufficient detail so that the tasks are clearly understood. Describe responsibilities of both Contractor and Client.]

    D. [Continue for all phases of project.]

    E. Contractor will travel [describe travel expected: destinations, organizations, expected results, time allocated, and justification].
        1. [Describe the expected results of travel. Include responsibilities of Contractor and Client.]
        2. [Describe additional issues related to travel.]

F. Contractor will conduct training [describe training expected: people, destinations, organizations, expected results, time allocated, and justification].

　　1. [Describe the expected results of training. Include responsibilities of Contractor and Client.]

　　2. [Describe additional issues related to training.]

G. Before completing this engagement, Contractor will give to Client:

　　1. [Describe project deliverables in relation to project goals and objectives.]

　　2. [Schedule for deliverables.]

　　3. [Recommendations, as needed.]

　　This work will be completed no later than [insert completion date] and will be conducted by Contractor's agent [insert consultant in charge of engagement].

　　It is understood that circumstances arising during the conduct of the consulting project may require the activities described earlier to be modified or changed. Such changes will be made with mutual agreement of both parties. The modifications may be recorded as an addendum to this agreement or in an exchange of letters between the parties proposing and accepting the changes. Products and deliverables produced during this engagement will become the property of the Client with the following exceptions: [insert a list of exceptions to be owned by the Contractor]. Changes will be made by mutual agreement.

2. Client agrees to:

A. Participate in consulting activities as requested. This includes arranging meetings, providing meeting venues and amenities, and providing information requested by Contractor. [Insert other specific items to be provided by Client including working space and access to data, as needed.]

B. Pay Contractor a fee not to exceed $ [insert maximum fee] plus expenses. Expenses to be billed include: [For each expense category or item, list rate of reimbursement and maximum allowable amount. Commonly reimbursed expenses include travel, meals, lodging, telephone, and any copying or mailing costs, excluding normal communications with Client.] All expenses will be documented with receipts. Requests for reimbursement will be submitted within 14 days of occurrence.

　　Payment for consulting services will be made in three installments: One-third [insert amount] on signing this contract, one-third [insert amount] upon completion of [insert a significant event approximately halfway through the project], and one-third [insert amount] upon completion of this project. The project will be considered complete when all deliverables have been submitted and accepted.

C. Authorize [insert name of Client representative] to accept Contractor's work and approve payment as specified in this Agreement.

D. Authorize [insert name of Client representative] to approve payment of expenses delineated in this Agreement or additional expenses as agreed upon by Contractor and Client.

3. Either party may terminate this agreement with written notice of 30 days. If the agreement is terminated, Contractor will present Client with a statement

of account showing all fees paid to that point and itemize all services rendered. If work performed exceeds fees paid to date, Client will pay Contractor for such work at the rate of $ [insert agreed upon rate] per hour. If fees paid exceed work performed to date, Contractor will return unearned fees to Client.

Signed:

for [Client]: _____ Date _____

for [Consultant]: _____ Date _____

Adapted from model prepared by Barbara Davis, 317 South Hamline, St. Paul, Minnesota 55105 and used with permission.

CHAPTER 22

Maintaining an Effective Human Resources Department

CHAPTER OBJECTIVES

After studying this chapter, readers will be able to:

- Describe the characteristics of an effective human resources department.
- Advise department managers how to approach human resources in a number of areas of concern.
- Know how senior managers can increase the value and strengthen the effectiveness of human resources services.
- Suggest some future options for human resources.

▶ Chapter Summary

The purpose of this chapter is to provide closure for the material presented in the preceding 21 chapters. It offers a summary of important points addressed in this book and offers strategies for optimizing the utility of a human resources (HR) department and the services it provides.

HR provides needed services for an organization. Human resources does not generate revenue, although the nature of the services it renders more than compensates for the lack of direct revenue contribution. Senior managers who support and fully utilize their HR department are usually more successful than those who do not.

Managers should approach HR as a partner, helping HR by providing data in a timely manner and complying with deadlines and schedules as necessary. Human resources should be consulted when job descriptions are prepared, when employee performance is reviewed, and whenever significant disciplinary action must be taken. Working in partnership with managers, HR should provide accurate and timely information. Such actions often reduce the extent to which informal channels

🔍 *CASE STUDY: Alarm Bells*

Feedback Specialists has just announced that Jamie Durango will be assuming the duties of chief executive officer in 6 weeks. Her selection culminated a nationwide search to replace Ed Worthington in the position. Jamie scheduled meetings with her senior managers to get better acquainted with them and to better understand the organization. Feedback Specialists conducts surveys and other research for companies throughout the region. Although its clients are drawn from all sectors of the economy, Feedback specializes in hospitals. Nearly 1000 employees work for the firm.

Jamie's first meeting was with Ed Worthington. She asked him about the company. After 10 minutes of conversation, she realized that HR had not yet been mentioned. "Ed, how are the employees served? You haven't mentioned human resources at all. Are HR operations outsourced?" asked Jamie.

Ed replied, "Payroll has been outsourced for almost 10 years. No major problems have ever arisen."

"What about other aspects, such as benefits and the usual HR services?"

"I believe in equality. Everyone receives the same benefits package. It really is quite generous. The supervisors assume all of the other responsibilities that HR often provides. This is doubly cost effective. Extra employees are not needed, and concern about the lack of revenue generated by an HR department is avoided," said Ed, with a satisfied smile.

Alarm bells started to ring in Jamie's head. What thoughts would you offer to Jamie at this point? Why? What would be your first suggestion to her? Why?

of communication are utilized among employees by rendering them unneeded; in other words, if employees are kept informed of what is happening throughout the organization, there will be less incidence of rumor and speculation.

▶ An Effective Human Resources Department

Users evaluate the effectiveness of HR departments. When viewing an effective HR department, managers should see evidence of concern for people as valued assets and as individuals rather than as disposable commodities. Senior management should support HR and its programs, and HR leaders should be members of an organizational administrative team.

Compensation throughout an organization should be competitive within similar industries in the immediate region and should recognize and reward performance. Benefits options offered to employees should be able to accommodate their different needs.

Training and development activities should be effective and constructively focused, and employees should have opportunities for growth and promotion within the organization. These opportunities should be supported by organization-wide policies. Open and candid communications allow employees to feel included and informed about what is happening within their organization. Effective HR operations are a positive influence on the organization's ability to retain employees. This is customarily supported by employee turnover rates that are less than the regional average for the industry. Finally, employee participation is encouraged, and input is valued.

Visible weaknesses in any of the aforementioned areas should be interpreted as signs of needed improvement. In an effective organizational environment, no management employee should hesitate to bring apparent weaknesses to the attention of HR management. If HR cannot resolve the issue, it should be able to begin to seek a remedy once a need has been identified.

Every department manager has needs that can be addressed entirely or in part by HR, but only if HR is made aware of the needs and the extent of the assistance required. Department managers in need of assistance should not wait for HR to offer help; rather, they should be proactive and challenge HR to provide needed assistance. Human resources personnel appreciate being treated as professionals. They are usually willing to negotiate reasonable deadlines, and they appreciate timely and professional follow-up.

Involve HR in Compensation Questions

Always bring HR into the process of resolving wage complaints, especially those involving real or perceived inequalities of wage scales and apparent pay inequities among employees who are otherwise similarly situated. Specific questions about errors on an employee's paycheck can be addressed either by HR or by the payroll section of the finance department, depending on an organization's payroll system.

Get Answers for Employees

Employees who have questions about HR-related matters that cannot be answered within the department in which they arise should be referred to HR. Rather than simply sending employees to HR, effective managers accompany them. They better prepare themselves to respond to subsequent employee questions, and they also demonstrate an interest in employee concerns.

Address Recruitment Issues

Review applications and résumés for possible interviews promptly and return them to HR with preferences noted. Such prompt reply accomplishes two important objectives: It accelerates the process of scheduling interviews and prompts HR to respond in timely fashion. This pattern of interaction acknowledges the professional standing of all involved parties and avoids complacency and procrastination.

When working with HR recruiters to fill a position, request additional candidates if those provided have been inappropriate. Providing a reason for rejecting specific candidates will help the HR recruiter focus on the organization's real needs. Managers should not go through numerous applicants looking for a "perfect" candidate. If HR is doing the job it ought to be doing, all of the applicants referred will possess the minimum qualifications for the position. One can understand why a department manager might wish to find a fully qualified and experienced applicant who can "hit the ground running" when hired, but the truly perfect candidate is a rarity.

After selecting a suitable candidate and agreeing with HR on a tentative offer, stay in close contact with HR until all requirements are satisfied. Active interest keeps the process moving.

Insist on Current Job Descriptions

Effective managers keep the job descriptions for their departments' positions up to date and ensure that HR retains current copies. Positions must be graded according to the organization's job evaluation process and associated with the appropriate pay scales. Position descriptions must be reviewed whenever there is a change in method, procedure, or equipment affecting the performance of any particular job. A job description should be updated at the time changes occur and not left until an up-to-date job description is needed for recruiting, performance appraisal, or some other immediate purpose.

Use HR for Support on Disciplinary Actions

Human resources assistance should be used in disciplinary actions. Human resources does not directly discipline employees except those in the HR chain of command as necessary; however, HR should be available for guidance regarding the consistency, appropriateness, and legality of disciplinary actions. All disciplinary actions of any consequence should be reviewed with HR before implementation. Department managers should seek and receive advice and guidance from HR. The ultimate decision in a disciplinary action resides with the department manager, but HR is charged with ensuring that any disciplinary action taken is both fair and legal.

Human resources should have a process for invalidating or removing past disciplinary actions in employee personnel files. There should be a time limit on how long the record of a specific infraction should remain in an employee's personnel file. Employees who do not repeat the same infractions should reasonably expect previous warnings to be removed after a reasonable period of time. For example, a facility may invalidate and remove a written warning if after a specific length of time (e.g., 22 months) no additional related infractions have occurred. A routine purge of personnel files for this purpose is impractical; however, whenever a particular file is reviewed or audited and an action older than 22 months is found, it should be removed. The objective of a warning is the correction of behavior, and invalidating and removing older warnings prevents an infraction from remaining a permanent mark on an employee's record. However, documents removed from personnel files should not be destroyed in case there is a need for them in future legal action; these should be retained in a separate confidential file.

Complete Performance Appraisals

If an organization's system calls for anniversary date appraisals, managers need to keep track of scheduled review dates for their departments' employees. Managers should be prepared to follow up with HR if appraisal forms and schedules are not forthcoming; in many organizations, HR is responsible for keeping the appraisal system moving, so there is no harm in following up if the process appears behind schedule. Avoiding or indefinitely delaying appraisals is not an option.

Human resources should periodically offer refresher training in how to conduct performance appraisals. This should be provided annually and whenever changes in the system are instituted. Managers should be required to complete refresher training in appraisal on a regular basis. At a fixed time in the appraisal cycle, HR should provide summary statistics of the results of the process to include information such as the range, mean, and standard deviation of appraisal scores. This should be available to individual departments and for the organization as a whole.

▶ Informal Channels of Communication

All organizations, indeed essentially all assemblages of people, have informal channels of communication; that is, they all have a form of "the grapevine" or the "rumor mill," which might also be referred to as the informal communications network of the organization or group. Informal channels are natural; they will always be there. It is not possible to abolish the grapevine; therefore, every department manager should learn how to work with it.

There are two positive aspects to the grapevine. First, it is fast; whether accurate or grossly inaccurate, information moves more rapidly than with most other means (with "bad news" often traveling faster than "good news"). Second, it is depth of penetration; some employees who avoid employee meetings, never look at an employee newsletter, or never even glance at a bulletin board, will nevertheless participate in the grapevine by listening and reacting and usually passing what they have heard along to others.

Since a manager cannot stamp out the "rumor mill" or prevent the department's employees from speaking with each other, the manager's most realistic approach to this informal communications system is to work with it. If the manager's relationship with the department's employees is healthy, some employees will repeat grapevine comments to the manager and ask about the quality of the information. The manager should take every such opportunity to "set the record straight" if possible or to assure employees that every effort will be made to find out the truth from within the organizational hierarchy.

In attempting to manage the grapevine or rumor mill, do not simply participate by repeating what you hear without checking it out; when you hear something you know to be wrong, correct it; and if what you hear raises questions for employees, do your best to answer these or promise to seek answers.

A manager's relative strength or potential for success in addressing the informal communications network ultimately depends on that manager's relationship with each employee in the group. The effective, participative manager who has developed and maintained a healthy one-to-one relationship with each employee is going to hear what is traveling on the grapevine; the employees will bring the rumors and tales to the manager.

Take Training Needs to HR

Managers are advised to approach HR with training needs if the organization is lacking a separate training or education department. HR can often provide some forms of training or can perhaps broker training arrangements with known sources of training.

Provide Current Information to HR

Professionals in the HR department will ordinarily be doing their best to fulfill the needs of line departments. To do so, however, HR must hear about these needs on a regular basis. Human resources staff members appreciate learning from the departments about the policies and procedures requiring revision as well as receiving recommendations related to recruiting, retention, and retraining. Feedback about employee attitudes toward pay, benefits, and other conditions of employment is always useful.

Encourage Human Resources to Prove Its Worth

Human resources services are often characterized as "soft" because they do not generate revenue, and not all HR services are readily quantifiable. A few key indicators of employment activity, such as average cost per hire and average time required to fill a position, can be quantified fairly easily. Employee retention can be measured by addressing turnover within specific departments, the organization as a whole, or within job titles or by month, quarter, or year. Human resources can be compared with standards used throughout the organization—for example, measuring HR cost as a percentage of total expenses or staffing as a ratio of HR workers to the total number of employees.

The effectiveness of training can sometimes be assessed by comparing scores obtained through pre-training and post-training testing. Human resources is usually able to establish benchmarks or baselines for measuring its own performance; comparing these with established industry benchmarks enables comparisons over time.

▶ HR and Optimal Organizational Efficiency

The fundamental nature of an organization's human resources department should always be of concern to the organization's leaders. Is HR reactionary, waiting for problems to develop or a crisis to occur before acting? Restating this question, has the HR made a sufficient systematic assessment of the organization's needs to identify potential problems in advance?

Human resources professionals are most effectively utilized when they work as internal consultants to management, involved in strategic planning and serving as part of the executive team. Organizations waste a resource when they use HR as simply a source of information to call upon when there are problems. Top management should insist on linking plans for recruitment, retention, training and development, performance appraisal, and compensation and benefits to the overall strategies of the organization. Human resources activities should be an integral part of an organization's strategic planning process, with management insisting on close cooperation between HR planning and corporate planning.

Executive managers should insist that both HR professionals and line managers be involved in designing HR programs; they should always insist that line managers be involved to the maximum extent possible when implementing HR programs. The approach that allows top management to receive the best from an organization's HR department is to insist that HR managers be proactive. To facilitate this goal, executives must provide visible support for the HR department.

Human resources provides benefits to individual employees and to the organization as a whole. An HR department exists to protect the rights of employees at all organizational levels. It assumes these responsibilities not simply because there are laws requiring the organization to do so but because safeguarding the rights of individuals is the ethical path to follow. Human resources strives to protect the organization by minimizing exposure to legal risk.

By extension, every manager of people becomes a practitioner of human resources. This department called human resources is a staff support activity, existing to provide services that support and enhance the efficient operation of the organization. Successful managers ensure that in their interactions with HR they support HR while making the best possible use of the services offered.

▶ Future Directions for Human Resources

The future is always uncertain, yet we can consider a few observations concerning what the future may hold for HR:

- Both the size and scope of responsibility of HR are likely to change. Consistent with other sectors of business and industry, demands and responsibilities are likely to increase while employee resources are likely to remain static. However, the importance of HR is highly likely to increase.
- More outsourcing of routine HR services can be expected. Owing to a number of factors, organizations are likely to increase managerial spans of control. As budgets become tight, education and training activities may be discontinued. (It has been very nearly traditional that when budget cuts are necessary, education is among the first to be cut.) The trend toward increased automation in creating, maintaining, and retrieving records is likely to continue. We may expect to see personnel records interface with increasing numbers of other data sources. Electronic security will necessarily have to be increased.
- The use of merit-based systems of compensation (also known as pay-for-performance) is highly likely to increase. This will most likely occur in tandem with a decline in automatic raises or so-called cost-of-living increases.
- In benefits, expect to see a dramatically diminishing number of defined benefit retirement plans as more defined contribution retirement plans are instituted and more cafeteria benefits programs are made available. Employee choice is becoming an important factor in recruitment and retention.
- Organizations are likely to pay more attention to employee attitudes as they seek to increase levels of employee interest and involvement in organizational management.
- We will likely see a renewed emphasis on productivity enhancement programs as organizations continue trying to do more with less and provide quality products and services with constrained and restricted resources.
- Finally, we expect to witness increasing concern for organizational values. Employees who become more attuned to their organizational cultures are more likely to advance and experience professional and personal satisfaction. For their part, we expect employees to be more attuned to the mission, vision, goals, and objectives of the organizations for which they work and upon which they depend for their continued economic livelihood.

▶ Conclusion

Organizations receive necessary services from HR. An HR department does not generate revenue, but the essential services it provides more than compensate for the function's lack of direct revenue contribution. Organizations in which senior managers support their HR departments stand a better chance of long-run success than those that do not.

Managers at all levels and human resources should form active partnerships. Within such partnerships, management assists HR by providing data in a timely manner and meeting deadlines and schedules. Human resources should be consulted whenever job descriptions are prepared, employees are reviewed, or significant disciplinary actions are contemplated for employees. Human resources and managers working together should provide accurate and timely information, lessening the perceived need for employees to turn to their informal channels for information.

🔍 CASE STUDY: Resolution

Responding to her ringing alarm bells, Jamie immediately rescheduled the appointments she had made for the next 2 days. She called a respected consulting firm that specialized in human resources issues and requested a meeting for the next day. "Yes, it's that important," she replied to the surprised principal of the consulting firm who had responded to her call. Establishing and launching an HR department became her first and greatest priority.

After agreeing on the general structure of a new HR department for Feedback Specialists, Jamie resumed her meetings with senior members of the management team. She expressed concern over the absence of an HR department. She also asked the senior managers to help construct the new department. She emphasized the need to establish partnerships with HR.

An HR manager was identified within the ranks of Feedback Specialists, and four additional employees were hired for HR.

"Consider this to be a beginning. Let me know if you need additional help," Jamie remarked to the new members of HR 2 months later.

During lunch with a first-line manager a year later, Jamie learned that employees had been talking about forming a union before she arrived. The union talk had stopped within a month after the new HR department began operation. The manager told her that the rumor mills had essentially stopped. The flow of accurate and timely information from managers and HR had made the rumor mills unnecessary.

Jamie enjoyed her dessert that day.

 SPOTLIGHT ON CUSTOMER SERVICE

The Contribution of Customer Service to Maintaining an Effective HR Department

As organizational departments go, human resources has relatively few employees. These individuals are responsible for processing large numbers of documents, maintaining records mandated by statutes, and regularly reviewing and updating many organizational documents; keeping position descriptions current provides a convenient example.

Human resources employees must provide good customer service, just like all other employees are expected to do. The recipients of their customer service efforts may be both internal customers (employees) and external customers (applicants and others).

Effective and caring customer service is always appreciated. Future conditions may dictate that customer service will become increasingly more important. Customer service is a timeless commodity.

Questions for Review and Discussion

1. Why must an HR department occasionally have to be prodded to ensure that it operates on a proactive basis?
2. How could a department manager help HR to resolve an organizational issue?
3. Why is the response "go talk to HR" not always appropriate when employees ask questions related to human resources?
4. Why might a department manager have to remind HR about an aspect of the performance appraisal process?
5. Why do many organizations require that significant disciplinary actions be cleared with HR before they are implemented?
6. How can department managers help to ensure that organizational job descriptions are current and complete?
7. How can an HR department assist department managers to control rumors?
8. Why should a supervisor insist that HR provides statistics related to turnover, cost per hire, and average time to fill a position?
9. Why should an individual manager be interested in supporting HR?
10. In your opinion, how will HR change in the future? Why?

Resources

Books

Aspatore Books Staff. (2005). *Human resources leadership strategies: 15 ways to enhance HR value in your company.* Boston, MA: Aspatore Books.

Jackson, S. J., & Schuler, R. S. (2005). *Managing human resources through strategic partnerships* (9th ed.). Mason, OH: Thomson South-Western.

Lussier, R. (2019). *Human resource management* (3rd ed.). Newbury Park, CA: Sage Publications.

Niles, N. J. (2013). *Basic concepts of health care human resource management.* Burlington, MA: Jones & Bartlett Learning.

Swart, J., Mann, C., Brown, S., & Price, A. (2005). *Human resource development: Strategy and tactics.* Burlington, MA: Elsevier.

Periodicals

Cohn, J. M., Khurana, R., & Reeves, L. (2005). Growing talent as if your business depended on it. *Harvard Business Review, 83*(10), 62–70, 155.

Coonan, P. R. (2005). Succession planning: Aligning strategic goals and leadership behaviors. *Nursing Leadership Forum, 9*(3), 92–97.

Datta, D. K., Guthrie, J. P., & Wright, P. M. (2005). Human resource management and labor productivity: Does industry matter? *Academy of Management Journal, 48*(1), 135–145.

Vermeeren, M., Steijn, B., Tummers, L., Lankhaar, M., Poerstamper, R., & van Beek, S. (2014). HRM and its effects on employee, organizational and financial outcomes in health care organizations. *Human Resources for Health, 12*, 35.

Index

Note: Tables and exhibits are denoted by *t* and *e*, respectively.